Medical Response to Weapons of Mass Destruction

Medical Response to Weapons of Mass Destruction

Editor
Phil Currance, EMT-P, RHSP

Senior Paramedic
Lakewood Fire Department (Ret.)
Hazardous Materials Emergency Response Training Coordinator
Rocky Mountain Training Center
Lakewood, Colorado
Deputy Commander, Central U.S. National Medical Response Team—Weapons of
Mass Destruction and the Colorado 2 Disaster Medical Assistance Team
Denver, Colorado

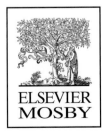

ELSEVIER
MOSBY

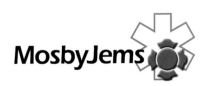

**ELSEVIER
MOSBY**

11830 Westline Industrial Drive
St. Louis, Missouri 63146

MEDICAL RESPONSE TO WEAPONS OF MASS DESTRUCTION   0-323-02331-2
Copyright © 2005 by Mosby, Inc.

NOTICE

EMS is an ever-changing field. Standard safety precautions must be followed, but as new research and clinical experience broaden our knowledge, changes in treatment and drug therapy may become necessary or appropriate. Readers are advised to check the most current product information provided by the manufacturer of each drug to be administered to verify the recommended dose, the method and duration of administration, and contraindications. It is the responsibility of the licensed prescriber, relying on experience and knowledge of the patient, to determine dosages and the best treatment for each individual patient. Neither the publisher nor the author assumes any liability for any injury and/or damage to persons or property arising from this publication.

International Standard Book Number 0-323-02331-2

Acquisitions Editor: Linda Honeycutt
Developmental Editor: Laura Bayless
Publishing Services Manager: Patricia Tannian
Project Manager: Kristine Feeherty
Designer: Kathi Gosche

Printed in China

Last digit is the print number: 9 8 7 6 5 4 3 2 1

Disclaimers

The views and opinions expressed in this text and related materials are solely those of the authors and do not reflect the positions or official policy of any local jurisdiction, state agency, department of the U.S. government, or affiliated agencies.

Information contained in this text in no way authorizes anyone to perform any of the procedures or protocols listed. Operating protocols, standing orders, and verbal orders must be established by local emergency medical service physician control. This text is based on current research, and the information, drug indications, dosages, and precautions are current, to the best of the author's ability, as of publication. The reader is urged to consult the package information provided by the manufacturer for the latest changes.

Do not enter hazardous environments or carry out decontamination procedures without proper protective equipment. It is beyond the scope of this text to advise you on the exact type of protective equipment needed. Other resources and chemical compatibility charts must be checked. Training in the proper use of protective equipment is essential to your safety.

The use of any product or equipment names in this text is for illustrative purposes only. It in no way endorses or promotes the use of any specific product or company.

Although the authors, editors, publisher, and their agents have made every effort to ensure the accuracy of information contained in this work, they cannot be held responsible for any errors found in the text. The authors, editors, publisher, and their agents do not bear any responsibility or liability for the information contained in this text or for any uses to which it may be put.

To the men and women who make up the National Disaster Medical System (NDMS)

NDMS teams provide medical and associated response during times of natural and man-made disasters. The full-time management staff and the nearly 7000 volunteers who make up the medical response teams are committed to providing an exceptional level of care. It is an honor to be associated with people of this caliber.

Reviewers

James B. Anderson II ("J.B."), AAS, NPQB
Training and Exercise Coordinator
Center for National Response Consequence Management and
    Counter-Terrorism Training
Fairfax, Virginia

Christian E. Cailsen, Jr., LP
Division Commander
Austin–Travis County Emergency Medical Services
Austin, Texas

Attila J. Hertelendy, BHSC, CCEMT-P, NREMT-P
Instructor
University of Mississippi Medical Center
Jackson, Mississippi

Paul E. Phrampus, MD
Assistant Professor of Emergency Medicine
Department of Emergency Medicine
University of Pittsburgh
Pittsburgh, Pennsylvania

John Michael Pickett, BS, BA
Professor Emeritus
San Antonio College
Retired Firefigher
San Antonio, Texas

James L. Schneider
NFPA Instructor II/III
Morristown Volunteer Fire Department
Morristown, Indiana

Contributors

Lana Blackwell, RN, BSN
Director of Emergency and Trauma Services
Parker Adventist Hospital
Parker, Colorado
Clinical Nursing Supervisor
Central U.S. National Medical Response Team—Weapons of
    Mass Destruction and the Colorado 2 Disaster Medical
    Assistance Team
Denver, Colorado

Gary Christman, EMT
Technician/Specialist
City of St. Louis Department of Public Safety, City Emergency
    Management Agency;
Deputy Commander
Missouri 1 Disaster Medical Assistance Team
St. Louis, Missouri

Bruce Clements, MPH
Associate Director
Saint Louis University School of Public Health, Center for the
    Study of Bioterrorism and Emerging Infections;
Safety Officer
Missouri 1 Disaster Medical Assistance Team
St. Louis, Missouri

Alan Colon, EMT
WMD Coordinator
Commerce City Police Department
Commerce City, Colorado
Security Supervisor
Central U.S. National Medical Response Team—Weapons of
    Mass Destruction and the Colorado 2 Disaster Medical
    Assistance Team
Denver, Colorado

Phil Currance, EMT-P, RHSP
Senior Paramedic
Lakewood Fire Department (Ret.);
Hazardous Materials Emergency Response Training
    Coordinator
Rocky Mountain Training Center
Lakewood, Colorado
Deputy Commander
Central U.S. National Medical Response Team—Weapons of
    Mass Destruction and the Colorado 2 Disaster Medical
    Assistance Team
Denver, Colorado

Patrick F. DeMarco, PhD, BCETS, KCStS
Licensed Psychologist, Private Practice
Allied Health Staff at McKee Medical Center
Loveland, Colorado
Consultant
Comprehensive Spine and Rehabilitation Center
Loveland, Colorado; Fort Collins, Colorado
Senior Mental Health Officer and Team Psychologist
Central U.S. National Medical Response Team—Weapons of
    Mass Destruction and the Colorado 2 Disaster Medical
    Assistance Team
Denver, Colorado

Wendy Hout, RN, BSN
Clinical Coordinator for Special Projects
Aurora South Medical Center
Aurora, Colorado
Administrative Officer
Central U.S. National Medical Response Team—Weapons of
    Mass Destruction and the Colorado 2 Disaster Medical
    Assistance Team
Denver, Colorado

Chris Mailliard, NREMT-P
Firefighter/Paramedic/Tactical Medic
West Metro Fire Department
Lakewood, Colorado
Operations Section Chief
Central U.S. National Medical Response Team—Weapons of
    Mass Destruction and the Colorado 2 Disaster Medical
    Assistance Team
Denver, Colorado

Tom Pedigo, PA-C, NREMT-P
EMS Administrator/Assistant Chief
Thornton Fire Department
Thornton, Colorado
Non-Ambulatory Decontamination Team Leader
Physician's Assistant
Central U.S. National Medical Response Team—Weapons of
    Mass Destruction and the Colorado 2 Disaster Medical
    Assistance Team
Denver, Colorado

The views and opinions expressed in this text and related
materials are solely those of the authors and do not reflect the
positions or official policy of any local jurisdiction, state agency,
department of the U.S. government, or affiliated agencies.

Foreword

Weapons of mass destruction are nothing new to humankind. The first weapon of mass destruction was probably a volley of stones hurled at an enemy. Volleys of spears and later arrows likely followed. The use of chemical weapons dates as far back as 423 BC during the Peloponnesian War when the forces of Sparta forced smoke from lighted coals, sulfur, and pitch into an Athenian fort through a hollow beam. Biological weapons were described as early as the sixth century BC when the Assyrians were purported to have poisoned enemy wells with rye ergot.

As technology and the understanding of biological concepts advanced, so did the weaponry of the day, the destructive power of these devices increasing exponentially. In the mid-1300s, plague-infested corpses were catapulted over city walls. Smallpox-contaminated clothing was proffered to South American native populations in the fifteenth century. The use of chlorine gas in the trenches of World War I is well known. Sulfur mustard was used in 1917 and caused some 200,000 casualties in a single attack near Ypres, Belgium. In the 1930s, nerve agents were first synthesized as industrial chemicals. The evolution of these weapons culminated in the most awesome of all armaments—the nuclear bomb.

Today we are faced with the specter of terrorists deploying nuclear, biological, and chemical weapons of mass destruction to assault and panic civilian populations and nations and to disrupt our way of life. In his January 1961 presidential inauguration speech, John F. Kennedy declared, "We shall pay any price, bear any burden, meet any hardship" to assure the survival of our liberty. Knowledge is among the most important factors in achieving that goal. We must prepare ourselves to rapidly recognize the deployment of these weapons, as well as to diagnose, treat, and otherwise mitigate the consequences of the weapons that might be employed against us.

This book comprehensively examines the spectrum of weapons of mass destruction and the ways in which we can preplan for and respond to their use. It details the mechanisms by which they cause injury and, most important, the methods and equipment that can be used to protect us from their effects and to treat their victims by employing the most up-to-date medical technology. Anyone involved with disaster response or wanting in-depth knowledge of weapons of mass destruction will find this text an invaluable source of cogent and practical information. It is an important tool in our quest for that elusive goal of total preparedness.

Charles Goldstein, DO, FACEP
Commander, Central U.S. National Medical Response
Team—Weapons of Mass Destruction
Commander, Colorado 2 Disaster Medical Assistance Team

Preface

A new age of emergency response is upon us. Responders must now be concerned with mass casualty incidents caused by weapons of mass destruction. Biological, chemical, nuclear, incendiary, and explosive agents are the terrorist's weapons of choice. Responders will be faced not only with the large numbers of victims involved in these incidents, but also with great risk to personnel.

Firefighters, police, and emergency medical personnel have always been identified as the "first responders." The nature of incidents of mass destruction will expand on that identity. Hospital and medical personnel will probably be the first to see casualties from attacks that involve biological agents. In addition, they must be prepared for the large number of patients who will make their own way to nearby hospitals. Many of these patients will not have been contacted or decontaminated by on-scene resources. Public health and environmental professionals will also find themselves on the front lines of many of these incidents.

Information and uniformity in training are needed to mount an effective and safe response. Research and development are ongoing, and what is considered current "state of the art" and standard care is constantly changing. This text is designed to present information and ideas to medical providers at all levels and to provide a common foundation upon which we can build and improve our capabilities.

We are faced with a massive challenge. History has demonstrated the effectiveness of weapons of mass destruction. Current intelligence suggests that terrorists are planning and perfecting new ways to use them. The outcome may be far beyond what most of us would consider a worst case scenario. We must take every step possible to prepare. My hope is that this text will assist in achieving that goal.

Phil Currance

Acknowledgments

I would like to thank all the people who helped with the production of this text. First, the contributors:

Lana Blackwell
Gary Christman
Bruce Clements
Alan Colon
Pat DeMarco
Wendy Hout
Chris Mailliard
Tom Pedigo

These people have not only the knowledge, but also the drive to put it down on paper, despite all their other commitments. This book could not have been completed without them.

I believe that any educational effort is made easier with visual input. The following photographers lent their talents to improve the quality of this text:

David Johnsrud
T. Schumacher (Veterans Administration)
All the authors who also took photos

I owe a major thanks to the people at Elsevier:

Andrew Allen
Linda Honeycutt
Kristin Armstrong
Claire Merrick
Kristine Feeherty
Joe Selby

They are truly dedicated to improving the level of health care through education. I thank them for supporting me in the past and allowing me to produce this text.

Contents

Introduction and Training Requirements

Phil Currance

CHAPTER OBJECTIVES

At the conclusion of this chapter the student will be able to:

- Identify the need for specialized weapons of mass destruction (WMD) training.
- Identify the need for interagency cooperation and cross training.
- Identify training regulations regarding Emergency Medical Services (EMS) response to hazardous materials and WMD, as well as the contact agencies that may provide additional information.
- Discuss Occupational Safety and Health Administration (OSHA) regulations regarding emergency response to hazardous materials incidents.
- Discuss National Fire Protection Association (NFPA) standards regarding emergency response to hazardous materials incidents, particularly NFPA 473.

CASE STUDY

An explosive device has been detonated at a local restaurant. Many patrons are injured and are not ambulatory. Numerous agencies are responding to the scene.

How has the threat of terrorism changed the way we respond to emergencies?

What types of weapons might terrorists use?

What problems must we solve to mount a safe and efficient response?

What types of training do responders need to cope with this problem?

EMERGENCY RESPONSE TO TERRORISM

TERRORISM THREAT

The world has changed and so have the mechanics of emergency response. Terrorism has reached where we work and live. The intentional attack on civilians has become an accepted part of warfare for some organizations. We are left with mounting an effective response to an overwhelming problem.

In the past, most terrorists have used explosive and incendiary devices as their weapons of choice. These weapons caused multiple casualties and safety concerns for the responders because of the nature of the attack and because of the possibility of secondary devices. In the present day the stakes have grown to enormous proportions because of the threat posed by chemical, biological, and radiological weapons.

TERMINOLOGY

The new threat and weapons are known by different terms, depending on the response agency. Popular names include nuclear, biological, and chemical (NBC) weapons; biological, nuclear, incendiary, chemical, and explosive (BNICE) weapons; and chemical, biological, and nuclear (CBN) weapons. The most popular term, and the one that we will use throughout this text, is weapons of mass destruction (WMD). Some authorities point out that the term *weapons of mass effect* (WME) may be more appropriate because it can include attacks such as cyberterrorism and effects such as mental health concerns. Such attacks can be devastating even without mass destruction to physical structures.

Whatever term you choose to use, the idea is clear. We are in a new era of emergency response. Multiple casualty results can instantly be replaced with mass casualties, possibly numbering in the thousands. Covert attacks using biological or radiological agents can result in sickness days after exposure, leading to mass confusion and overwhelmed medical resources. Explosive secondary devices can release invisible vapors that affect responders at a sizable distance from the initial damage.

Injury profiles and treatment modalities are also changing. Trauma care may need to be supplemented with mass decontamination procedures and antidote therapy. Crime scene protocols and preservation of evidence become vital concerns in preventing the next incident. We now find ourselves in a response pattern that combines multiple and mass medical response, hazardous materials concerns, and crime scene protocols all in one event.

RESPONSE ASSETS

FEDERAL AGENCIES

Many agencies and groups will play a part in a WMD response. Federal agencies include the Federal Bureau of Investigation (FBI), Federal Emergency Management Agency (FEMA), Coast Guard, Environmental Protection Agency (EPA), Food and Drug Administration (FDA), Centers for Disease Control and Prevention (CDC), Department of Defense (DOD), Department of Veterans Affairs (VA), numerous medical response teams, and many others.

DEPARTMENT OF HOMELAND SECURITY

Many of these agencies have been moved to the Department of Homeland Security (DHS) to better coordinate the response. The formation of DHS has streamlined information analysis and response by placing agencies with terrorism response and prevention responsibilities under one agency. This organization allows for improved threat analysis, response activities, equipment acquisition, training, and administrative support.

NATIONAL DISASTER MEDICAL SYSTEM (NDMS)

The federal medical response to WMD incidents is conducted through DHS under the National Disaster Medical System (NDMS). The NDMS medical response includes field units, coordination of patient transportation, and provision of hospital beds. The field component comprises volunteer teams of medical professionals. Disaster Medical Assistance Teams (DMATs) (Fig. 1-1) are field-deployable hospital teams that include physicians, nurses, emergency medical technicians, and other medical and nonmedical support personnel. There are also specialty DMATs that concentrate on specific medical areas such as burns, pediatrics, and mental health.

National Medical Response Teams for Weapons of Mass Destruction (NMRT-WMD) are quick-response specialty teams that are trained and equipped to provide mass casualty decontamination and patient care after the release of a chemical, biological, or radiological agent (Fig. 1-2). There are four NMRTs in the nation. One team is stationary and is based in Washington, D.C.; the other three are nationally deployable teams based on the East Coast, central United States, and West Coast.

International Medical-Surgical Response Teams (IMSuRTs) are specialty surgical teams that can respond both domestically and internationally. They respond with staff and a portable operating suite to provide advanced medical and surgical services. There are three IMSuRTs in the United States.

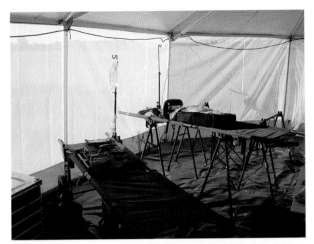

Fig. 1-1
Disaster Medical Assistance Team (DMAT) field hospital.

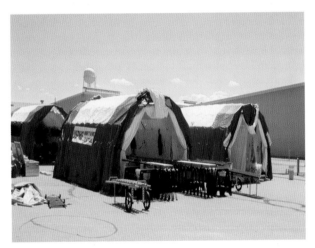

Fig. 1-2
National Medical Response Team for weapons of mass destruction (NMRT-WMD).

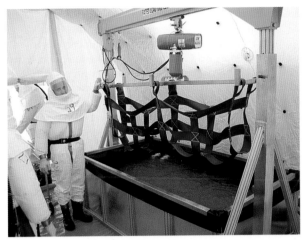

Fig. 1-3
Weapons of mass destruction (WMD) Disaster Mortuary Operational Response Team (DMORT) with special fatality decontamination system.

Disaster Mortuary Operational Response Teams (DMORTs) are made up of forensic and mortuary professionals who are trained to deal with human remains after disaster situations. There are 10 DMORTs. One DMORT-WMD is specially trained and equipped to provide services if the bodies are contaminated (Fig. 1-3).

Veterinary Medical Assistance Teams (VMATs) provide animal care and assistance during disasters. They also provide care for search and service dogs and expert consultation for biological attack clues occurring in animal populations. There are four VMATs in the nation.

STATE AND LOCAL AGENCIES

METROPOLITAN MEDICAL RESPONSE SYSTEM

State and local agencies include public health departments, environmental health agencies, mental health agencies, and emergency response agencies such as EMS, fire, police, and the Metropolitan Medical Response System (MMRS). The MMRS is designed around the 120 cities with the largest populations in the United States. Funding was established to provide training and equipment to these cities to allow them to improve a multidisciplined response to a terrorist attack that used a weapon of mass destruction. Each city was allowed to select the type of equipment that would be necessary to upgrade its level of response. Typical equipment additions include mass decontamination equipment, antidote stockpiles, personal protective equipment, and detection equipment. Training under the Domestic Preparedness Program (DPP) was conducted for Operations Level responders, hazardous materials technicians, incident commanders, EMS responders, and hospital personnel.

CROSS-TRAINING OF ALL RESPONSE DISCIPLINES

Responders from all disciplines—including law enforcement, emergency medical response, fire, hospital, mental health, and public health—are finding that interdisciplinary cooperation and cross-training are becoming mandatory. Law enforcement personnel need new personal protective equipment to carry out their duties. Medical and hospital personnel must be able to manage mass decontamination procedures. Fire personnel must recognize evidence and crime scene concerns when conducting rescue operations. Public health personnel are becoming new detectives in recognizing and controlling the effects of a covert attack. Mental health professionals need to deal with mass casualties over a wide area.

EQUIPMENT CONCERNS

Enhancement of skills and knowledge isn't the only challenge that we face. Current equipment stocks may not be adequate for the problem. Protective equipment regulations may need to be changed to provide for adequate responder protection and still allow mission flexibility when dealing with these threats. Additional and specialized detection equipment may need to be obtained. Most field and hospital decontamination systems will be quickly overwhelmed when dealing with patients by the hundreds or even thousands. Medication stockpiles must be purchased and maintained. New, more efficient surveillance systems must be developed to identify exposures as early as possible. All of these problems require combinations of research, development, training, and funding to develop effective solutions.

A major problem is the deadline that we must meet in obtaining these new skills and equipment. Many years of complacency have left us underprepared. The problem has caught up to us and we are quite literally out of time. Research and development have shifted into high gear, and even the equipment purchased very recently may be inadequate or inappropriate.

TRAINING PROGRAMS

Training programs have to address this new threat and be adaptable and flexible. Subjects that must be addressed include the following:
- Agency cooperation and use of an effective incident management system
- Threat assessment and preplanning concerns
- Identification and management of incidents involving explosive and incendiary devices
- Identification and management of chemical, biological, and radiological threats
- Problems posed by large gatherings
- Use and limitations of detection devices
- Use and limitations of personal protective equipment
- Effective scene management and control at WMD incident sites
- Effective hospital management of WMD casualties
- Mass casualty triage concerns, especially in the face of WMD threats
- Effective mass decontamination procedures
- Public health and mental health needs resulting from a WMD incident
- Crime scene and evidence preservation concerns

HAZARDOUS WASTE OPERATIONS AND EMERGENCY RESPONSE

Fortunately there are many training programs that are starting to address the needs of a WMD response. OSHA 29 CFR 1910.120 and EPA 40 CFR 311 Hazardous Waste Operations and Emergency Response (HAZWOPER) training and response regulations are focused on standard hazardous materials problems but are the backbone of a safe and efficient WMD training program. These OSHA and EPA rules provide for the safety of personnel who work on hazardous waste cleanup sites, who work on hazardous waste treatment storage and disposal sites, or who respond to hazardous materials

emergencies no matter where they occur. The requirements of the HAZWOPER law include the following:
- Training
- Hazard identification and characterization
- Personal protective equipment
- Decontamination procedures
- Safe work or response practices
- Medical monitoring of personnel

Because federal OSHA rules exempt federal and local government personnel, the EPA passed 40 CFR 311. This "mirror standard" was designed to protect workers exempted from the OSHA standard. Because federal OSHA standards do not apply to state or local government workers, many states have passed state OSHA regulations that cover all workers in the state no matter whom they work for.

LEVELS OF TRAINING

The EPA and specific state standards require training for all personnel who respond to any emergency incident that involves hazardous materials. For emergency responders, the standards require that the training be based on their expected activities. The regulations break the training down to five levels. These levels of training are Awareness, Operations, Technician, Specialist, and Incident Command.

Awareness Level. Responders at a WMD incident, at a minimum, must be trained to the Awareness Level. Some states require that EMS personnel be trained to the Operations Level because they respond to protect life and safety at a hazardous materials emergency. In some areas, EMS agencies have decided to take an active role in hazardous materials response and have trained their responders to the Technician Level.

First responders at the Awareness Level (Fig. 1-4) are personnel who are likely to witness or discover a release of hazardous materials and are trained to initiate an emergency response.[1] Awareness Level responders are limited to tasks that involve isolating the scene and calling for assistance. They must remain in a safe area.

Operations Level. First responders at the Operations Level (Fig. 1-5) are those who respond to releases, or potential releases, of WMD as part of the initial response to protect people, property, and the environment from the effects of the release.[2] Operations Level first responders are trained to take defensive actions rather than try to stop the release or take offensive actions. OSHA considers any activity that can be carried out without making direct contact with the substance to be defensive. The function of Operations Level first responders is to contain the release from a safe distance, keep it from spreading, and prevent exposures.

While the entire Operations Level curriculum may not be appropriate for all responders, certain tasks in this level are appropriate for many WMD field activities. WMD responders should be trained to the Operations Level with a program that is specialized to their needs.

Technician Level. Hazardous materials technicians (Fig. 1-6) are personnel who respond to releases or potential releases of WMD for the purpose of stopping the release.[2] Personnel trained to the Technician Level assume a more

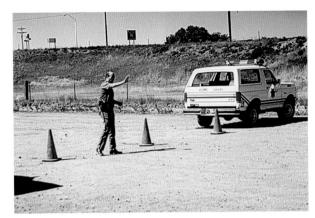
Fig. 1-4
Awareness Level responder.

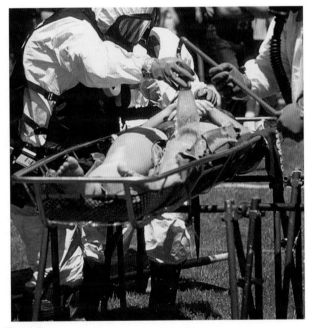
Fig. 1-5
EMS responders trained to the Operations Level
conducting patient decontamination.

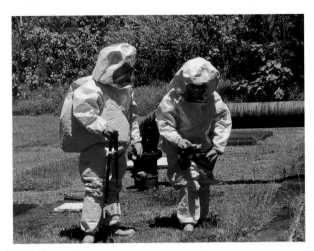
Fig. 1-6
Technician Level responders conducting air monitoring
in a contaminated area.

parallel those of hazardous materials technicians, but personnel trained to the Specialist Level are required to have more direct or specific knowledge of the various substances they may be called on to contain.[2] They also act as senior leaders of hazardous materials teams and may act as site liaisons with federal, state, and local governments regarding site activities according to OSHA 29 CFR 1910.120.

Incident Command Level. Incident Command Level responders (Fig. 1-8) assume control of the incident scene beyond the first-responder Awareness Level.[2] They must be able to implement their employer's incident command system and emergency response plan. They must also be able to coordinate local, state, and federal emergency response.

NATIONAL FIRE PROTECTION ASSOCIATION (NFPA)

In addition to the OSHA and EPA regulations, the National Fire Protection Association (NFPA) has developed voluntary training competencies for personnel who respond to hazardous materials incidents. The NFPA is a privatized agency that provides standards that local authorities can adopt as codes or ordinances. *NFPA 471* sets competency standards for hazardous materials emergency response. *NFPA 472* sets training standards for emergency response personnel. *NFPA 472* standards parallel the OSHA and EPA regulations but add more detail and description.

NFPA 473

Of special interest to EMS responders is *NFPA 473*. This standard is designed for EMS personnel who respond to hazardous materials incidents. It designates two levels of training, Level 1 and Level 2.

Emergency medical services personnel at EMS Hazardous Materials (HM) Level 1 may, in the course of their normal duties, be called upon to perform patient care activities in the

aggressive role than first responders at the Operations Level. They carry out offensive activities such as approaching the point of release to plug, patch, or otherwise stop the release of a hazardous substance. Like the Operations Level, the Technician Level includes some competencies, such as advanced control and containment practices, that may not be appropriate for every WMD responder, such as EMS responders. A program can be designed that parallels the Technician Level and gives specific response group information.

Specialist Level. Hazardous materials specialists (Fig. 1-7) are senior experienced responders who respond with, and provide support to, hazardous materials technicians. Their duties

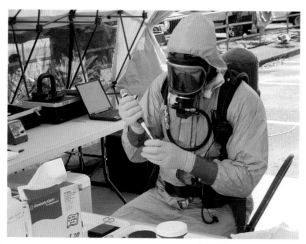

Fig. 1-7
Hazardous materials specialist conducting laboratory analysis in the field.

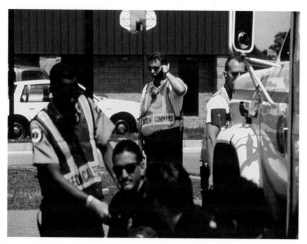

Fig. 1-8
Incident commander at a WMD incident site.

cold zone at a hazardous materials site.[1] The incident's cold zone is the area that contains the command post and other support functions. In other documents it is referred to as the *clean zone* or *support zone*. This zone should be free of contamination; response activities in this area represent a minimal risk. The role of the EMS HM Level 1 responder is to provide care only to those persons who no longer pose a significant risk of secondary contamination (that is, a risk of contaminating others, including those providing care).[1]

EMS personnel at EMS HM Level 2 (Fig. 1-9) may be called upon to perform patient care activities during decontamination procedures in the *warm zone* (the area where personnel and equipment decontamination takes place) at hazardous materials sites. Personnel in this zone have a greater chance of being exposed to the hazardous material and are at higher risk than personnel in the cold zone.[1] The EMS HM Level 2 response personnel may provide care to persons who still pose a significant risk of secondary contamination.

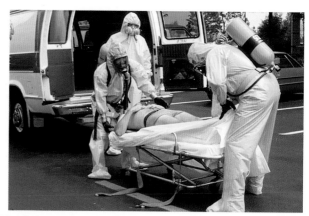

Fig. 1-9
EMS HM Level 2 responders transferring decontaminated patient to EMS HM Level 1 responders.

Using EMS responders trained in hazardous materials activities to assist in decontamination procedures will result in a higher level of care and the ability to provide effective and efficient patient assessment and prehospital care to exposed and contaminated patients.[1] Because of the detailed competencies and requirements expected of EMS HM Level 2 responders, they should attend specially designed training that parallels that for the basic duties of the hazardous materials technician.

DOMESTIC PREPAREDNESS PROGRAM

The OSHA, EPA, and NFPA standards will provide necessary skills in safe response practices, personal protective equipment use, and basic decontamination practices. There are also programs that are more specific to WMD response. The Domestic Preparedness Program training has been presented to scores of emergency responders across the country. It offers specific training for various levels of fire and hazardous materials response, emergency medical response, and hospital providers. Other programs, such as the Noble Training Center in Alabama, programs from Texas A & M University and Louisiana State University, and many others are helping us to come up to speed quickly in this vital area. Because of the rapidly changing face of this response need, more high-quality training programs and texts are becoming available.

CHAPTER SUMMARY

WMD and hazardous materials incidents are among the most dangerous and complex that you will respond to. Please keep these points in mind: This text is intended to be used as a supplemental resource, not a replacement for any of your training. It was produced to share information, but it is up to you to judge the merits of the philosophies and techniques.

Always follow your standard operating procedures. They were developed for your specific problems, equipment, and personnel. Remember that personnel should never attempt to carry out procedures unless they have received specific training for those procedures.

In the field, decisions should be based on everything that the responder has learned and experienced. Never rely on just one source of information.

It is important to remember that research and development are continuing at a rapid pace, and new information is becoming available daily. It is imperative that we continue to seek new ideas and second options, adapt response procedures, cooperate with outside agencies, and improve our efficiency and safety.

REFERENCES

1. National Fire Protection Association: *NFPA 473, Standard for professional competence of EMS responders to hazardous materials incidents*, Quincy, Mass, 2002, National Fire Protection Association.
2. Occupational Safety and Health Administration: *29 CFR 1910.120, Hazardous Waste Operations and Emergency Response, Final Rule, March 6, 1989*, Washington, DC, 1989, US Government Printing Office.

BIBLIOGRAPHY

Agency for Toxic Substances and Disease Registry: *Managing hazardous materials incidents, emergency medical services: a planning guide for the management of contaminated patients*, Atlanta, 2001, U.S. Department of Health and Human Services.

Andrews LP, editor: *Emergency responder training manual for the hazardous materials technician*, New York, 1992, Van Nostrand Reinhold.

Bronstein AC, Currance PL: Module 4: emergency medical operations. In Ayers S, Christopher J, editors: *Medical response to chemical emergencies*, Washington, DC, 1994, Chemical Manufacturers Association.

Buck G: *Preparing for biological terrorism*, Albany, NY, 2002, Delmar.

Coleman RJ, Williams KH: *Hazardous materials dictionary*, Lancaster, Pa, 1988, Technomic Publishing.

Currance PL: *Hazmat for EMS (videotape and guidebook)*, St Louis, 1995, Mosby–Year Book.

Currance PL, Bronstein AC: *Hazardous materials for EMS*, St Louis, 1999, Mosby.

Hawley C: *Hazardous materials incidents*, Albany, NY, 2002, Delmar.

Laughlin J, Trebisacci DG, editors: *Hazardous materials response handbook*, ed 2, Quincy, Mass, 2002, National Fire Protection Association.

National Fire Protection Association: *NFPA 471, Recommended practice for responding to hazardous materials incidents*, Quincy, Mass, 2002, National Fire Protection Association.

National Fire Protection Association: *NFPA 472, Standard for professional competence of responders to hazardous materials incidents*, Quincy, Mass, 2002, National Fire Protection Association.

Noll GG, Hildebrand MS, Yvorra JG: *Hazardous materials—managing the incident*, ed 2, Stillwater, Okla, 1995, Fire Protection Publications.

Strong CB, Irvin TR: *Emergency response and hazardous chemical management—principles and practices*, Delray Beach, Fla, 1996, St Lucie Press.

United States Fire Administration: *Guidelines for public sector hazardous materials training*, Emmitsburg, Md, 1998, Federal Emergency Management Agency.

Basic Principles of Chemistry and Toxicology

PHIL CURRANCE

CHAPTER OBJECTIVES

At the conclusion of this chapter the student will be able to:

- Discuss the importance of determining the state of matter involved in the incident.
- Given physical properties of a specific chemical, identify the state of matter and describe the probable movement pattern.
- Discuss how water solubility and vapor pressure relate to a patient's chemical exposure.
- Identify five types of chemical hazard potential.
- Determine the fire, corrosive, reactive, and toxicity potentials of a chemical.
- Identify common types of radiation exposure and discuss how they relate to patient management.
- Discuss protection measures to guard against radiation exposure.

CASE STUDY

Terrorists have successfully detonated an explosive device in the protective dome of a 90-ton railcar of liquefied chlorine at a large metropolitan wastewater treatment facility. A large amount of chlorine gas is escaping and may threaten people stuck in rush hour traffic and in the downtown area.

If the product is liquefied chlorine, why is so much vapor present?

What hazards does chlorine gas present?

How far downwind will the cloud go?

Where will the cloud go?

How toxic is chlorine?

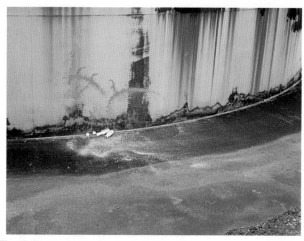

Fig. 2-1
Solid chemical release.

Safe and efficient response to the intentional or unintentional release of a biological, radiological, or, especially, chemical agent mandates a basic knowledge of chemistry and toxicology. The knowledge of where the agent will go and what it can do is essential. Responders need this information so they can predict exposure patterns and levels and anticipate the potential injuries that may occur with specific products.

This chapter provides the responder with the basic information necessary to understand movement and potential hazards of chemicals, including a brief overview of radiation and toxicology. More detailed information can be found in the chapters on chemical, biological, and radiological hazards.

PREDICTING MOVEMENT OF CHEMICALS

A very important issue for responders is being able to predict movement of chemicals. This allows the responders to stage equipment in a safe area and to predict the pattern of exposure.

STATES OF MATTER

The state of matter of the chemical has a direct impact on the type of victim exposure. Chemicals can occur in solid, liquid, or gas (vapor) form.

Atoms in solids have a high molecular attraction for one another and do not usually move farther than their volume allows. Physical means such as wind, ventilation systems, and people can cause a solid product to move. Solids, when mobile, can present an inhalation, ingestion, or skin-contact hazard (Fig. 2-1).

Liquids are more mobile than solids. They are affected by gravity and therefore flow and expand over flat surfaces. Liquids

can also evaporate and turn to vapor, creating a larger problem. Liquids can present an inhalation, ingestion, skin-contact, or skin-absorption hazard (Fig. 2-2).

Gases and vapors present the greatest hazard. They move with air currents, diluting and expanding as they go. This dispersal may result in a wide exposure pattern. Exposure to gases usually results in inhalation, skin-contact, and possibly skin-absorption hazards (Fig. 2-3).

DETERMINING THE STATE OF MATTER

Assessing the melting and boiling point of a material allows the responder to determine the agent's state of matter. At the melting point, a solid turns to a liquid; at the boiling point, a liquid chemical produces maximum vapor. (The vapor pressure equals atmospheric pressure.) By assessing these properties and the ambient temperature, the responder can predict the state of matter of a known material that was released.

The temperature of the product also has a direct impact on the number and type of injuries. For example, as temperature increases, so does the evaporation rate of a liquid, which results in an increase of vapors and in the extent of inhalation exposures.

State of matter is solid, liquid, or gas. States are separated by the melting point and the boiling point.

Melting point is the temperature at which a solid changes to a liquid. An example is ice melting to water at 32° F (0° C).

Boiling point is the temperature at which the vapor pressure of the material being heated equals atmospheric pressure (760 mm Hg). Water boils to steam at 212° F (100° C). Sarin boils at 316° F (157° C). VX boils at 569° F (298° C).

Solution is a mixture in which all of the ingredients are completely dissolved. An example is adding sugar to coffee. Solid agents are often dissolved in a hydrocarbon such as xylene to form a solution that can be sprayed.

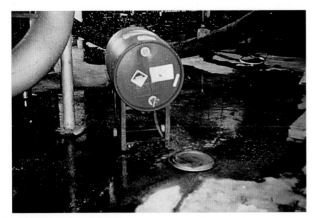

Fig. 2-2
Liquid chemical release.

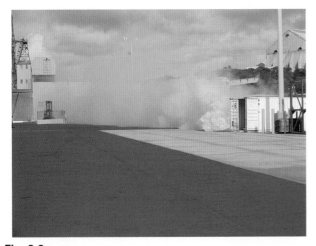

Fig. 2-3
Vapor release.

PHYSICAL PROPERTIES OF MATTER

Once the state of matter has been identified, movement of the agent can be predicted by assessing physical properties. Movement of a liquid contaminant in water can be predicted by looking at the chemical's specific gravity and water solubility. How quickly the chemical will evaporate and pose an inhalation hazard can be assessed by looking at the chemical's vapor pressure and sublimation ability.

Specific gravity is the ratio of a liquid's weight compared to an equal volume of water. Water is given a constant value of 1. Materials with a specific gravity of less than 1.0 float on water, and materials with a specific gravity greater than 1.0 sink. Most hydrocarbons, gasoline for example, float on water (Fig. 2-4).

Water solubility is the degree to which a material or its vapor dissolves in water. Materials that are completely soluble in water are called *miscible* or *polar* solvents. Alcohols are miscible in water. Insoluble materials are called *immiscible* or *nonpolar* solvents.

Viscosity is a measure of the thickness of a liquid. Viscosity determines how quickly a substance flows. Liquids with high viscosity are not very fluid and do not flow or absorb easily. Persistent agents such as mustard and VX have a high viscosity (similar to that of motor oil). Liquids with low viscosity spread easily, increasing the size of the endangered area. Low-viscosity liquids also present a greater risk of skin absorption.

Volatility is a measure of how quickly a material passes into the vapor or gas state. The greater the volatility, the greater the rate of evaporation. Vapor pressure is a measure of volatility. An example is gasoline and diesel fuel: Gasoline is more volatile and evaporates faster than diesel fuel does.

Vapor pressure is the pressure exerted by a vapor against the sides of a closed container. It is temperature dependent: As the temperature increases, so does vapor

Specific Gravity

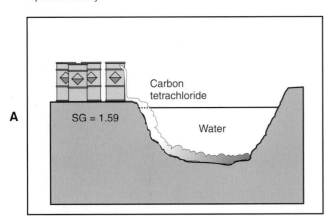

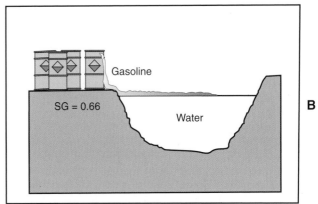

A

Carbon tetrachloride

SG = 1.59

Water

Gasoline

SG = 0.66

Water

B

Fig. 2-4
Liquid chemicals will either float or sink in water depending on their specific gravity.

pressure, and thus more liquid evaporates or vaporizes. Values for vapor pressure are most often given as millimeters of mercury (mm Hg) at a specific temperature. Vapor pressure is used as an indication of how quickly a liquid will evaporate. Water has a vapor pressure of approximately 20 mm Hg at 70° F (21° C) and will evaporate slowly at room temperature. If a chemical has a higher vapor pressure, it will evaporate faster and present an increased inhalation hazard. Sometimes a chemical's vapor pressure is listed in atmospheres (atm). One atmosphere is equal to 760 mm Hg. Chemicals with vapor pressures in excess of 1 atm will turn to vapor almost immediately after being released from their container. Chlorine, for example, has a vapor pressure of 6.8 atm and will evaporate immediately once it leaves its container.

Sublimation is a change of state from solid directly to gas without becoming a liquid first. As temperature increases, so does the rate of sublimation. Dry ice turning directly into carbon dioxide is an example of sublimation.

Of special importance to medical responders are the properties of water solubility and vapor pressure. Inhaled chemicals that are highly water soluble cause upper airway symptoms; chemicals with lower solubility have a tendency to cause lower airway symptoms. Chemicals with a high vapor pressure evaporate very quickly, causing an increased risk of inhalation.

The importance of these properties cannot be underestimated. The Tokyo subway incident is an excellent example. This attack did not cause more fatalities because a form of sarin with a very low vapor pressure was used. Although many people identify sarin and other chemicals in the same class as nerve *gases,* they are in fact liquids at room temperature; they have low vapor pressures, and as a result they evaporate slowly unless they are heated. Sarin has a vapor pressure of 2 mm Hg at 70° F (21° C) and evaporates more slowly than water, resulting in a relatively small amount of vapor in the air. This low vapor pressure causes another problem, however. When these agents are sprayed in a mist or droplet form, they leave liquid on the skin, allowing easy skin absorption and increasing the chance of secondary exposure to care givers.

The military uses terms such as *persistent* and *nonpersistent* to describe chemical warfare agents. This relates directly to their vapor pressure. Many people think that a nonpersistent agent will evaporate almost immediately and will not remain on skin and clothing or cause secondary exposure to caregivers. According to the military definition, a nonpersistent agent is one that will evaporate in less than 24 hours under moderate outdoor conditions. Persistent agents are those that remain for an extended period of time. Sarin, which has a vapor pressure of 2 mm Hg at 70° F (21° C), is a nonpersistent agent; VX, which has a vapor pressure of 0.0001 mm Hg at 70° F (21° C), is a persistent agent.

Boiling point and vapor pressure are closely related. Vapor pressure controls the product's boiling point. This is the reason materials such as chlorine, ammonia, and petroleum gas are kept in a liquid state inside a container even though the

temperature is well above the material's boiling point. Liquefied gases usually have an extremely high expansion ratio. The expansion ratio determines how much vapor will result when liquids evaporate (e.g., 100 cubic feet of gas to 1 cubic foot of liquid is an expansion ratio of 100 to 1). Liquefied petroleum gas (LPG) expands 270 to 1, chlorine 450 to 1, and anhydrous ammonia 840 to 1. Once a liquefied gas is released from its container it will form an extremely large vapor cloud.

When containers of liquids and liquefied gases under pressure are suddenly breached, the product can rapidly boil and expand. If the product is flammable, it can produce a large fireball; this is known as a boiling liquid expanding vapor explosion (BLEVE) (Fig. 2-5). Even nonflammable products can present a BLEVE hazard. The increase in pressure can cause the container to violently rupture, resulting in a large vapor release. The container or projectiles from it can travel great distances.

In most cases BLEVEs are caused by thermal stress. A fire on the outside of the container heats the product inside, causing an increase in vapor pressure. If the container is equipped with a pressure relief valve, the valve usually reduces the pressure and the risk of a BLEVE. However, if the pressure exceeds the ability of the relief valve to adequately reduce the pressure, or if the strength of the container is reduced by heat, a BLEVE can occur. Other factors besides thermal stress can cause a BLEVE, such as mechanical damage to the container or chemical reaction inside the container.

Physical properties can also be used to predict the movement of gases and vapors. The property of vapor density is similar to specific gravity. With vapor density, the chemical's density is compared to the density of air. Assessing a chemical's vapor density will determine if it will float or sink compared with air. With this information the responder can better predict dispersion patterns and exposure risk.

Vapor density is the weight of a volume of pure gas compared to the weight of an equal volume of pure dry air. Air is given a constant value of 1. Materials with a vapor density less than 1.0 are lighter than air and will rise. Materials with a vapor density greater than 1.0 are heavier than air and will sink. Most vapors have

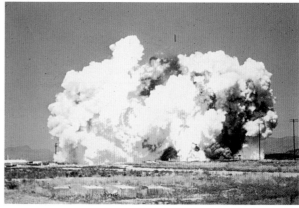

Fig. 2-5
Boiling liquid expanding vapor explosion.

densities greater than 1.0. Heavier vapors can flow and settle in low areas, presenting a greater risk of exposure and fire should they reach an ignition source (Fig. 2-6).

PREDICTING HAZARD POTENTIAL

PREPARING FOR INJURIES AT HAZARDOUS MATERIALS INCIDENTS

To properly prepare for injuries they might have to treat, responders must be able to predict the type of damage a chemical can do. Responders should always assess the hazard potential of a chemical by checking the chemical properties. Responders should assess the flammability, corrosivity, reactivity, radioactivity, and toxicity.

FLAMMABILITY

To date, most terrorist incidents have involved the use of explosives and incendiaries. These can cause traumatic injuries and burns. A chemical's flammability (Fig. 2-7) can be assessed by knowing its flash point, fire point, autoignition temperature, lower flammable limit, and upper flammable limit.

Flash point is the minimum temperature at which a substance evaporates fast enough to form an ignitable mixture with air near the surface of the substance.

Fire point is the temperature at which a liquid gives off sufficient vapor for the air-vapor mixture to contain enough fuel to continue burning after ignition.

Autoignition point is the temperature at which a material will ignite and burn without an ignition source.

Lower flammable limit (LFL) or lower explosive limit (LEL) is the minimum concentration of fuel in the air that will ignite. Below this point there is too much oxygen and not enough fuel to burn (the mixture is too lean).

Upper flammable limit (UFL) or upper explosive limit (UEL) is the concentration of fuel in the air above which the vapors cannot be ignited. Above this point there is too much fuel and not enough oxygen to burn (the mixture is too rich).

Flammable range is the concentration of fuel and air between the LEL (or LFL) and the UEL (or UFL) (Fig. 2-8). The mixture of fuel and air in the flammable range supports combustion.

Chemicals are often classified by their flash point. Many people use terms like *flammable, combustible,* and *noncombustible* without understanding the true definition of these terms. By definition, the difference among a flammable liquid, a combustible liquid, and a noncombustible liquid is the flash point of the chemical. It is not the liquid that burns; the vapors that come off the liquid present the flammability risk. At a chemical's flash point there are enough vapors to create a fire hazard. Flammable chemicals have a flash point below 140° F. Combustible products have a flash point between 140° F and 200° F. Noncombustible products have a flash point at temperatures greater than 200° F. If a noncombustible product is spilled onto a surface that has been heated to a temperature higher than its flash point and an ignition source is present, the product will burn.

At its *autoignition* temperature, a chemical will burn without an ignition source. Some chemicals have autoignition temperatures below room temperature. The chemical's flammable range is also an indication of its inherent flammability. The *flammable range* is the concentration of vapors that exists between the LFL (or LEL) and the UFL (or UEL) and contains enough oxygen and fuel for combustion if an ignition source is present. The wider the flammable range, the easier it is to find an ignition source and a flammable mixture. At the point of release, the mixture may be too rich to burn, but as vapors disperse and mix with air, the flammable range may be found at a distance from the point of release.

Vapor Density

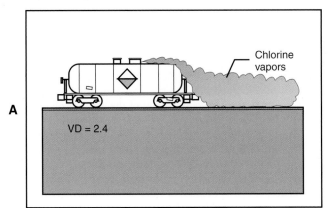
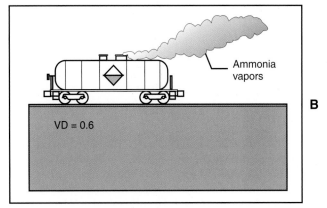

Fig. 2-6
Gases and vapors will either rise or sink to the ground depending on their vapor density.

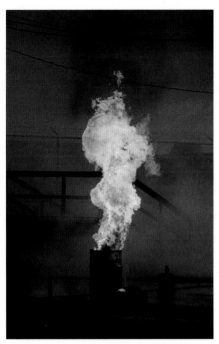

Fig. 2-7
Many chemicals present a flammability hazard.

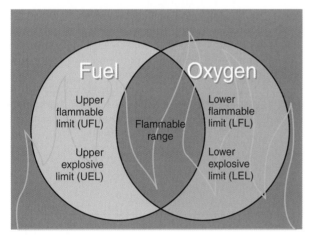

Fig. 2-8
The flammable range is the concentration between the LEL and the UEL.

CORROSIVITY

Another injury hazard is corrosivity. The Department of Transportation defines a corrosive product as one that damages human tissue or has a severe corrosion rate on steel. A more in-depth assessment of a corrosive can be accomplished by determining the chemical's pH. The pH scale (Fig. 2-9) is used to define corrosivity and determine if the product is an acid or base. A material with a pH of 7 is neutral, neither acidic nor alkaline.

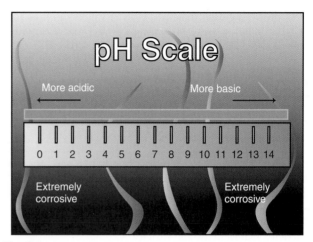

Fig. 2-9
Acids have a pH value of less than 7 and bases have a pH value greater than 7.

Acids are materials with a pH value less than 7. Examples include hydrochloric acid and sulfuric acid.

Bases or alkalis are materials with a pH value greater than 7. Examples include sodium hydroxide and potassium hydroxide.

Understanding how the pH scale works will allow responders to assess the potential hazards associated with the chemical.

The pH scale is an inverse logarithmic representation of the amount of hydrogen ions that are available. This is an important factor in assessing a corrosive chemical's strength. On the pH scale, 7 is neutral. Because the pH scale is inverse or opposite, the lower the number, the greater the amount of hydrogen ions and the stronger the acid. The higher numbers on the scale represent decreasing amounts of hydrogen ions but increasing amounts of hydroxide ions. The more hydroxide ions in the material, the more alkaline or basic the material is. The U.S. Environmental Protection Agency (EPA) defines an extremely corrosive product as one with a pH value of 2 or less or a pH value of 12.5 or greater. Both strong acids and strong alkalis will cause extensive tissue damage. Because the pH scale is a logarithmic scale, for each number change up or down from 7, the strength of the acid or alkali increases by 10 times (pH 6 is 10 times stronger than pH 7; pH 5 is 100 times stronger than pH7; and so on).

Strength describes the corrosiveness of a solution. It refers to the amount of hydrogen or hydroxide ions that are available to go into solution in water.

Concentration is a comparison of the amount of corrosive to the amount of water that is present in a solution. Concentration is not the same as strength. It is possible to have a high concentration of a weak acid or a low concentration of a strong acid.

Both sides of the scale are corrosive. Strong alkalis usually cause deeper burns because of their ability to penetrate tissue. When assessing the hazards of a corrosive chemical, vapor pressure should also be assessed. Chemicals with high vapor pressure will evaporate, and the corrosive vapors will cause inhalation exposure and tissue damage.

Hazardous materials response teams frequently neutralize corrosive chemicals. Although this is an effective way to deal with the released chemical on the ground, corrosive chemicals on skin should *never* be neutralized. Neutralization causes an exothermic (release of heat) reaction, and the tremendous amount of heat released increases the amount of tissue damage. Immediate flushing with copious amounts of water is the treatment of choice.

Neutralization reaction is the process of counteracting an acid or base to form a salt and water. This reaction can produce an enormous amount of heat.

REACTIVITY

Chemicals can present a reactivity hazard. Chemicals may interact to produce heat or increased corrosivity, causing container failure or increasing toxicity when mixed with other chemicals. Some chemicals ignite and burn when exposed to air or water; others can give off oxygen. Chemical compounds can break down into component parts with a tremendous release of energy. Chemicals also frequently become more toxic when they decompose under fire or heat conditions (toxic products of combustion). Fig. 2-10 shows the NFPA 704 marking system for hazardous materials.

Water-reactive materials violently decompose or burn vigorously when they come into contact with moisture. Sodium reacts with water to form sodium hydroxide and hydrogen. Sulfuric acid reacts violently with water due to the heat of solution generated, which can form vapor clouds of steam and sulfuric acid. Terrorists are rumored to have mixed a flammable liquid Molotov cocktail with a water-reactive agent to be thrown on police officers. When water was used to extinguish the fire, the water-reactive chemical would cause even more extensive burns.

Air-reactive materials react with atmospheric moisture and rapidly decompose. White phosphorous found in WP grenades will react and burn in air at temperatures higher than 85° F. Chlorosulfonic acid reacts violently with moisture in the air, creating heat and a vapor cloud and forming hydrochloric acid and sulfuric acid.

Pyrophorics are substances that form self-ignitable flammable vapors when in contact with air.

Oxidation ability is the ability of a substance to release oxygen readily to stimulate combustion. Many chemicals (e.g., nitric acid, chlorine, bromine, hydrogen peroxide, benzoyl peroxide) act as oxidizers.

Polymerization is a chemical reaction in which two or more smaller molecules chemically combine to form larger molecules. The reaction is often violent. If it takes place inside a closed container, the container usually fails.

Inhibitors are chemicals that are added to products to control chemical reactions. Inhibitors are commonly added to monomers to keep them from polymerizing. Inhibitors may be time sensitive or heat sensitive. If an inhibitor loses its effectiveness, polymerization may occur, resulting in container failure.

Catalysts are products that control the rate of a chemical reaction. Catalysts can either speed up or slow down a chemical reaction without being used up or becoming part of the end product. If chemical reaction speed is increased, pressure may build up, causing container failure.

Unstable materials in the pure state vigorously polymerize, decompose, condense, or become self-reactive and undergo other violent chemical changes. For example, ether decomposes to form peroxides, which are shock sensitive. Benzoyl peroxide decomposes explosively at 176° F (80° C).

PREDICTING REACTIVITY

Because so many chemicals are available, predicting reactivity can be a major problem. Labeling systems do not always accurately relate reactivity hazards. The yellow section on the NFPA 704 marking (see Fig. 2-10) indicates reactivity but uses strict criteria. The NFPA reactive criteria include reaction with water and the ability to explode. The NFPA marking might not reflect reactivity when multiple chemicals are mixed.

Some reactivity can be assessed from an understanding of the chemical structure. Organic materials are derived from living or once-living materials. Organic compounds are formed by covalent bonding. In covalent bonding, the elements combine into compounds by sharing of electrons. Covalent bonding can produce very complicated chemical compounds.

CHEMICAL STRUCTURE

HYDROCARBONS

Hydrocarbons are organic chemicals that contain chains of carbon and hydrogen atoms. Most organic materials react with oxidizers and are flammable or combustible. There are three kinds of hydrocarbons: saturated, unsaturated, and aromatic. In many cases their reactivity differs.

Saturated hydrocarbons (alkanes) are straight chain or branched hydrocarbons with only single covalent bonds. In

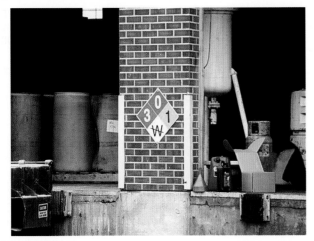

Fig. 2-10
NFPA 704 marking system for hazardous materials.

other words, all of the carbons are saturated with hydrogen. This saturation generally makes the chemical fairly stable. Hydrocarbons that end in "ane" (e.g., methane, pentane, butane) are examples of saturated hydrocarbons.

Unsaturated hydrocarbons (alkenes and alkynes) have double or triple bonds between some of the carbon atoms in the molecule. In other words, not all of the carbon molecules are saturated with hydrogen. Generally speaking, these double or triple bonds are weaker than single bonds and make the chemical more reactive than saturated hydrocarbons. Hydrocarbons that end in "ene" (e.g., pentene, butene) and "yne" (e.g., ethyne) are examples of unsaturated hydrocarbons.

Aromatic hydrocarbons contain a benzene ring. Benzene, toluene, and xylene are examples of aromatic hydrocarbons. They are fairly nonreactive solvents, but some, such as benzene, can be toxic.

Another term that you may hear is *halogenated hydrocarbon.* A halogenated hydrocarbon has an element from the halogen group (chlorine, fluorine, bromine, iodine) attached in place of a hydrogen atom. Many solvents contain halogenated hydrocarbons (e.g., carbon tetrachloride, trichloroethylene, trichloroethane). Halogenated hydrocarbons are usually more toxic than nonhalogenated hydrocarbons.

INORGANIC COMPOUNDS

Inorganic compounds do not usually contain carbon. Some may contain carbon atoms, but they lack carbon chains. Inorganic compounds form by ionic bonding. In ionic bonding, elements form compounds by giving off or taking on an electron. This type of bonding limits the size of the chemical structure. Inorganic compounds range from extremely stable (e.g., water) to some that are extremely reactive with water (e.g., sulfuric acid, lithium hydride) and with air (e.g., phosphine, silane).

RADIOACTIVITY

Responders may come into contact with radioactive substances. A terrorist might use a radiological agent as a simple exposure device, a radioactive agent placed in a location where many people may gather. Another major threat is a *dirty bomb,* a radioactive agent coupled with a conventional explosive device. The explosive is used to spread the radioactive agent over a large area. A third threat is a nuclear device, which could be detonated with devastating effects.

TYPES OF RADIATION

Radioactivity is the spontaneous disintegration of unstable nuclei accompanied by the emission of nuclear radiation. Ionizing radiation can be particles, or it can be pure energy that produces changes in matter by creating ion pairs. Responders or patients exposed to electromagnetic radiation sources emitting gamma rays will be irradiated. They are not contaminated and pose no risk of secondary contamination. Conversely, exposure to particle radiation sources (alpha and beta particles, neutrons, protons, and positrons) in the form of dusts, liquids, or gases do result in contamination and present a secondary contamination risk. The most common types of

radioactive sources (Fig. 2-11) encountered are alpha particles, beta particles, and gamma rays.

Alpha particles are the largest of the radioactive particles. They are the same size as the nucleus of the helium atom, can travel less than 10 inches (25 cm), and can be stopped by a sheet of paper.

Beta particles are the same size as an electron. They can travel approximately 10 feet (3 m) and can be stopped by a piece of aluminum that is 1-mm thick.

Gamma rays are weightless forms of pure energy. They can travel great distances and are stopped by heavy shielding such as lead.

Neutron radiation is very penetrating radiation that can result in whole-body irradiation. There are few natural emitters, but neutron radiation can be found in reactors and research accelerators and after nuclear detonations.

Half-life is a measure of the rate of decay of a radioactive material. It indicates the time needed for one-half of a given amount of a radioactive material to change to another nuclear form or element.

PROTECTION FROM RADIATION

Time, distance, and shielding are means of protection against ionizing radioactive materials. The exact amounts of time, distance, and thickness of shielding depend on the type and amount of radioactive source. Radiation experts, using special detection equipment, can assist with these decisions. In all cases, the shorter the exposure time, the greater the distance from the source, and the greater the shielding, the lower the dose. A detailed discussion can be found in Chapter 4.

TOXICOLOGY

Toxicity is a major concern when dealing with weapons of mass destruction. Just as the other hazards can be identified by assessing chemical properties, the agent's level of toxicity can be assessed by dose and exposure attributes.

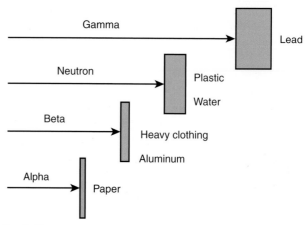

Fig. 2-11
Alpha, beta, neutron, and gamma radiation.

DOSE-RESPONSE RELATIONSHIP

The most important concept in toxicology is the *dose-response relationship*. Paracelsus (1493-1541) noted that all substances known to man are poisons, and only the amount or dose determines the effect. This idea led to the concept of the dose-response relationship: The larger the dose, the greater the response; the smaller the dose, the less the response. Thus the toxic effects of a chemical exposure can be estimated based on the level of exposure.

One measure of toxicity is the *lethal dose system*. This system is based on animal research studies that determine fatal exposures with oral, dermal, and inhalation exposures. Table 2-1 shows the lethal doses and concentrations of nerve agents.

Lethal Dose 50% (LD_{50}) is the median lethal dose; that is, the oral or dermal exposure dose that will kill 50% of the exposed animal population in two weeks.

Lethal Concentration 50% (LC_{50}) is the air concentration of a substance that will kill 50% of the exposed animal population. This is also commonly seen as LCt_{50}. This denotes the concentration (C) and the length of exposure time (t) that will result in fatality in 50% of the exposed animal population.

This system can be used to compare toxicity of chemicals, but it has limitations. The results are based on data from animals, not humans, and the studies are based on lethal effects, not the amount of agent that would cause harm or injury.

Whereas the LD_{50} and LC_{50} are based on a lethal endpoint, other dose-response systems provide guidelines for safe occupational exposures. These levels have been established by government, industry, and private groups to identify potentially dangerous levels of exposure. In the United States the most often used exposure limits are published by the National Institute of Occupational Safety and Health (NIOSH), the Occupational Safety and Health Administration (OSHA), and the American Conference of Governmental and Industrial Hygienists (ACGIH).

Recommended exposure limit (REL) is the time-weighted average (TWA) for an 8-hour day and a 40-hour work week during which nearly all workers may be repeatedly exposed without adverse effects. These levels are established by NIOSH and are not legally enforceable. RELs are given as time-weighted average (REL-TWA), short-term exposure limits (REL-STEL), and ceiling limits (REL-C).

Threshold limit value (TLV) is established by the ACGIH. TLV refers to the airborne concentrations of a substance and represents conditions under which it is believed that nearly all workers may be repeatedly exposed day after day without adverse effects. TLVs are given as time-weighted average (TLV-TWA), short-term exposure limits (TLV-STEL), and ceiling limits (TLV-C).

Permissible exposure limit (PEL) is the allowable air concentration of a substance in the workplace 8 hours a day, 40 hours a week, as established by OSHA. These values are legally enforceable. PELs are given as time-weighted average (PEL-TWA), short-term exposure limits (PEL-STEL), and ceiling limits (PEL-C).

Time-weighted average (TWA) is the average concentration of a substance for a normal 8-hour work day and a 40-hour work week to which nearly all workers may be repeatedly exposed, day after day, without adverse effect.

Short-term exposure limit (STEL) is an exposure level safe to work in for short periods of time (15 minutes), 4 times a day, with at least 60 minutes between each exposure. No irritation or other adverse effects should be experienced. This level is in addition to exposure at the TWA.

Ceiling limit (C) is the concentration that should never be exceeded during any part of the working exposure. This value has been established as the maximum level to be used in computing the TWA and STEL limits.

IDLH (immediately dangerous to life or health) is the maximum environmental air concentration of a substance from which a person could escape within 30 minutes without symptoms of impairment or irreversible health effects. This level was established by the EPA and NIOSH and was originally developed for respirator selection. Because the IDLH was designed for acute emergency exposures that could result in death, the 30-minute window is arbitrary. Immediate evacuation and the use of high levels of PPE must be emphasized.

There are other exposure limits besides the RELs, PELs, and TLVs. Many private companies establish their own in-house exposure limits.

These exposure levels have been developed with the healthy adult subject in mind. The safe level of exposure may vary from agency to agency, so the lowest established level should be used. However, these levels do not take into consideration individual differences such as age, sensitivity, or medical conditions. Some people experience adverse effects at or below the established limits. In addition, the limits are developed for the workplace, where exposure is limited, not for the home, where people spend many more hours.

These limits are usually reported in parts per million (ppm) (parts of gas or vapor per million parts of air) or parts per billion (ppb) (parts of gas or vapor per billion parts of air) for gases and vapors. These are obviously very small amounts. One ppm can be visualized as one drop of water in a swimming pool. The limits can also be given in mg/m^3 (milligrams of a substance per cubic meter of air) for substances that would be respirable as a liquid mist or solid particle mass.

Table 2-1
Nerve Agent Toxicity

Agent	LC_{50} (Inhalation) mg/min/m^2	LD_{50} (Skin) mg/person
Tabun (GA)	200	4000
Sarin (GB)	100	1700
Soman (GD)	100	300
VX	50	10

Carcinogens. Some chemicals are known or suspected to cause cancer. These chemicals are *carcinogens.* The ACGIH rates carcinogens with the following system:
• A1: Confirmed human carcinogen
• A2: Suspected human carcinogen
• A3: Animal carcinogen
• A4: Not classifiable as a human carcinogen
• A5: Not suspected as a human carcinogen
NIOSH and OSHA indicate potential carcinogenic chemicals with a "Ca" notation.

RESPONSE GUIDELINES

Because of the inadequacies of PELs and TLVs in assessing exposures in the general population and home environments, special exposure limits have been established. Emergency Response Planning Guidelines (ERPG), short-term public emergency guidance levels (SPEGL), and the level of concern (LOC) are designed to aid the emergency responder in making decisions regarding nonworkplace exposures.

Emergency Response Planning Guidelines (ERPG) are published by the American Industrial Hygiene Association. These exposure limits are designed for emergency planning. There are three levels of ERPG: ERPG-3 is the level to which persons could be exposed for 1 hour without experiencing or developing life-threatening effects; ERPG-2 is the level for a 1-hour exposure that should not cause irreversible adverse or other serious health effects or symptoms that could impair an individual's ability to take protective action; ERPG-1 is the level for a 1-hour exposure that should not result in health effects more severe than sensory perception or mild irritation. Only a few ERPGs are established.

Short-term public emergency guidance levels (SPEGLs) are established by the National Research Council. These are concentrations considered acceptable for public exposures during emergencies. Only a few SPEGLs are established.

Level of concern is established by the EPA for public exposures to chemicals that have established IDLH limits. This level is set at one tenth the level of the IDLH. The level of concern was developed as an interim level until more appropriate exposure limits are developed to protect the public during short-term exposures.

DURATION OF EXPOSURE

The duration of the chemical exposure is another important part in assessing the level of toxic threat. The shorter the exposure, the lower the dose and presumably the lower the response. Exposures are commonly referred to as *acute* and *chronic.*

Acute exposure is an exposure that occurs over a short time (less than 24 hours). It usually occurs when there has been a spill or release.

Chronic exposure is an exposure to low concentrations over a long period of time. These exposures usually occur on a day-to-day basis in the workplace.

Care must be taken to avoid confusing exposure with onset of symptoms. Acute exposures often, but not always, result in the immediate onset of exposure symptoms. Acute exposures can also result in a delayed onset that occurs hours to days later, or they can produce long-term symptoms that do not show up until years later. Exposure to vesicants such as mustard (H) is an example of an acute exposure with a delayed onset of symptoms.

ROUTES OF EXPOSURE

The *route of exposure* through which the agent enters the body is also an important concept in evaluating an agent's toxicity potential. Damage may be *local* (confined to the exposed area), *systemic,* or both.

Local damage is present at the point of chemical contact.

Systemic damage is remote to the site of exposure or absorption.

Hazardous agents usually enter the body by inhalation, ingestion, skin or eye absorption, or injection (subcutaneous, intramuscular, or intravenous).

Inhalation. Inhalation is the quickest and most common route of chemical exposure. The human pulmonary system has an enormous surface area available for absorption. The average adult lung surface area available for chemical absorption measures 140 to 150 square meters. In comparison, the skin surface of the average adult is about 2 square meters. The respiratory system has many times more surface area available for chemical absorption than the skin does.

Many different chemical forms are respirable. Gases and vapors are the states most often encountered. Solid particles and liquid drops may also be respirable. For particulate matter, the size of the particle is extremely important.

Gases are substances that distribute uniformly in a container at room temperature.

Vapor is the gaseous state of a chemical that is a solid or liquid at room temperature (70° F, 21° C) and standard pressure (760 mm Hg).

Dust is solid particulate matter of varying size.

Aerosol is a suspension of liquids or solids in air.

Mist and fog are condensation of liquid droplets on particles. Mists are created by the combustion of vapors.

The respiratory tract is divided into the *upper* and *lower* respiratory tract.

Upper respiratory tract consists of the nasal cavity, oral cavity, pharynx, larynx, and trachea.

Lower respiratory tract consists of the lower trachea, air passages (bronchial tubes), and alveoli.

The air passages subdivide into main bronchi, secondary bronchi, terminal bronchioles, respiratory bronchioles, alveolar ducts, and the alveolar sacs, where oxygen and carbon dioxide exchange takes place. The system decreases in size from top to bottom, acting as an increasingly fine filter. This filter determines where particles will deposit in the lower respiratory tract (Fig. 2-12). Generally, particles from 5 to 30 μm are deposited in the upper airway. Particles in the 3 to 5 μm range make it into the lower respiratory tract. Particles must be 1 μm or smaller to be deposited in the alveoli. One of the

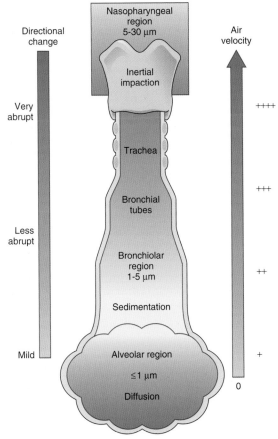

Fig. 2-12
Particles can be deposited throughout the respiratory tract.

features of weaponized anthrax spores is a size that allows the spores to reach the lower respiratory tract.

Gas, vapor, and liquid water solubility determines how far into the respiratory tract the substance will reach and the onset of symptoms. Agents such as ammonia that are highly water soluble will react with water in the upper respiratory tract. This reaction causes upper airway irritation and damage, with immediate onset of symptoms such as coughing. Agents that are less water soluble, such as phosgene, usually penetrate into the lower respiratory tract. This usually causes direct lung damage leading to pulmonary edema, often with a delayed onset. Other chemicals, such as hydrogen fluoride, may cause delayed onset of symptoms because of their systemic toxicity.

Another kind of inhalation toxicity is caused by *asphyxiants*. Asphyxiants are chemicals that impair the body's ability to either get or use oxygen. Asphyxiants are divided into two general classes: *simple* and *chemical*.

Simple asphyxiants are inert gases and vapors that displace oxygen in inspired air. Examples include carbon dioxide and nitrogen.

Chemical asphyxiants are chemicals that prevent the transportation of oxygen to the cells or the utilization of oxygen at the cellular level. Examples include carbon

monoxide, hydrogen cyanide (AC), cyanogen chloride (CK), and hydrogen sulfide.

Ingestion. Although ingestion is not the most common way for hazardous chemicals to enter the body, it is certainly possible in an intentional release. Food or water supplies may be contaminated by biological, chemical, or radiological agents. A group in The Dalles, Oregon, used *Salmonella* to contaminate salad bars in an attempt to sway a local election. Ingestion may also occur when victims or responders fail to decontaminate before smoking, eating, or drinking. Ingestion may also occur when particulate matter is breathed in, impacts in the oropharynx, and then is swallowed.

Absorption. Unlike the respiratory and gastrointestinal systems, intact skin is usually an effective barrier to many toxic agents. However, many agents, such as corrosives, can cause skin and eye damage. If the chemical is absorbable across the skin and eye membranes, it may cause systemic toxicity. Some chemicals, such as nerve and blister agents, can easily pass through the skin.

Certain parts of the body absorb chemicals faster than other areas. For example, the eyes, scalp, and groin area absorb chemicals many times faster than the feet or hands do. Skin absorption is increased in hot weather and in cases of skin damage.

Once a chemical is absorbed across a body membrane (e.g., lungs, skin, eyes, or gastrointestinal tract) it is distributed throughout the body. It can then be metabolized, be stored in organs or adipose (fat) tissue, and cause damage to specific organs where it is stored or from which it is excreted. Chemicals are usually metabolized by the liver. The byproducts of this metabolism may be more toxic than the original compound. Chemicals can be stored in organs or adipose tissue and released over an extended period. Excretion occurs by the lungs, kidneys, skin, and gastrointestinal system. Specific organs that can be damaged are referred to as target organs. Typical target organs include the brain, heart, lungs, liver, and kidneys.

CHAPTER SUMMARY

Although responders do not have to be chemists or toxicologists, they must have an understanding of how chemicals move and what type of harm they cause. A thorough grasp of this material is vital to safe response and patient management. By assessing the chemical and physical properties of a hazardous agent, responders will have a better idea of what they are facing during a WMD event. Physical properties such as boiling and melting point, specific gravity, and vapor density can help responders predict movement of hazardous chemicals and predict injury patterns. Knowledge of chemical properties will assist responders in identifying the harm that a chemical can do. Flash point, fire point, autoignition temperature, and upper and lower explosive limits can indicate flammability risk. To assess a chemical's corrosive potential, pH should be assessed. Chemical structure can help to determine a chemical's reactive potential. Radioactivity threat and protective measures can be assessed by identifying the type of radiation hazard present. Lastly, the potential toxicological effects can be assessed by a responder who has an understanding of the dose-response relationship, duration of exposure, and route of exposure.

BIBLIOGRAPHY

Agency for Toxic Substances and Disease Registry: *Managing hazardous materials incidents, emergency medical services: a planning guide for the management of contaminated patients,* Atlanta, 2001, United States Department of Health and Human Services.

Andrews LP, editor: *Emergency responder training manual for the hazardous materials technician,* New York, 1992, Van Nostrand Reinhold.

Bowen JE: *Emergency management of hazardous materials incidents,* Quincy, Mass, 1995, National Fire Protection Association.

Bronstein AC, Currance PL: *Emergency care for hazardous materials exposure,* ed 2, St Louis, 1994, Mosby.

Coleman RJ, Williams KH: *Hazardous materials dictionary,* Lancaster, Pa, 1988, Technomic Publishing.

Currance PL, Bronstein AC: *Hazardous materials for EMS,* St Louis, 1999, Mosby.

Hawley C: *Hazardous materials incidents,* Albany, NY, 2002, Delmar.

Laughlin J, Trebisacci DG, editors: *Hazardous materials response handbook,* ed 2, Quincy, Mass, 2002, National Fire Protection Association.

National Fire Protection Association: *NFPA 471, Recommended practice for responding to hazardous materials incidents,* Quincy, Mass, 2002, National Fire Protection Association.

Noll GG, Hildebrand MS, Yvorra JG: *Hazardous materials—managing the incident,* ed 2, Stillwater, Okla, 1995, Fire Protection Publications.

Strong CB, Irvin TR: *Emergency response and hazardous chemical management—principles and practices,* Delray Beach, Fla, 1996, St Lucie Press.

Sullivan JB, Kreiger GR, editors: *Hazardous material toxicology, clinical principles of environmental health,* Baltimore, 1992, Williams & Wilkins.

Varela J, editor: *Hazardous materials handbook for emergency responders,* New York, 1996, Van Nostrand Reinhold.

Explosives and Incendiary Devices

GARY CHRISTMAN

CHAPTER OBJECTIVES

At the conclusion of this chapter the student will be able to:

- Explain why terrorists use explosive devices.
- Discuss what makes up an explosive device.
- Define improvised explosive device (IED).
- Describe detonators that are used to detonate IEDs.
- Describe a secondary device and the use of such devices.
- Describe incendiary devices.
- Describe blast injuries and the human response.

CASE STUDY

On routine patrol an officer notices a heavy odor of fuel in the atmosphere. She also notices a rental truck sitting in front of the federal building in downtown St. Louis. Because these trucks have been used in the past for explosive devices and because it is parked in front of the federal building, the officer calls for a supervisor and bomb and arson squads to respond. She decides to set up a perimeter and warn the federal officers about the truck. With this done, the decision to pull the fire alarm to evacuate the building is made. When the officers pull the fire alarm, a secondary device detonates that in turn sets off the primary device that was concealed in the rental truck. The explosion causes a large amount of damage to the building, the surrounding buildings, the street and the tunnels below. There are numerous fatalities and injured patients. Many of the patients are still trapped in the building. The utilities in the area are damaged with flooding in the tunnels due to broken water mains, which will hamper fire suppression.

What are some of the things that you will need to worry about besides search and rescue, fire suppression, and evidence preservation on the scene?

How will treatment protocols be changed if another component—such as a chemical, biological, or radiological agent—had been added to the bomb?

What are the chances that additional secondary devices have been planted at the scene?

HISTORY OF TERRORIST BOMBINGS

History shows that to date, more than 90% of terrorist attacks have used explosive or incendiary devices. A history of high-profile events in the United States includes:
- Bombing of the World Trade Center in New York in 1993
- Attempted bombing of an IRS building in 1995
- Bombing of the Murrah Building in Oklahoma City in 1995
- Bombing of the FBI field office in Texas in 1996
- Bombing of a women's health clinic in Atlanta in 1996 (secondary devices used)
- Bombing in Centennial Park in Atlanta in 1996
- Bombs in Columbine High School in 1999 (secondary devices)
- Coordinated airplane attacks on the World Trade Center in New York and the Pentagon in Washington in 2001

EXPLOSIVE DEVICES

Explosives and incendiaries have been the terrorist weapon of choice for many reasons. The components and instructions for bomb making are readily available. The effects of a bomb are immediate and deadly.

Explosive materials and accessories are cheap to buy or they can be stolen. Components for explosive devices can be purchased in farming supplies stores, hardware stores, or gun stores, and they can be made from materials and products found in most homes. From 1993 to 1997, more than 50,000 pounds of explosives and blasting agents and more than 30,000 detonators were reported stolen in the United States.[1]

Many books have been written on the subject of bomb making. Add to this the vast resource that the Internet provides. Members of many terrorist organizations or local militia groups have received military training in the United States or abroad.

The history of the explosive devices that have been deployed in the United States shows that when an explosive device is deployed properly, it will cause a number of injuries and fatalities, and the number of injuries is going to be high. There will also be an overwhelming psychological effect on citizens at the scene and at home watching on TV. This same effect will be felt by first responders.

Explosive devices produce immediate results. With explosive devices, the terrorist knows that there will be immediate and high-profile damage. This will catch people off guard and send a lot of resources into a small area. This could be the perfect setup for a secondary device. Past responses such as the first World Trade Center attack and the Oklahoma City bombing have shown responders rushing to help. Had secondary devices been deployed, the death toll may have been much, much higher. We need to consider that every explosion may be a possible WMD attack until proved otherwise.

Explosive devices can be detonated in different ways, and they can be detonated at the scene or by radio, phone, or pager from a long distance away. This can allow the bomber to be far away before the device is activated. In some countries, suicide bombers are a common way to deliver and detonate a bomb.

TYPES OF EXPLOSIVE DEVICES

Explosive devices are energetic material and come in three different forms: pyrotechnics, propellants, and explosives.

PYROTECHNICS

Pyrotechnics are created to make light, sound, and smoke for firework displays. Pyrotechnics are used for other devices that include road flares and thermite devices, which are used by railroad workers so they know a train is coming while they are working on the tracks.

PROPELLANTS

Propellants are designed to move an object. Propellants give a bullet the power to fire from the gun. A gas buildup is caused by the chemical release and becomes a propellant. This gas buildup is a controlled one designed to perform a job.

EXPLOSIVES

Explosives are designed to provide a rapid expansion of gas. Explosives are classified as *low explosives* or *high explosives.*

Low Explosives. Low explosives are made to deflagrate, or rapidly burn, not explode. Unless the low explosive is confined, no pressure wave is created. Two common low explosives are *black powder* and *smokeless powder.* Black powder was the first powder used as a propellant for ammunition. Rifle enthusiasts still use this powder for black powder weapons (muzzleloaders). Black powder is extremely durable and does not deteriorate with age or when submerged in water. Smokeless powder is now the leading powder for firearm use and rockets.

High Explosives. High explosives detonate (burn faster than the speed of sound). Detonation, unlike deflagration, is accompanied by a pressure wave. These explosives are not as easy to set off as low explosives and typically require a detonator.

IMPROVISED EXPLOSIVE DEVICES

Improvised explosive devices (IEDs) are relatively easy to make and hard to detect. The IED is limited only by the bomber's imagination. The most common type of IED has always been the pipe bomb. This type of IED is not complicated but can cause substantial damage, casualties, and possibly fatalities. This shows that the IED does not have to be sophisticated, it just has to be designed to destroy whatever is near. IEDs are usually used because the bomber doesn't have access to military explosives. IEDs can be found in the form of car bombs, boat bombs, and package bombs, or they can be delivered by suicide bombers wearing the explosive in vests, belts, or shoes.

BOOK BOMB

A book bomb is a book with the pages glued together and an area large enough for explosive material, wires, and power supply cut out. This can be triggered by a number of different switches. The most common switch for this IED is a pressure switch that detonates when the book is opened (Fig. 3-1).

LETTER BOMB

Letter bombs can be made out of any type of envelope, package, or box. The most common type is the package bomb, but letters or greeting cards have been used. Greeting cards may be used because of the setup of the card. Greeting cards that play music when they are opened are already an explosive device minus the explosive. The card has the power supply, wires, and switch (Fig. 3-2).

DRY ICE BOMB

Dry ice has been used in a number of different ways to keep products cold and to produce "smoke" at events. Dry ice can be used as an explosive device. The bomber places dry ice in a glass bottle, adds hot water, caps the bottle, and runs. This device explodes in as little as a few seconds or as long as a few hours. Although the mixture itself is not usually deadly, it can be combined with projectiles such as nails or screws to add to the lethality of the device. This information is found on a number of sites on the Internet and is commonly used by adolescents to blow up mailboxes.

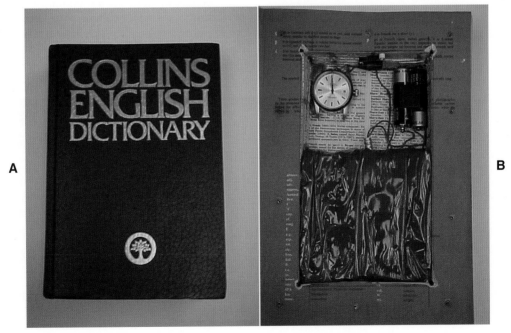

Fig. 3-1
Book bomb.

VCR TAPE BOMB

A VHS tape cassette can be opened and the tape replaced with an explosive charge and a small power supply. When the tape is introduced into the machine, the VCR opens the tape, triggers the power supply, and detonates the device (Fig. 3-3).

PIPE BOMB

Pipe bombs can be made from any type of PVC (polyvinyl chloride), galvanized steel, or metal pipe. Components include a pipe around a foot long with threaded end caps, an explosive agent, a power supply, and a switch (Figs. 3-4 and 3-5). The switch can be a watch, alarm clock, pager, cell phone, or mercury switch or a combination of any of these. The traditional fuse for a pipe bomb is a standard burning fuse.

FIRST AID KIT BOMB

For many years there has been a concern of an explosive device left on the scene of a medical or trauma emergency to be

picked up by an EMS unit and transported to the hospital or back to the EMS station. Fig. 3-6 shows a first aid kit made into an explosive device. This type of device can be hidden in a flashlight, trauma kit, or airway bag. On the scene of an emergency it is difficult to keep track of all of your equipment. Mark your equipment and double check it before the unit leaves to be sure that no extra equipment is picked up. This explosive could be wired to explode by remote, timer, shaker, or switch hooked to the lid, zipper, or an on/off switch.

TRUCK OR CAR BOMB

Truck bombs and car bombs are used frequently in bombings and assassinations. Most of these explosives are made from ammonium nitrate and a fuel such as diesel fuel (ammonium nitrate–fuel oil, ANFO). This is the explosive that was used in the Oklahoma City bombing. The first attack on the New York World Trade Center used urea nitrate (a similar fertilizer) and fuel oil. ANFO is a common explosive that has been used for years. Two different types of ammonium nitrate are sold: One is fertilizer grade and the other is explosive grade. The fertilizer grade can be turned into explosive grade and used in an IED.

These are just a few of the many different types of IEDs. Remember that the type of IED is limited only by the bomber's imagination. IEDs look like a regular item and can be detonated by a number of different detonators. Most of them can be made at home or purchased legally or through underground channels. IEDs can also incorporate conventional military explosives, as Fig. 3-7 shows.

TNT (TRINITROTOLUENE)

TNT is a military explosive but is also used in commercial applications. TNT burns (detonates) at a velocity of 22,000 feet per second (fps). As the burning rate of an explosive increases, so does the amount of pressure developed. The explosive yield of all other high explosives is compared against TNT. Some of the other military explosives that may find their way into terrorist hands include RDX (cyclotrimeth-

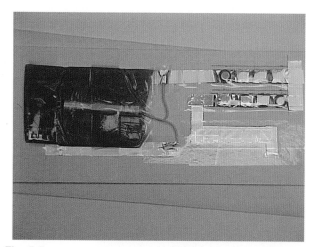

Fig. 3-2
Letter bomb.

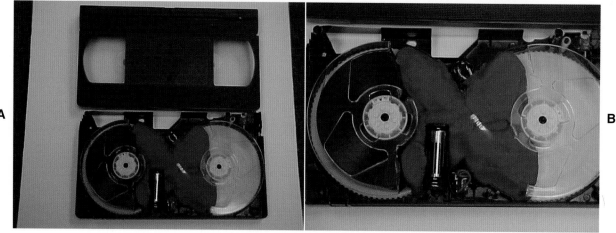

Fig. 3-3
VCR bomb.

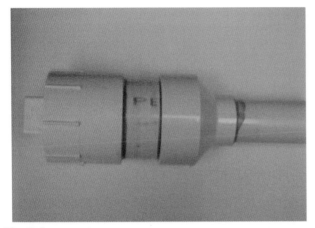

Fig. 3-4
PVC pipe bomb.

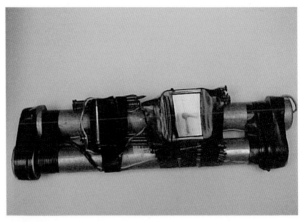

Fig. 3-5
Galvanized steel pipe bomb.

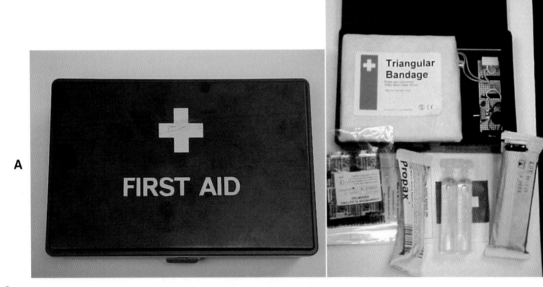

Fig. 3-6
First aid kit bomb.

ylenetrinitramine, 26,800 fps), HMX (high melting point explosive, 29,900 fps), PETN (pentaerythritoltetranitrate, 27,200 fps), and Semtex (a compound of RDX and PETN, 26,400 fps).

DETONATORS

There are many different ways to detonate explosive devices or IEDs. The imagination is the only limit. A few of the detonators that have been used include a basic fuse, clocks (wrist watch, timers, and alarm clocks), pressure switch, compression switch, on/off switch, mercury switch, sensor switches (used on alarm systems and outside lighting), remote control, garage door opener, cell phone, and pager.

SECONDARY DEVICES

The Atlanta women's health clinic bombing brought the concept of the secondary device into the minds of U.S. responders. The first device was in the building itself. This secondary device went off on the scene after the first responders were set up and working the first explosion. The secondary device was placed at a location commonly used as a staging area for emergency responders answering calls at the clinic.

Secondary devices have been used in other incidents such as the Otherside Lounge bombing in Atlanta and the Columbine High School shooting in Jefferson County, Colorado. Secondary devices have been a standard method of operation

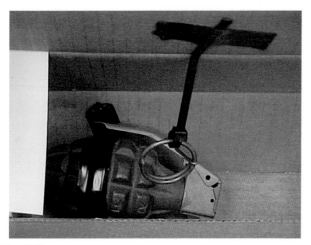

Fig. 3-7
Improvised explosive device using a military grenade.

in other parts of the world. Most secondary devices in the past have been explosive devices, but they can be a number of different weapons including chemical, biological, or nuclear devices, and possibly a sniper waiting for the first responders to arrive on the scene.

Many different hazards may be present at a bombing scene. If the bomb is made with a plastic explosive, there could be pieces of undetonated plastic explosive scattered about the area. These pieces of plastic explosive can be detonated with an impact, such as a responder stepping on the material. Be suspicious of secondary devices when approaching the scene. Also be aware of the damage the explosive device will cause (gas leaks, fires, and building damage). Remember that primary or secondary devices could contain other weapons of mass destruction such as biological, chemical, and radiological material.

One major concern now is the dirty bomb, a conventional explosive device used to disperse radiological, chemical, or biological weapons. The effectiveness of the technique depends on the bomb and the agent selected. Highly volatile chemicals will be destroyed by the blast. For example cyanide was used in the bomb at the first New York World Trade Center bombing. Because of the high volatility of cyanide, most of the chemical was destroyed by the explosion and only trace amounts were found. This is not always the case. Explosive devices can be effectively used as dispersal devices. Typically these devices use a low explosive directional charge designed to propel the agent into the atmosphere. This is been the standard military design used since World War I.

INCENDIARY DEVICES

MOLOTOV COCKTAIL

The most popular incendiary device throughout history has been the Molotov cocktail. A Molotov cocktail is made by filling a glass bottle with gasoline or other flammable liquid. A fuel-soaked rag is used to plug the bottle. The rag is ignited and the bottle is thrown at a target. A glass bottle is used so the glass will break on impact and spread the fuel. A Molotov cocktail has about a 2% failure rate. Several different mixtures can be used. These devices can also be used to disperse other agents. When other chemicals are added, the damage potential can be significantly increased. Adding a chemical that reacts with water will increase the damage when sprinkler systems are activated or the fire department attempts to put out the fire.

CHEMICAL FIRE BOTTLE

A chemical fire bottle is an advanced type of Molotov cocktail. This does not need to be fused by a rag dipped in a flammable liquid. The bottle is filled with a mixture of gasoline and other chemicals to create a device that will burst like an explosive device. This device does not need to be lit like the standard Molotov cocktail. It will burst and ignite on its own due to the reaction of the chemical mixture. The device is thrown just like a Molotov cocktail and will burst into flames upon impact.

Incendiary devices are used for arsons as well as assassination and terrorist attacks. Molotov cocktails have to be thrown at the target, which means the person throwing the bottle must be close to the area thus risks being apprehended. Another possibility is to have chemicals react, causing the ignition. This can be used as a delayed fuse of sorts. A common type is one chemical in a glass jar and a second in a Styrofoam cup over the mouth of the glass jar. The chemical in the cup dissolves the cup, leaks into the glass jar, and causes a chemical reaction. A number of different chemicals can be used in this type of device. Be aware when you respond to these incidents that some of these chemicals can be extremely toxic.

BLAST INJURIES AND THE HUMAN RESPONSE TO BLAST EFFECTS

Medical responders must have an understanding of the types of injuries that explosives can cause. Effective triage principles can be based on these specific effects. Four classes of injury are commonly seen at blast locations. When treating patients, keep in mind that patient clothing and anything that is removed from the patient's body is evidence and will need to be documented and turned over to law enforcement agencies.

PRIMARY BLAST INJURY

Explosive devices when detonated turn from a solid into a superheated gas in 0.0001 sec. These gases expand at a rate of 13,000 mph (Mach 17.6). After the device explodes, waves of pressure called *blast waves* are sent out from the seat of the blast. These are the first to cause injury by smashing and shattering anything in the way. Blast waves cause death or injury, depending on the victim's distance from the explosive device (Boxes 3-1 and 3-2). Four target organs are mainly affected by this wave: ears, lungs, gastrointestinal tract, and central nervous system.

Blast Wave Injuries — Box 3-1

Lethal blast injuries usually result from a blast that develops more than 100 psi. The following is the spectrum of injuries based on pressure increase:
- 1 psi: Knock down
- 5 psi: Eardrum damage
- 15 psi: Eardrum rupture
- 30 psi: Lung damage
- 75 psi: Lung damage and complications
- 100 psi: Death

psi, Pounds per square inch.

Oklahoma City Bombing Blast Pressures — Box 3-2

The blast from the Oklahoma City bombing was caused by approximately 4800 pounds of ammonium nitrate and fuel oil. The following are the estimated pressures from the blast by distance from the source:
- 25 feet: 373 psi
- 45 feet: 106 psi
- 55 feet: 67 psi
- 75 feet: 33 psi
- 100 feet: 18 psi
- 125 feet: 11 psi
- 550 feet: 1.07 psi

psi, Pounds per square inch.

EARS

The ears are the most sensitive of all the organs to a blast. The eardrums will be damaged at 5 pounds per square inch (psi). At 15 psi there is a 50% chance of rupture. When the eardrums rupture, you see bleeding from the ears and the patient experiences extreme pain and loss of hearing.

LUNGS

The lungs are damaged at 30 psi and are severely damaged at 75 psi. The signs and symptoms will be difficulty breathing, cyanosis, chest pain, restlessness, and pain in the upper abdomen due to impaired diaphragm movement. This type of injury may cause rapid death from air emboli.

GASTROINTESTINAL TRACT

Injury to the gastrointestinal tract typically is caused by a blast in an enclosed place. It is also a common injury in underwater blasts. It is uncommon in open-air blasts. The large intestine is affected the most by increased pressure because it has more air space than the rest of the tract. The signs and symptoms are abdominal pain and guarding, rebound tenderness, absent bowel sounds, and bright red rectal bleeding.

CENTRAL NERVOUS SYSTEM

This injury is common from blast waves of 145 psi. The signs and symptoms are progressive mental deterioration, headache, neck stiffness, and blurred vision.

SECONDARY INJURIES

Secondary injuries are caused by shrapnel from the fragments of the device and from things that have been attached to the device. This trauma is just like any other penetrating trauma. The patient may also have bruising, bleeding, broken bones, and shock.

TERTIARY INJURIES

Tertiary injuries are caused when the patient is thrown like a projectile. These injuries are similar to injuries from falls or motor vehicle accidents, and treatment is the same as for these injuries. Patients with tertiary injuries may also have primary and secondary blast injuries.

TYPE IV (MISCELLANEOUS) INJURIES

Type IV injuries are all the other injuries caused by the event. Burns and psychological injures are the most common kinds of type IV injuries. The symptoms from the psychological trauma may not be evident for months or even years.

Patients do not need to be close to the blast to suffer damage. Injuries differ from person to person due to their location when the device went off. The blast wave can ricochet off a flat surface, causing a double injury. In a closed room, the overpressure of the explosion causes more damage than an outdoor blast does.

TRIAGE

Triage in blast injuries is performed in the same manner as any mass casualty incident, but there are a few differences to consider. Any patient with ear trauma has sustained exposure to the pressure increase and may have much more significant internal injuries. The psychological trauma from the blast may mask other signs and symptoms. Patients who were in the vicinity of the blast may need to be observed for a delayed onset of symptoms. Remember that another component may have been added to the bomb. There may be chemical, biological, or radiological exposure and contamination.

RESPONSE PRACTICES

Responders should consider any explosion a possible WMD event. Responders should use proper protective equipment in case a chemical, biological, or radiological agent has been added to the device. Detection devices can be used to determine the presence of chemical or radiological agents. All radios, cell phones, and computers within 500 feet of the scene should be shut off.

Consider using different staging areas at locations that you frequently respond to. Responders should be on the lookout for secondary devices. Injured patients should be rapidly removed from the immediate area. A triage and treatment area should be established in an area that has been checked for secondary devices. Transport patients from the area as quickly as possible. Patients' clothing and personal items need to be preserved as evidence.

REFERENCE

1. U.S. Department of Justice: *A guide for explosion and bombing scene investigation*, NCJ Research Report No. 181869, Washington, DC, 2000, National Institute of Justice.

BIBLIOGRAPHY

St. Louis Metropolitan Police Department, Bomb and Arson Squad.

St. Louis Office of the Federal Bureau of Investigations.

U.S. Department of Defense: WMD awareness course.

U.S. Department of Energy: *High explosives* (WMD web-based training course).

U.S. Department of Justice: *Emergency response to terrorist bombing* (training course), St Louis, November 25-26, 2002.

U.S. Department of Justice: *A guide for explosion and bombing scene investigation*, NCJ Research Report No. 181869, Washington, DC, 2000, National Institute of Justice.

Radiological Weapons

TOM PEDIGO

CHAPTER OBJECTIVES

At the conclusion of this chapter the student will be able to:

- Review the four sources of radiation and their significance.
- Review the effects of radiation on the human body, both somatic and genetic.
- Identify concerns for initial responders.
- Describe methods available for the detection of different types of radiation.
- Describe the primary methods available for the decontamination of alpha, beta, and gamma radiation.
- Describe the concerns for prehospital, hospital, and public health personnel.
- Identify particular concerns that exist with large-scale radiological events.

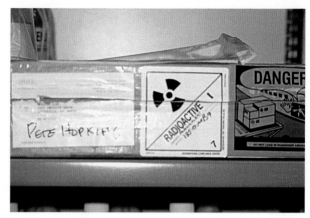

Fig. 4-1
Radioactive shipping box.

of radiation illnesses can be the key to recognizing the extent of the exposure and the possible prognosis of victims.

Responders must recognize the dangers and clues peculiar to the initial response while collecting the appropriate information that will help them treat exposed persons. Detection and decontamination equipment must be appropriately accessed and used to ensure that further exposure is minimized. Decontamination must also be considered with the application of any treatment, be it prehospital or at the emergency department. Self-referred victims of a radiological incident should be expected and prepared for by any nearby hospital. Public health personnel will need to rely on incident data to control any possible contamination of food and water supplies and to prevent or prepare for the treatment of future diseases and illnesses within the affected regions.

SOURCES OF RADIATION

The source of radiation is an important component in determining how severe the effects will be on victims. Sources of radiation fall into four categories: medical, artificial, background, and nuclear.

Medical radiation sources are used for therapeutic or diagnostic purposes. These sources include x-rays used in emergency departments, radiation therapy for cancer, fluoroscopy used in the cardiac catheterization lab, and other types of imaging (Fig. 4-2). Radiation sources used for medical purposes can cause significant exposure when the doses are prolonged and repetitive over months to years.

Artificial radiation is emitted from equipment used by businesses or the general public. Examples of artificial radiation sources include microwave ovens, televisions, and computers. These pose very little threat to persons who are exposed on a repetitive, daily basis.

Background radiation results from the normal breakdown of naturally existing elements. Background radiation can take many forms. Cosmic radiation from the sun is filtered out by the atmosphere, but it can be a concern for astronauts with prolonged exposure. Gradual breakdown of rock, soil, and

Of all the potential weapons of mass destruction, none strike fear as quickly as the thought of a nuclear holocaust. During the Cold War era of the 1980s, nuclear weapons were thought to be a *deterrent*, or a method of maintaining peace by way of threatening the unthinkable retaliation. As modern technology has progressed, so have the utilities (and therefore terrorist uses) of radioactive materials. A variety of radioactive materials now exist, and they are used for a variety of applications, not the least of which include medical diagnostics, chemotherapy and the production of energy (Fig. 4-1). Many of these sources provide the terrorist with a weapon capable of causing mass morbidity or mortality.

The effects of radiation also vary. Direct exposures may cause radiation burns, trauma, or whole-body irradiation. Ingestion via consumption, absorption, or inhalation can enhance the acute and chronic effects of radiation exposure. The signs and symptoms that appear during the various phases

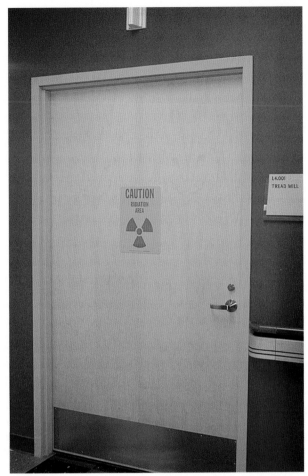

Fig. 4-2
Radiation sources can be found in many locations.

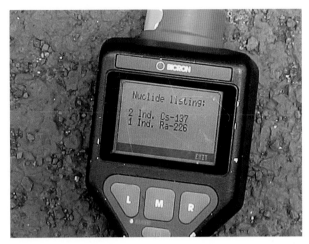

Fig. 4-3
Some radiation monitors can identify the specific radioactive isotope.

vegetable matter also causes the emission of radiation. Radon is an example of background radiation that is of concern to homeowners. Radon is derived from the decay of the natural element uranium found in the rock or soil under the house. Amounts vary from one house to another, and radiation to the occupants can range from very little to quite significant over years. Overall, background radiation accounts for nearly 60% of the total yearly radiation exposure for the average person.

Nuclear radiation is emitted from radioactive isotopes. Stability of these isotopes varies, but they can release significant amounts of energy (Fig. 4-3). Examples include the radiation emitted from nuclear power plants, radioactive waste, and uranium mines. Nuclear radiation from detonation of a nuclear weapon is the result of either a fission process or a fission-fusion chain reaction. The fission process was first used in the notorious atom bombs dropped on Nagasaki and Hiroshima. The fission-fusion reaction is the current method used in the nuclear warheads of intercontinental ballistic missiles (ICBMs) or aircraft-delivered munitions and is approximately 100 to 1000 times stronger than the fission process alone.

RADIATION DOSAGE

When determining the dosage absorbed by a victim, radiation is measured in terms of radiation absorbed dose (rad) or Roentgen equivalent in man (rem). The two are related, though not the same. Many texts and resources use one or the other to measure radiation exposure. The two measures are related in this equation:

$$\frac{rem}{(QF \times DF)} = rad$$

where *QF* is the qualitative factor and *DF* is the distribution factor. The distribution and qualitative factors vary with the type of radioactive material. The QF varies with the type of radioactive particle (electron, neutron), and the DF varies with the type of tissues exposed and whether the exposure is internal or external. Whereas rem is a useful measurement relative to the total effect of radioactive energy on a particular biological entity, rads are pure expressions of radiation dosage and therefore are used as the primary measurement in this chapter.

MEASURING RADIATION IN THE FIELD

In the field, radiation is typically measured in milliroentgens or Roentgens per hour. Some instruments measure millisieverts per hour. These units express an exposure rate, or the amount of radiation that a person would be exposed to at the point of measurement. Alpha and beta radiation detectors typically measure in counts per minute. Both counts per minute and milliroentgens are functionally related.

TYPES OF RADIATION EXPOSURE

EXTERNAL RADIATION EXPOSURE

A person who is exposed to large amounts of gamma or neutron radiation should be considered to have *external radiation exposure.* These persons are generally not any danger to health care providers. The few exceptions concern the exposure to specific neutron-originating radiation. Thus it remains important to determine the type of radioactive material that caused the exposure. Fortunately, neutron-originating radiation rarely exists, and therefore the primary contamination concern should be that of external particle contamination.

EXTERNAL PARTICLE CONTAMINATION

Alpha and beta particles can remain on the skin and clothing and can be spread by contact with the patient or by moving the patient through an area. All such areas or contact must be considered contaminated, because these particles pose a radiation threat to nonexposed persons.

INTERNAL PARTICLE CONTAMINATION

Radiation can also be communicated to internal organs by consumption, inhalation, and absorption or through an open wound. Generic decontamination methods will not rid the patient's body of these particles. Instead, the patient should be evaluated for possible internal decontamination treatment as discussed later in this chapter.

EFFECTS OF RADIATION

Various types of radiation exposure can cause different injuries. Generally speaking, radiation injuries are grouped into two categories, somatic and genetic. *Somatic injuries* refer to those incurred directly by the individual exposed. These can be further classified as *local radiation injuries* and generalized *whole-body irradiation.* Local radiation injuries are a result of a direct contact between a person's body and a radiated material, such as spilling a radioactive liquid on the arm. Whole-body irradiation is a generalized exposure of the person's body to a large dose of radiation. The severity of the injury is directly related to the duration of exposure, the amount of exposure, and the type of radioactive material (Table 4-1).

Table 4-1
Survival Rates by Radiation Dose

Measure	Dose (Rads)
LD$_{50/30}$ without treatment	250-325
LD$_{50/30}$ with treatment	350-400
LD$_{50/60}$ without treatment	300-350
LD$_{50/60}$ with treatment	450-500
LD$_{95}$ without treatment	500
LD$_{95}$ with treatment	700

LD$_{50/30}$, Estimated dose that will cause death in 50% of those exposed within 30 days; *LD$_{50/60}$,* estimated dose that will cause death in 50% of those exposed within 60 days; *LD$_{95}$,* estimated dose that will cause death in 95% of those exposed.

Genetic injuries represent the effects brought about in future generations or the exposed population as a result of mutated genes. Examples of this is illustrated by the higher rate of cancers and birth defects evident in the survivors of the Hiroshima and Nagasaki atomic bombs and the Chernobyl reactor fire.

Although genetic injuries can affect an entire population or region, it is the somatic injuries that acute care facilities and responders can have an immediate impact upon. The responder or hospital worker must be aware of the types of somatic effects associated with different levels of radiation.

SOMATIC INJURIES CAUSED BY LOCAL RADIATION

Local radiation injuries are frequently identified as burns. Like thermal burns, radiation burns must be quickly assessed and treated to prevent infections. Unlike thermal burns, radiation burns affect deeper tissues than the extent of the surface burn and can prevent the natural healing process. Tissues that are exposed to radiation are therefore more apt to become infected. Local radiation injuries can be grouped into one of four categories and should be treated accordingly. The doses listed are relative to healthy persons without comorbid medical conditions such as diabetes or immunocompromising syndromes.

ACUTE TYPE 1

Acute type 1 is the least severe of local radiation burns. In most cases, an initial phase occurs with mild warmth, redness, and itching. A latent phase of several weeks is then followed by the final illness, during which the skin may redden and desquamate. Type 1 injuries typically occur with a local exposure of 600 to 800 rads, and patients usually recover with no permanent impairment.

ACUTE TYPE 2

After an initial phase that mimics that of type 1 radiation burns, type 2 burns typically return in the final stages as second-degree burns. These injuries usually occur with a local exposure of 800 to 2000 rads. They remain much longer than typical second-degree thermal burns, are extremely painful, and often become infected due to the radiation damage that has occurred in the deeper tissues.

ACUTE TYPE 3

The acute type 3 level of injury begins quickly, with very excruciating pain and erythema that quickly progresses to blistering and desquamation. The apparent injury includes subdermal tissue, but the radiation damage is quite extensive and may require skin grafting and ultimately amputation of extremities to prevent death from infection. These injuries are caused by a dose of greater than 2000 rads.

CHRONIC TYPE 1

These injuries manifest very slowly as red, irritated skin that progresses to ulceration. Due to the chronic nature of the exposure, high doses of radiation can be absorbed over a long period, causing these ulcers to develop cancers or infection.

WHOLE BODY IRRADIATION

When a person's whole body is exposed to radiation, he or she exhibits four phases as the illness progresses. The *prodromal phase* is the initial phase of acute illness. This phase typically lasts 1 or 2 days, and depending on the dose it could range from undetectable to generalized flulike symptoms, changes in skin sensation, and skin burns. The *latent phase* is a dormant period in which there are no symptoms. This phase may last

hours to weeks depending on the severity of the dose. Following the latent phase is the *manifest illness phase*. This is where the severity of the exposure is revealed. Laboratory values and affected organs will demonstrate the level of damage. The final stage is either *recovery* or *death*. The last two phases may be affected by rapid intervention and acute intensive care treatment.

To determine the severity of the illness, the patient's symptoms throughout the four phases and the dose of irradiation can assist the health care provider in predicting what type of supportive therapy will be needed. These levels of severity are outlined in Box 4-1. As with local radiation

---

Somatic Whole-Body Irradiation Levels

Box 4-1

Type 1*

Exposure level: 50-150 rads
Prodromal phase: Ranges from absence of symptoms to nausea and vomiting for up to 1 day
Latent phase: Ranges from one day to several weeks; may not be noticeably different from prodromal phase
Manifest illness phase: May not materialize; can show generalized weakness, nausea and vomiting, temporary hair loss
Recovery or death: Recovery
Laboratory values: Minimal to no changes

Type 2†

Exposure level: 150-400 rads
Prodromal phase: Nausea, vomiting, diarrhea, fatigue and weakness for up to 2 days
Latent phase: Ranges from 1 to 3 weeks
Manifest illness phase: Immunosuppression, leukopenia, thrombocytopenia, hair loss
Recovery or death: Recovery is possible with supportive care and intervention; some patients progress to death
Laboratory values: Decreased leukocyte counts, decreased platelet counts, anemia

Type 3

Exposure level: 400-600 rads
Prodromal phase: Same as type 2 prodromal phase
Latent phase: Typically shorter than type 2 latent phase
Manifest illness phase: Bleeding diathesis, sepsis, immunosuppression, blood disorders, permanent hair loss
Recovery or death: Death without supportive care, isolation, and antibiotics
Laboratory values: Severe leukopenia, thrombocytopenia, anemia

Type 4

Exposure level: 600-1500 rads
Prodromal phase: Severe nausea, vomiting, diarrhea; significantly shorter period than lower types
Latent phase: Very short, usually only several days at most
Manifest illness phase: Gastrointestinal syndrome, immunosuppression, sepsis, blood disorders
Recovery or death: Varies with individual's response to supportive care
Laboratory values: Electrolyte imbalances associated with diarrhea and fluid loss; type 3 laboratory values

Type 5

Exposure level: 1500 rads or more
Prodromal phase: Almost immediate severe nausea, vomiting
Latent phase: Nonexistent
Manifest illness phase: Acute neurological syndrome, cardiovascular collapse
Recovery or death: Death occurs within 48 hours
Laboratory values: These do not alter the outcome for this patient

---

*Type 1 systemic exposure may appear to the health care provider to be a viral syndrome that recurs in several weeks and then gradually fades.
†Type 2 exposures appear within several weeks with signs of immunosuppression or hematopoietic syndrome.

injuries, these groupings assume that the persons exposed are otherwise generally healthy and without any comorbid illnesses.

Their presenting illness may resemble general malaise or an infection. Type 2 patients at the upper range of exposure (250 to 350 rads) have a 50% chance of death within the first 60 days if they are left untreated ($LD_{50/60}$). As discussed later, intervention and supportive therapy may have a significant impact on these patients. The type 3 whole-body exposure patient will certainly progress to death without intervention and might do so despite aggressive therapy. These patients present with immunosuppression, bleeding diatheses, sepsis, and permanent bone marrow suppression (Box 4-2).

The type 4 patient will present with a more acute, more severe illness identified as a *gastrointestinal syndrome* (Box 4-3). In this syndrome, the epithelial layer of the gastrointestinal tract erodes and leaves a denuded mucosa. This denuding causes severe diarrhea and a loss of the normal flora from the gastrointestinal tract. These patients will also likely experience severe immunosuppression and an accompanying hematopoietic syndrome. (See Box 4-2.) They fall under the category $LD_{50/60}$ in spite of aggressive supportive therapy at a dose of between 1000 and 1200 rads.

Type 5 patients have typically received 1500 rads or more. They exhibit a rapid onset of severe nausea and vomiting. This progresses to an acute neurological syndrome (Box 4-4) and cardiovascular collapse. Death usually occurs within 48 hours. These patients should be made as comfortable as possible throughout their illness.

FURTHER SOMATIC EFFECTS

With some radioactive incidents, other types of injuries can occur. These include thermal and blast injuries. *Thermal injuries* are caused by heat released from reactions or explosions. They may or may not be related to radioactivity,

depending on the type of attack. As in the case example, a dirty bomb may cause thermal and blast injuries without the use of fission or fusion as an explosive trigger. *Blast injuries* result from the pressure waves or projectiles that occur after an explosion. These injuries can include blunt trauma, penetrating trauma, and vision loss.

GENETIC EFFECTS

Genetic effects of radiation exposure can be broken down into two categories, primary and secondary. Primary genetic effects cause the growth of cancers as a result of mutations of affected genes. Secondary genetic effects are represented by birth defects, connective tissue disorders, and a higher incidence of cancers in future generations that are the offspring of the exposed population. While these effects are important to recognize for purposes of research and chronic public health issues, the focus of emergency care remains on the initial radiation exposure.

CONCERNS FOR RESPONDERS

Two decades ago, the primary concerns of a responder's radiological incident training revolved around one of two types of nuclear incidents. The first was the apocalyptic explosion of a nuclear missile. The second was the fear of a repeat of Three Mile Island or a Chernobyl-like nuclear reactor meltdown. These days, with the world's realization of a variety of radioactive agents, other possibilities must remain in the back of the responder's mind when approaching a scene. The emergency responder's awareness of what to look for and how can have an immediate impact on the safety of the responders as well as the safety and treatment of the patients.

INDICATIONS OF A NUCLEAR ATTACK

Like many disasters, large-scale nuclear attacks have certain indicators that the trained emergency responder should look for in the area while responding to the epicenter of the incident. Depending on the type of attack, the indications may be immediate and obvious (e.g., damage to buildings from a nuclear bomb explosion) or insidious and long-term (e.g.,

Hematopoietic Syndrome   Box 4-2

Depending on the dose, temporary or permanent damage of the bone marrow can occur. At a dose of 700 rads, permanent loss of marrow occurs. Deficiencies of all types of cells occur at this point. Resulting presentations include hemorrhage, infection, and anemia. Death occurs at higher doses within the first 1 to 2 months.

Gastrointestinal Syndrome   Box 4-3

Desquamation of the mucosal layer of the gastrointestinal tract results in significant nausea, vomiting, diarrhea, and dehydration. Although death is not definite with gastrointestinal syndrome, it becomes significantly more likely, and it typically occurs within several weeks. A dose of 600 rads or more is associated with this syndrome.

Central Nervous System Syndrome (Acute Neurological Syndrome)   Box 4-4

The patient exposed to an acute dose of up to 2000 rads or more usually suffers ataxia, seizures, lethargy, and coma. These symptoms occur within minutes of an acute exposure. Presentation of this syndrome is prognostic for death within days to weeks. Neuronal axons are the most highly differentiated cellular tissues, making it difficult for lower radiation doses to affect them. As a result, they are the last to be affected. Neurological syndromes therefore indicate a dose high enough to cause permanent damage to multiple organ systems.

multiple sick or dying animals from a contaminated water source). The key to recognizing early warnings of a radiological attack lies with the emergency responder's ability to do a rapid scene assessment. As with any hazardous materials situation, the scene assessment of a radiological event must be made with the highest index of suspicion, beginning with the initial dispatch and continuing until arriving at the scene of the incident.

BUILDINGS AND GROUNDS

Begin by noticing any signs of debris or explosions. Damage to windows may be the most obvious sign around the outer perimeter of an explosion. Structural collapse and unusual metal debris may be found closer to the initial site. Although it is rare, it is possible to see radioluminescence of highly radioactive material such as components of a bomb, destroyed building, or other solid materials. Any unusual sources of heat should also arouse suspicion, because heat may be a result of radioactivity. Keep an eye out for placards or other signs consistent with radioactive materials.

ATMOSPHERIC CHANGES

When approaching a large chlorine spill, responders typically begin surveying the sky for unusual green clouds before arriving at the spill site. Likewise, unusual radioluminescent clouds may accompany a large radiological incident. This phenomenon, reported during the reactor fire at Chernobyl, is a clear sign of immense amounts of radioactive particles and should indicate imminent danger to the responder and any life in the surrounding region.

PEOPLE AND LIVESTOCK

Unusual numbers of sick or injured people or animals should indicate the possibility of a radiological incident. Further indicators include signs of acute radiation poisoning such as nausea, vomiting, and radiation burns. Multiple dead or dying animals provide a strong clue to the responder about the hazards that lie ahead.

When encountering any of these signs, the responder must quickly recognize the clues before arriving at the location. Safety measures should be taken and detection equipment must be brought to the area (Box 4-5). Time, distance, and shielding are means of protection against ionizing radioactive materials. The exact periods of time, distance, and thickness of shielding depend on the type and amount of radioactive source. Radiation experts using special detection equipment can assist with these decisions (Fig. 4-4). In all cases, the shorter the exposure time, the greater the distance from the source, and the greater the shielding, the lower the dose.

TYPES OF INCIDENT SCENES

Although some of the following events may strike the responder as accidents, it is important to remember that any site with nuclear capability, weapons, or waste is a potential target for sabotage, theft, or detonation.

Approach to a Radiological Incident   Box 4-5

The following steps should always be taken by any responder who recognizes the potential radiological incident:
1. Don the appropriate protective equipment immediately. Cover all exposed skin and use the appropriate respiratory protection. (See Chapter 12.)
2. Maximize distance from the site of radiation, preferably withdrawing to a location that offers protection.
3. Notify specialized experts to respond with advanced protection, decontamination, and detection equipment.
4. Deploy the appropriate radiological detection equipment if it is available.
5. When you are appropriately protected, approach the incident site from upwind.
6. Should the incident be contained within a building or structure, remain outside until the appropriate detection and protection equipment is available.
7. Evacuate any civilians within your immediate area to a decontamination site.

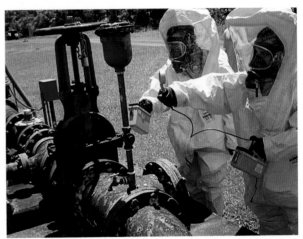

Fig. 4-4
Responders using radiological monitoring equipment.

NUCLEAR REACTORS

Among the first sites identified in the United States as potential terrorist targets in 2002 were the nuclear reactor sites that provide energy for various industries and cities (Fig. 4-5). Incidents at nuclear reactors are likely to be obvious, as the request for first responders will direct them toward the site. Even so, it is important to remember several factors unique to nuclear reactors.

First, responders should attempt to determine if the incident is contained within the site or poses a threat to the surrounding region. Any threat to the region should be relayed immediately to the local emergency management agencies so they can prepare for evacuation or sheltering and can request

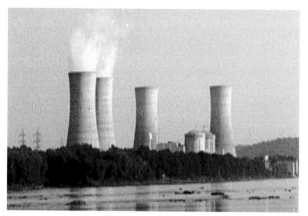

Fig. 4-5
Nuclear power plants are potential terrorist targets.

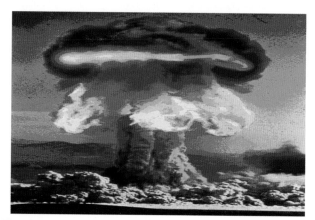

Information to Collect at a Nuclear Reactor Site **Box 4-6**

Several key pieces of information must be collected as soon as possible when responding to incidents at nuclear reactors:
- Was the incident accidental or intentional?
- What type of nuclear fuel is used at the facility?
- How much radioactive material was released?
- If the release was intentional, how was the material released? (Was an explosive involved?)

Fig. 4-6
Nuclear explosion.

additional resources. *Sheltering* refers to the containment of personnel within their current homes and structures to minimize exposure to the immediate atmospheric fallout. Determining the use of sheltering is a complex issue that should be left to the radiological emergency experts.

Emergency responders should recognize the likelihood that they will encounter people leaving the facility or general site with varying degrees of radiation exposure. Until proved otherwise, the responder should assume that everyone could be contaminated both internally and externally and will therefore require some form of external decontamination. Appropriate detection and decontamination should take place as soon as possible. A nuclear reactor incident will likely contain radioactive isotopes that are of a different nature than those of conventional nuclear weapons (Box 4-6). The treatment may vary in some cases, as will be discussed later. It is important to consider the potential for secondary devices, explosives, or even hostile persons when concerned with a possible intentional attack on a nuclear reactor.

ATOMIC WEAPONS

The atom bombs dropped on Hiroshima and Nagasaki at the end of World War II caused widespread death and destruction as well as thousands of injured or chronically contaminated people and contaminated food and water sources. In the event an atomic weapon is detonated, responders can expect to find multiple hazards during response. Responders in the immediate area are likely to suffer severe injuries and possibly death, depending on the proximity to the explosion (Fig. 4-6).

Responders caught within 10 kilometers of a 10 kiloton bomb should consider themselves victims and not responders. Decontamination and treatment will be necessary. Electronic equipment, including vehicles and communications equipment, might be incapacitated by the electromagnetic pulse emanating from the explosion.

Responders moving into the detonation area should consider awaiting clearance from rapid response radiological teams and existing emergency management personnel. Any initial responders should weigh entering the site of a nuclear detonation seriously. Rioting, secondary explosions, and

nuclear fallout are among the inherent dangers encountered in such situations. The responder can make several key preparations while awaiting the "all clear" to enter the area.

Shelter Preparation. Preparation of shelters will allow persons in the immediate area to escape the fallout from the explosion. Because up to 99% of the fallout's strength is within the first 48 hours, it is critical to minimize the exposure during this time. Examples of good shelters include underground buildings, basements, or reinforced windowless buildings.

Decontamination. Decontamination areas should be established to minimize the external contamination on the victims' bodies and clothing. Decontamination is discussed in more detail later.

Storage of Supplies. Sheltering involves a period of protection from fallout, so collection of up to 14 days' worth of food, water, and medical supplies will assist those sheltered in place. Battery-powered radios with extra batteries will assist with communication attempts to other responders.

Medical Care. Victims of the blast and those with radioactive burns require immediate life-saving intervention. Stabilization of critical injuries and relocation to the appropriate facilities are essential for these patients. Consider the possibility that some area hospitals may also have been affected by either the blast or the electromagnetic pulse emanating from the detonation.

Depending on the responder's proximity and role, one or all of these preparations may be necessary. The detonation of an atomic weapon will be no less than a major catastrophe, requiring the resources of a variety of agencies and municipalities. Recall that radiation illnesses are a result of two components: level of radiation and duration of exposure. Neither can be reduced by the emergency responder's hasty response into the area of a detonation. Await appropriate resources and make preparations for those survivors who will be making their way out of the site.

RADIOACTIVE WASTE AND CONTAMINATION

Management of an accidental leakage of radioactive waste is discussed in many hazardous materials training courses. The intentional use of radioactive waste or other purposeful contamination with radioactive material must be recognized as a different type of hazardous situation. The responder should look for clues about what was contaminated and how. Water supplies, food storage areas, and atmospheric plumes must be considered potential sources for radiation.

Clues should be evident during the response to the area. Multiple complaints of nausea and vomiting may be the initial clues to a contaminated source. Death of local vegetation and animal life provide additional clues. Although contaminated food and water sources present a threat to those who consume them, the vegetation itself and affected people and animals are not likely to present any radioactive threat to the responder. Fluids, solids, and particulate forms must be considered with this type of incident. Radioactive materials remain a potential target for theft or attack when they are removed from a storage site.

DIRTY BOMBS

Imagine that the first responder to the Oklahoma City bombing arrives on scene and surveys the damage. She immediately renders aid to the injured parties and evacuates those on the adjacent streets. Minutes or hours later she is told that the HAZMAT team has detected a radiological component in the explosion. This responder has just become victim to the most cloaked radiological exposure possible.

It is imperative that the emergency responder consider each intentional explosive device a potential radiological dispersal device or dirty bomb. Although it is not likely to affect a large group beyond the immediate blast area, the dirty bomb is becoming an increasingly likely possibility as a terrorist maneuver. Depending on the level of radiation attached to the bomb, responders may have little or no long-term effects provided they leave the area and decontaminate as soon as possible. It is primarily the persons within the initial blast radius who are most likely to be affected. Still, appropriate detection equipment should be brought in to ensure the safety of responders and medical providers.

DETECTION OF RADIATION

Detection of radiation is a necessary step in the treatment of injured and irradiated victims. It is imperative that the emergency responder and hospital personnel recognize the role of detection equipment in the treatment of radiation incident victims. (Detection equipment is covered in more detail in Chapter 11.)

Initial examination of the exposed victim should include radiation survey for gamma, beta, and alpha radiation. Emphasis should be placed on beta and alpha particle detection, as these particles can easily lie in the skin folds of the patient's axillae, in inguinal folds, or in hair follicles (Fig. 4-7). Because alpha and beta particles can be consumed and hence increase the acuteness of the exposure, the responder should use appropriate detection equipment before and after decontamination to determine the level of exposure to these particles.

Several hand-held cameras provide portable means of rapid detection. Care should be taken in using these instruments, because inappropriate use can result in false negative values, missing the radioactive particles. Instruments available include ionizing chambers and Geiger counters. Ionizing chambers detect gamma radiation and some beta radiation. Geiger counters can serve to detect all types of radiation provided they are scaled to measure for the appropriate radioactive material. Only two types of radiation, H-3 and Fe-55, cannot be detected by Geiger counters.

The key to radiation detection equipment in the prehospital and emergency department settings is to be familiar with how the equipment must be operated to detect the appropriate radiation particles. An operator who is not familiar with the detection equipment will likely miss contamination that could cause further harm to the patient or providers.

DECONTAMINATION

Recall the patients from the dirty bomb example at the beginning of the chapter. Once it is determined that decontamination must be initiated, what should the prehospital provider consider to be an appropriate decontamination method (Fig. 4-8)? The method of decontamination is relatively simple, but it requires a rapid assessment of the patient for any immediate life-threatening

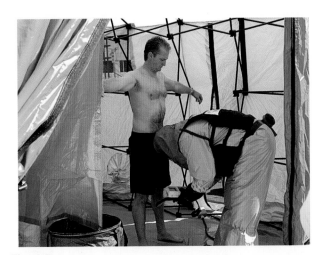

Fig. 4-7
Responders in a training drill monitor patients for radiation contamination.

injuries or any open wounds (Box 4-7). These steps are for external decontamination. (Internal decontamination is discussed later.)

For additional decontamination, the responder may also consider using Lava soap, detergent paste, or a combination of one-half detergent and one-half cornmeal. These last two options can be somewhat abrasive to the skin, and they should be used by personnel familiar with decontamination procedures. Other, more abrasive solutions are readily available, but they should be used only by decontamination technicians with expertise in the arena of radiation decontamination.

Once the appropriate decontamination has taken place, responders should doff their protective equipment as described in Chapter 13, double bag it, and label it with the responder's name, location relative to the incident, and type of radioisotope, if known.

PREHOSPITAL TREATMENT

GENERAL CONSIDERATIONS

Radiation injuries can result from a variety of sources. Explosions can cause immediate trauma secondary to blast injuries, in addition to the radiation damage. Once decontamination has been completed, the most immediate life-threatening injuries should be addressed. Prompt attention should be paid to the primary survey of the injured victim, as well as any major sites of trauma. Spinal precautions should be taken when the provider is concerned about a significant blast or fall during the incident.

LOCAL RADIATION INJURIES

Local acute radiation injuries should be treated as burns. Burns greater than 18% of the total body surface area are considered major burns and warrant emergency transfer to the appropriate facility. The responder should monitor the patient en route for symptoms of acute radiation sickness extending beyond the local injury. Prompt inquiry into the type, duration, and amount of radiation exposure may be helpful to

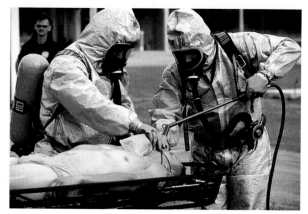

Fig. 4-8
Responders carrying out patient decontamination.

hospital providers. The responder should not attempt to gain access or collect samples from the radiation source. Allow minor bleeds to ooze for several minutes prior to decontaminating and covering the burn site.

WHOLE-BODY IRRADIATION

Treatment for whole-body irradiation depends upon the symptoms present. The neurologic syndrome may indicate immediately fatal irradiation.

Patients exhibiting neurological deficits should be closely monitored for airway and respiratory compromise. High-flow

---

Decontamination   Box 4-7

Basic decontamination of the radiation victim can easily be completed, provided that there are no open wounds. (Don't forget to use the appropriate PPE for decontamination!)

1. Remove clothing that may contain radiation particles. Turn clothing inside out as it is being removed from the victim to prevent further spread of the particles.
2. Place articles of clothing in a double bag, and label the bag "Hazardous: Radioactive Material."
3. Label the bag with the victim's name, location at the event, date, and the identity of the radioactive material, if known.
4. Using appropriate detection equipment, survey the victim for radiation particles on the skin surface, taking particular care to examine skin folds, hair follicles, and inguinal and axillary regions.
5. Flush contaminated areas with soap and warm water. Use caution to avoid spreading contamination to areas that are not already contaminated, especially mucosal regions and skin folds.
6. Clip fingernails and toenails when contamination is found beneath the nails, and scrub the fingers and toes with soap and warm water.
7. Swab any sites that appear to have some decontamination in difficult-to-examine areas such as the nostrils, eyes, ears, or other hard-to-reach areas. Nasal and oral swabs may assist in determining if any significant amounts of radiation particles were ingested.

Decontamination of the patient with open wounds should be handled with more attention paid to the wound site. In the event of an active bleed, ensure the following steps are completed:

1. Allow any slow to moderate bleeding to continue for several minutes. This will decrease the amount of contamination absorbed into the site.
2. Irrigate the wound with soap and warm water to reduce particle levels.
3. Survey the victim for radiation particles as described above.
4. Careful simple debridement of the wound may be attempted by qualified medical personnel to decrease the amount of necrotic or severely injured skin.
5. Cover the wound site with a waterproof dressing.
6. Continue decontaminating the rest of the victim's body as described above.

oxygen, intravenous access, and cardiac monitoring are necessary for all patients exhibiting immediate signs of radiation-induced sickness. Advanced airway adjuncts and antiseizure medications should be readily available for the patient with impending neuroleptic syndrome. Patients with less-severe reactions of nausea and vomiting should be given antiemetics and intravenous fluids.

Patients exhibiting cardiovascular symptoms should be treated symptomatically and should be closely monitored for cardiovascular failure.

Patients exhibiting immediate severe symptoms of nausea, vomiting, seizures, or cardiovascular compromise have likely received fatal doses. Care should be directed toward ensuring comfort and immediate transport to an acute care facility for closer monitoring. Patients with mild to no symptoms upon arrival of emergency personnel may or may not have received fatal doses. After decontamination, the most important step in ensuring their survival will be at the hospital with weeks to months of supportive intervention.

HOSPITAL TREATMENT

Initial treatment at the hospital will be very similar to that initiated by emergency responders in the field. As in the 1995 sarin gas attack in the Tokyo subway, many people are likely to self-refer to the closest facility. Triage of these persons and decontamination of exposed persons will be necessary to ensure that acutely ill patients receive immediate care.

ON-SITE DECONTAMINATION

The hospital provider should recognize the potential for mass casualties and stage the appropriate resources outside the emergency department. Qualified personnel from local hazardous materials teams should establish a triage and decontamination point. All arriving patients should be scanned for radiation contamination and decontaminated appropriately. Additionally, a second point should be established for the acutely ill or nonambulatory patients arriving at the facility.

TRIAGE

Once decontamination has been completed, the patient population should initially be sorted into one of three categories: asymptomatic, mildly symptomatic, or unstable.

ASYMPTOMATIC (GREEN)

Although they may manifest illness over the course of the next 48 hours, asymptomatic patients may be treated as walking wounded and placed en masse in a holding area where progression of symptoms can be monitored.

MILDLY SYMPTOMATIC (YELLOW)

Mildly symptomatic patients have nausea, mild vomiting, or local radiation injuries. These patients require supportive therapy to decrease the morbidity and mortality associated with the early symptoms. Some of these patients will die, but

others may survive with aggressive supportive monitoring and intervention.

UNSTABLE (RED)

Unstable patients have severe refractory vomiting, diarrhea, hypotension, unconsciousness, neurologic syndrome, or cardiovascular compromise. These patients face an extremely poor prognosis if such symptoms occur within the first 48 hours. They initially require the most immediate care, with attention focused on basic life support. Overall mortality for this group approaches 100% after 30 days. After initial life support, measures should be focused on comfort care of the patient.

TREATMENT OF RADIATION VICTIMS

Hospital treatment of local radiation injuries mimics thermal burn treatment. After decontamination, simple wound debridement will be the initial step in the emergency department. It will take several weeks to determine if the injury is severe enough to cause permanent damage and warrant skin grafting. These patients will require routine follow-up, as well as serial lab tests described later, to ensure they have not received a more systemic dose. The primary focus will be determining the exact dosage received by the patient. Skin lesions in the second or third weeks may provide clues to the degree of local damage, but ultimately it is the overall dosage that should take priority.

PHYSICAL EXAMINATION

The initial examination may reveal only the obvious immediate skin damage. Care must be taken to ensure there are no signs of whole-body irradiation or consumption of radiation particles. When examining the head and neck, note any burns around the mucosal areas. Inspect the eyes for any contact burns, paying particular attention to the cornea, sclera, and conjunctivae.

Closely observe the skin for signs of irradiation. Erythema, inflammation, and necrosis must be recognized on initial exam. Hair loss is evident in most cases of local radiation exposure. Depending on the dose, future erythema or exudative necrosis may present, suggesting a severe local dose. Any irradiation greater than 18% of the body surface area (using the rule of nines) is considered a case of whole-body irradiation.

DIAGNOSTIC MODALITIES

The key to determining skin care is best centered on the dose and type of radiation, but several modalities exist that enable the practitioner to assess additional damage. Each of these modalities is more likely to be useful on an outpatient basis, as initial changes may not be evident. Scintigraphy and capillaroscopy may provide insight into the damage of local circulation. A magnetic resonance image (MRI) will assist with the early detection of radiation-induced injury, but it is seldom warranted in the initial emergency department evaluation.

DISPOSITION

All local injuries should be evaluated for further indication of whole-body irradiation. In the absence of whole-body irradiation, evidence of invasive burns, or obviously necrotic tissue, additional follow-up may be handled through the appropriate outpatient clinical setting. Some patients may eventually need skin grafting or more advanced wound care, but the prognosis will at least partially depend upon the resulting injuries. The degree of injury may not become evident for several weeks; hence referral outside of the emergency department is essential.

TREATMENT OF WHOLE-BODY IRRADIATION

Whole-body irradiation must be closely evaluated as a likely life-threatening exposure. Clues must be combined from the history of events, physical examination, reported and requested symptoms (review of systems), and laboratory values to ensure that an appropriate evaluation has been made.

REVIEW OF SYSTEMS

Review the following symptoms with each patient who presents to the emergency department, either initially or after several weeks to months.

General: Fever, malaise, lethargy, weight loss, dehydration
Head and neck: Headache, visual disturbances, mucosal irritation, dry mouth
Immunologic: Multiple illnesses, prolonged fever, rashes, and fungal infections
Gastrointestinal: Nausea, vomiting, bright red blood per rectum, bloody stool, and diarrhea
Cardiovascular: Chest pain, shortness of breath, sensation of chest fullness
Neurologic: Confusion, ataxia, memory loss, tremors, loss of sensation or strength
Dermatologic: Skin or hair changes, skin erythema or desquamation

PHYSICAL EXAMINATION

General: Assess the patient for any change in level of consciousness or hemodynamic instability.
Head and neck: Observe for changes in the eyes, vision, or mucosa.
Chest: Assess for unusual lung sounds, muffled heart tones, or irregular heartbeat.
Abdomen: Assess for distention, tenderness, and rigidity.
Pelvis: Obtain stool sample and assess for any blood present.
Extremities: Observe for any direct skin damage, hair loss, or necrosis. Pale skin or diaphoresis may also be apparent in the acutely ill patient.
Neurologic: A complete neurologic examination should be performed, including cranial nerves, cerebellar function, extremity strength, movement, sensation, and circulation. Ambulation should be demonstrated to detect any gait abnormalities. Seizures or tremors exist only in the fatally ill patient.

DIAGNOSTIC MODALITIES

An electrocardiogram can show evidence of severe cardiovascular collapse in the acute illness. Electrolyte imbalances are sometimes detected in the manifest illness phase.

Urine and stool samples and swabs of potential residual areas (e.g., nasal passages, inguinal folds) should be taken to help further determine radiation dose per patient.

Laboratory values are imperative in both the initial and the chronic evaluation of exposure victims. The complete blood count (CBC) with differential is the key laboratory assessment that indicates both dose and probable prognosis.

The first most critical value is the lymphocyte count. Serial lymphocytes should be monitored a minimum of every 24 hours and ideally every 6 hours. Decrease by 50% or more in the first 24 hours indicates a lethal injury. At 48 hours, the lymphocyte count should be reassessed. A lymphocyte count greater than 1500 is prognostic for probable survival, whereas a count less than 800 indicates the need for aggressive interventional therapy. A lymphocyte count less than 100 indicates a lethal exposure.

Neutrophil count, while not immediately useful, aids in determining likely infectious sequelae. A 50% decrease in neutrophils is consistent with an exposure likely to result in a hematopoietic syndrome. Platelets should be measured at the onset to provide a baseline. Unlike with the CBC, platelet counts will not show changes in the first several days, but they will provide necessary trends in the noninvasive evaluation of bone marrow suppression. Red cell counts are not useful in initial surveys unless bleeding occurs, as they do not indicate radiation injury for 6 to 8 weeks.

Chromosomal analysis is useful in determining the degree of radiation. However, this method may not be practical in the mass casualty situation because it requires staff and equipment. Chromosomal analysis should be reserved for those in whom it will help determine the appropriate therapy.

Bone marrow sampling can provide useful information when confirmation of hematopoietic suppression is necessary. Initially, bone marrow aspiration is both time consuming and unnecessary. This modality should be reserved for later follow-up decisions.

INTERNAL DECONTAMINATION

Determining the type of radiation can be key to the continued treatment of exposure victims. Victims with internal contamination may benefit from the use of specific agents that decrease the absorption of contaminants. Table 4-2 lists several radioactive materials that have specific therapies. A toxicologist or radiological emergency assistance clinician should be consulted before initiating any internal decontamination procedures. Specific internal decontamination procedures *must not* be used until identification of the radionuclide is made. Additional generic treatments may be employed to facilitate the expulsion of radioactive materials from the intestinal tract (Table 4-3).

Overall, key resources must be put to use before exercising invasive or internal decontamination procedures. The prehospital provider should never attempt any of these procedures. The emergency department clinician should do so only after reviewing the patient's symptoms, known dosage, material type, and initial laboratory values. Public health and primary care providers should avoid these methods because they are intended primarily for initial decontamination procedures.

Table 4-2
Specific Therapies by Type of Material

Material	Therapy	Modality
Strontium	Calcium gluconate, magnesium sulfate	Intravenous, oral
Multiple	Dimercaprol	Intravenous
Cesium	Diuretics	Intravenous
Iron	DTPA	Intravenous, topical
Lead	DTPA	Intravenous, topical
Plutonium	DTPA	Intravenous, topical, inhaled
Cobalt	DTPA	Intravenous, topical
Tritium	Hydration	Intravenous
Multiple	Penicillamine	Intravenous
Manganese	Potassium iodide	Oral or intravenous
Iodine	Prussian blue	Intravenous

DTPA, Diethylenetriamine pentaacetic acid.

Table 4-3
Generic Therapies by Type of Therapy

Medications	Category	Treatment Goal
Aluminum antacids	Miscellaneous	Reduce absorption
Barium sulfate	Miscellaneous	Reduce absorption
Activated charcoal	Ion exchange	Reduce absorption
Sodium phosphate	Saline cathartic	Reduce absorption
Bisacodyl	Laxative	Reduce absorption
Ipecac	Emetic	Reduce absorption
Potassium gluconate	Miscellaneous	Dilution
Zinc sulfate	Miscellaneous	Dilution
Calcium gluconate	Miscellaneous	Dilution
Potassium iodide	Iodides	Block uptake
Ammonium chloride	Expectorant	Mobilizing agent-respiratory
Propylthiouracil	Antithyroid	Mobilizing agent
Potassium thiocyanate	Antithyroid	Mobilizing agent
Lavage	Lung lavage	Reduce concentration
EDTA, DTPA	Chelating agents	Inactivate particular isotopes

EDTA, Ethylenediaminetetraacetic acid; *DTPA,* diethylenetriamine pentaacetic acid.

DISPOSITION: ADMISSION VERSUS OUTPATIENT THERAPY

Deciding which patients can be suitably treated with outpatient therapy is critical in the mass casualty situation. Key findings in support of discharge include the following:
- No symptoms after 24 to 48 hours
- Absence of local radiation burns exceeding 18% of total body surface area
- Lymphocyte count greater than 1500 mm^3 at 48 hours
- Less than 25% loss of neutrophil count at 48 hours
- Lack of exposure to areas known to have concentrated radiation doses

Key findings requiring admission include the following:
- Refractory nausea and vomiting
- Neurologic symptoms
- Cardiovascular compromise
- Radiation burns exceeding 18% of total body surface area
- High levels of alpha and beta particles at the time of initial decontamination
- Lymphocyte count below 1500 mm^3 at any time in the first 48 hours
- Conjunctival erythema or damage
- Diarrhea or bloody stool
- Neutrophil count less than 50%

On an outpatient basis, repeating the CBC, bleeding time, prothrombin time (PT), and activated partial thromboplastin time (aPTT) can aid in the evaluation of the chronic onset of hematopoietic syndrome. A basic metabolic panel will assist the practitioner in evaluating electrolyte and fluid loss in patients developing gastrointestinal syndromes. A complete review of systems should be performed weekly on any patient believed to have significant exposure. Before discharge, patients must be informed of the possibility of recurring symptoms in the prodromal and manifest illness stages. Education will be necessary to ensure they receive the appropriate follow-up care with public health or primary care providers.

LONG-TERM SUPPORTIVE CARE AND INTERVENTION

Hospitalized patients should be admitted to the ICU, hematology floor, burn unit, or clinical immunology department. In severe circumstances, hospital isolation and sterile environments should be provided for those experiencing severe immunocompromise. Skin grafts and bone marrow transplants, while controversial, may be used in such cases to provide maximum opportunity for recovery.

Mass casualty situations may dictate that long-term supportive care, and acute intensive care should be made available to patients who require aggressive therapy with hope of possible recovery. Patients showing clear signs of a lethal injury should be placed on comfort care. Clear signs of lethal injuries include one or more of the following:
- Lymphocyte count less than 100 mm^3 in the first 48 hours

- Neurologic syndrome, specifically seizures, ataxia, and confusion
- Refractory nausea and vomiting in the first 1 to 2 hours of exposure

Aggressive therapy will not affect the outcome for these patients.

PUBLIC HEALTH CONSIDERATIONS

In situations of mass contamination or mass casualty, public health officials need to begin assessing the type of radiation and dosage levels in the immediate vicinity. Plans should be enacted to prepare for chronic monitoring and appropriate referral for victims who show delayed signs weeks or months after the incident. The public should be notified of the signs and symptoms of prodromal and manifest illness to educate potential victims about their possible exposure. Evacuation, while not an initial step in a fallout situation, should be considered in locations whose food and water supplies are contaminated. Uncontaminated food, water, and medical supplies should be shipped to safe collection points.

CHAPTER SUMMARY

Although the Cold War era has ended, the threat of nuclear or radiological incidents remains as a potential terrorism threat. It is therefore essential that the prehospital provider, the hospital clinician, and the public health official maintain an awareness of the particular presentations and treatments of radiological illnesses and injuries. Care must be taken to ensure appropriate decontamination, followed by triage and treatment of the most immediate life-threatening injuries. Detection of the pertinent signs and symptoms, along with appropriate laboratory evaluation measures, will help the hospital clinician determine the necessary disposition and advanced treatment. Although there are a multitude of possible measures to treat contaminated and irradiated patients, the clinician should consult an expert in radiological medicine before instituting any situation-specific interventions. Finally, it is of utmost importance that all information possible be collected with regard to the radionuclide type, dose, and any other compounding factors that may aid in the further treatment of irradiated victims. Additional resources for the emergency provider are as follows:

Department of Energy, radiological assistance: 630-252-4800 (24 hours a day)

Radiation Emergency Assistance Center/Training Site (REAC/TS): 865-576-3131

U.S. Department of Energy Operations Center at Oak Ridge: 865-576-1005

BIBLIOGRAPHY

Basic radiological emergency response training and us, Minnesota Public Safety, http://www.dps.state.mn.us/emergmgt/rep/brert/radiation.htm, retrieved January 24, 2003.

Central Intelligence Agency: *Chemical, biological, radiological incident handbook*, http://www.odci.gov/cia/reports/cbr_handbook/cbrbook.htm, retrieved June 12, 2004.

Committee on Battlefield Radiation Exposure Criteria: *Potential radiation exposure in military operations: protecting the soldier before, during, and after*, National Academies Press, http://books.nap.edu/books/0309064392/html/, retrieved June 12, 2004.

Cruise R: *Nuclear disaster at Chernobyl*, Buena Park, Calif, 2000, Artesian Press.

Daugherty NM: *Radiation protection and emergency response*, Certified Health Physicist, Denver, 1998, Colorado Department of Public Health and Environment.

de Boer J, Dubouloz M: *Handbook of disaster medicine*, Nieuwegein, Netherlands, 2000, Hentenaar Boek.

Radiation accidents: guide for emergency medical personnel, Springfield, Ill, 1999, Department of Nuclear Safety, State of Illinois.

Radiation safety manual, Chicago, 1997, Environmental Health and Safety Office, Radiation Safety Section, University of Illinois at Chicago.

U.S. Department of State: *Document 22.6: Exposure to radiation in an emergency*, ES and H manual, http://www.travel.state.gov/nuclear-incidents.html, retrieved March 3, 2003.

U.S. Department of State: *Fact sheet: guidance for responding to radiological and nuclear incidents*, http://travel.state.gov/travel/nuclear_incidents.html, retrieved June 12, 2004.

Biological Weapons

Bruce Clements

CHAPTER OBJECTIVES

At the conclusion of this chapter the student will be able to:

- Define bioterrorism.
- Describe health surveillance systems used to identify outbreaks in their earliest stages.
- Identify the epidemiological clues that may indicate an act of bioterrorism is occurring.
- List the biological agents considered the most critical threats.
- Describe the common characteristics of high-threat biological agents.
- Identify diagnosis and treatment recommendations for critical agents.
- Describe infection-control precautions needed for bioterrorism agents.
- Identify reliable information resources for bioterrorism preparedness.

CASE STUDY

Several busy days of emergency medical services (EMS) activity and hospital admissions seem to signal the start of an unusually early and severe influenza season. Although many patients are younger and otherwise healthier than patients normally seen during typical flu seasons, little notice is initially taken of these differences. The diversity of the organizations and settings of care providing treatment to the ill make recognition of unusual trends difficult. The traditional processes of case reporting by physicians and collection and analysis of epidemiological information by the public health department are under way. These processes take time and delay the recognition of epidemiological trends that indicate this outbreak is not a natural event.

A physician noticing the unusually young ages of his severely ill "flu patients" orders additional lab tests. The initial results raise suspicions. Subsequent chest x-rays on several patients with worsening conditions show mediastinal widening, a hallmark of advanced inhalational anthrax disease. Confirmatory lab tests verify cases of anthrax.

The Federal Bureau of Investigation initiates a criminal investigation. At the same time, public health officials initiate an epidemiological investigation to identify additional cases and characterize the exposures. Federal health officials have initiated coordination with state public health authorities to deliver an initial push package from the Strategic National Stockpile (SNS). Federal and state officials are anxiously waiting to see if the doses of antibiotics, numbering in the hundreds of thousands, are adequate therapeutic supplies for the potentially large number of persons at risk. Local officials are hopeful that the mass care plans they have developed are effective. The public is waiting for answers and demanding action.

What epidemiological clues should raise the suspicions of public health and health care providers that this outbreak is not natural?

What health surveillance systems may quickly identify outbreaks?

Which biological agents would a terrorist use?

How might terrorists carry out attacks using biological agents?

What protective actions should EMS and health care providers take for high-risk biological threats?

Bioterrorism moved to the forefront of our national preparedness agenda following the discovery of four anthrax-tainted letters that circulated on the East Coast of the United States during the autumn of 2001. The letters caused 22 cases of anthrax disease and 5 deaths.[25] In addition, information shared throughout 2002 on the growing threat of smallpox as a biological weapon resulted in vigorous debates over who should receive smallpox vaccinations. Federal, state, and local terrorism preparedness efforts accelerated and led to the establishment of a new federal department, the Department of Homeland Security. The concern of the American people over these emerging threats has made our nation's preparedness a moral imperative.

Bioterrorism is one of the most complex preparedness challenges our nation is facing. There is no universally accepted definition of bioterrorism, but most agree it includes the use or threatened use of a biological agent as a weapon of terror. Current federal laws make the threat alone, even in the absence of possession or use of a biological weapon, a serious crime. The agent may be lethal or nonlethal, a common bacterium or virus, the toxic byproduct of a pathogen, a rare organism, or even a specially engineered organism never before diagnosed or treated.

Although most public concerns focus on the threat to humans, bioterrorists may also attack crops or livestock. Even a small attack on these resources could have serious economic consequences for any nation targeted. Regardless of the agent used or the focus of the attack, the ultimate goal of bioterrorism is the same as that of conventional terrorism. These acts are intended to instill fear in the targeted population.

THE PERCEPTIVE PROVIDER

The diversity of emerging terrorist threats is influencing substantial investments in public health and health care preparedness. This trend is likely to continue for many years. Much of this spending takes the form of high-tech solutions, including new software for epidemiological surveillance or new detection devices for air monitoring. Although this technology may complement many preparedness initiatives, no technological solution will ever replace the perceptive provider.

Throughout history, astute physicians and well-informed providers have been the sentinels of our nation's public health. Typically, they identify emerging problems for public health, rather than public health identifying the problems in advance for providers.[35] This was still true in 2001 when prepared clinicians and scientists diagnosed the index case of inhalational anthrax.[5] The education and training of health care providers stands out as one of our nation's most important preparedness measures. We must consistently hone the intuition and skill of our providers so they are able to recognize a bioterrorism attack early and take the appropriate actions.

BIOTERRORISM SURVEILLANCE

Disease surveillance is a common function of local and state public health agencies. This typically involves mandatory disease reporting by local health care providers, data entry and analysis by local or regional public health agencies, and additional analysis, reporting, and allocation of needed resources by state and federal public health agencies. However, the bioterrorism agents of concern have short incubation periods that require rapid identification to facilitate early treatment. Many existing local surveillance activities do not process and analyze information quickly enough to ensure a prompt response. They are also not sensitive enough to detect small changes in population health, and they are not specific enough to distinguish normal fluctuations in illness from unusual or suspicious cases.

There is no single answer to the question of effective surveillance systems. An ideal system will include a network of systems that can simultaneously analyze multiple variables, effectively compare changes and trends, and control confounders and background noise.[28] The realization of an effective, uniform system throughout the United States is years away. Until it is developed and implemented, we will continue to depend upon a patchwork of surveillance and detection systems.

APPROACHES TO BIOTERRORISM SURVEILLANCE

Bioterrorism surveillance has two basic approaches: epidemiological surveillance and standoff detection.

EPIDEMIOLOGICAL SURVEILLANCE

One example of active epidemiological surveillance is the comprehensive, symptomatic surveillance accomplished at the Olympic Games, the Super Bowl, political conventions, and other high-visibility events. This is a labor-intensive and expensive endeavor requiring additional staff placement in key points of health care delivery to gather information. The information collected focuses on respiratory, neurological, and dermatological clues that may quickly indicate that an intentional biological release has occurred. Although this may appear to be an ideal method for gathering accurate information in a timely manner, it is far too expensive to sustain every day.

Other surveillance approaches include monitoring available information in public health and health care databases. These data may include ambulance runs, chief complaints of 911 calls, hospital admissions, school or work absenteeism, or trends in pharmaceutical or laboratory demands.

The challenge of surveillance is twofold. First, the correct baseline is often difficult to determine. The success of surveillance depends upon the accurate determination of a trigger or threshold that signals an unusual event or trend. This is only successful if the numerous confounders in the data are controlled. For example, how can 911 calls or absenteeism trends distinguish between a suspicious event and the onset of cold and flu season, or how can sales trends in certain pharmaceuticals distinguish between an increase in flulike symptoms and price discounts for those products?

STANDOFF DETECTION

Another form of surveillance is environmental monitoring, often referred to as *standoff detection*. Detector research and development is a fast-moving area with enormous growth. Standoff detectors include everything from basic bioaerosol collectors to advanced laser particle analyzers. There are many point detector technologies under development. They include nucleic acid, antibody, whole cell, and mass spectrometry analysis technologies. These detectors may enhance preparedness for specific high-risk events or buildings, but they will always have inherent limitations.

DETECTION LIMITATIONS

The greatest limitation today is cost. This emerging technology is expensive and fiscally out of reach for most state and local agencies. The technology is also not always sensitive enough to detect the full range of biological threats at a low level or always specific enough to distinguish between normal background biological material in the air and the pathogens of greatest concern.

Instruments must be prepositioned, which requires accurate risk assessment of a community. This involves identifying the most likely targets in a community. The risk assessment may be accurate today, but the risk can shift depending upon community activities. Identifying the most likely points of a biological terrorism release and placing detectors in the expected path of release is an elusive undertaking. In addition, because detectors can cover only a limited area, a terrorist can simply move to a more vulnerable region to carry out a release.

In the future, standoff detection will serve a vital role in monitoring high-risk facilities and high-risk urban areas. However, whereas technology certainly plays a significant role in how we address bioterrorism threats in the future, it will never replace a well-trained physician or epidemiological surveillance.

EPIDEMIOLOGICAL CLUES

SALMONELLA IN THE DALLES, OREGON

Bioterrorism encompasses the intentional use of such a wide array of pathogens and pathogenic byproducts that it is impossible to define a typical bioterrorism event. In 1984 The Dalles, Oregon, experienced a large outbreak of *Salmonella* gastroenteritis. More than 700 people became ill after eating at 10 local salad bars. The epidemiological investigation could not identify a single food as the source of the illnesses. Months later, the criminal investigation identified the origin of the outbreak as intentional contamination of area salad bars by members of a religious cult.[36] In this case, the agent used was not lethal and initially appeared to be a large, but accidental, foodborne outbreak.

A bioterrorism scenario will unfold in a very different way if a lethal agent is used. If the agent is transmissible from person to person or if it is delivered by spraying it in the air, the footprint or focused area of an outbreak could expand across entire metropolitan areas or large regions of the United States. The diversity of the threats and the potential extent of bioterrorism attacks mandate the diligence of public health and health care workers. Everyone involved in direct patient encounters must maintain a high index of suspicion. Most illnesses resulting from an act of bioterrorism will have an incubation period. This allows a window of opportunity for prophylactic treatment, even for the most lethal agents. However, the only way this delayed onset can be used to the advantage of the patients is if providers are suspicious enough to recognize unusual trends early.

BIOTERRORISM CLUES

Clues that should raise the suspicion of providers include anything that is out of the ordinary. Every community has trends in seasonal illnesses, with some variation from year to year. There may be obvious differences emerging, such as out-of-season flulike outbreaks or more severe cases among groups that normally do not experience serious illness. An illness may be uncharacteristic for a particular region, such as plague in New Jersey, or the strain may be unusual or resistant to treatment. Clues that should raise suspicion may range from more subtle trends to the obvious clues that may be provided through claims made by aggressors or evidence identified by law enforcement authorities. However, no single clue will typically identify a bioterrorism event. Maintaining a high index of suspicion increases the likelihood of discovering an event sooner. The swift discovery of an event translates into more lives saved. A good summary of these clues, compiled by Dr. Julie Pavlin of the Walter Reed Army Institute of Research, is displayed in Box 5-1.

BIOTERRORISM AGENT THREAT LIST

Much of the bioterrorism preparedness training and planning initiated in 2001 focused on anthrax and smallpox. Although these two pathogens pose extraordinary public health threats, a terrorist has many other options. As weapons, pathogens each present unique risks and response challenges, making bioterrorism preparedness particularly difficult. In an effort to narrow our nation's bioterrorism preparedness focus, a group of military and civilian experts convened in 1999 to review a wide range of biological agent information resources and prioritize the biological threats based on each agent's potential public health impact.[29]

The resulting list includes three categories, A, B, and C (Table 5-1). Category A pathogens are highly lethal agents that are easily dispersed or transmitted from person to person. In the early Cold War era of the 1950s and 1960s, most of these organisms were successfully weaponized in the offensive biological weapons programs of the United States and the former Soviet Union. Category B pathogens are also somewhat easy to deliver as weapons but cause much lower morbidity

---

Bioterrorism Epidemiological Clues   Box 5-1

- A large epidemic, with greater case loads than expected, especially in a discrete population
- More severe disease than expected for a given pathogen, as well as unusual routes of exposure
- Unusual disease for a given geographic area, found outside the normal transmission season, or impossible to transmit naturally in the absence of the normal vector for transmission
- Multiple, simultaneous epidemics of different diseases
- A zoonotic disease outbreak as well as a human outbreak, because many of the potential threat agents are pathogenic to animals
- Unusual strains or variants, antimicrobial resistance patterns different from those circulating
- Higher attack rates in those exposed in certain areas, such as inside a building if the agent was released indoors, or lower rates in those inside a sealed building if an aerosol was released outdoors
- Intelligence that an adversary has access to a particular agent or agents
- Claims by a terrorist of the release of a biologic agent
- Direct evidence of the release of an agent, with findings of equipment, munitions, or tampering

Source: Pavlin JA: *Emerg Infec Dis* 5:528-530, 1999.

Table 5-1
Critical Biological Agents for Public Health Preparedness

Biological Agent(s)	Disease
Category A	
Variola major	Smallpox
Bacillus anthracis	Anthrax
Yersinia pestis	Plague
Clostridium botulinum (botulinum toxins)	Botulism
Francisella tularensis	Tularemia
Filoviruses and Arenaviruses (e.g., Ebola, Lassa fever)	Viral hemorrhagic fevers
Category B	
Coxiella burnetii	Q fever
Brucella spp.	Brucellosis
Burkholderia mallei	Glanders
Burkholderia pseudomallei	Melioidosis
Alphaviruses (VEE, EEE, WEE)	Encephalitis
Rickettsia prowazekii	Typhus fever
Toxins (e.g., ricin, staphylococcal enterotoxin B)	Toxic syndromes
Chlamydia psittaci	Psittacosis
Food safety threats (e.g., *Salmonella* spp., *Escherichia coli* O157:H7)	
Water safety threats (e.g., *Vibrio cholerae, Cryptosporidium parvum*)	
Category C	
Emerging threat agents (e.g., Nipah virus, hantavirus)	

Source: Centers for Disease Control and Prevention: *MMWR Morb Mortal Wkly Rep* 49(RR-4):1-14, 2000, http://www.cdc.gov/mmwr/preview/mmwrhtml/rr4904a1.htm, retrieved September 28, 2004.
EEE, Eastern equine encephalomyelitis virus; *VEE,* Venezuelan equine encephalomyelitis virus; *WEE,* western equine encephalomyelitis virus.

and mortality than Category A pathogens. Category C pathogens are emerging diseases that could be harnessed for use by bioterrorists at some point in the future.

EXAMPLES OF BIOTERRORISM THREATS

ANTHRAX

Anthrax disease is caused by the gram-positive, spore-forming bacterium *Bacillus anthracis* (Fig. 5-1). It occurs naturally as a zoonotic disease, and cases sometimes occur in humans due to occupational exposures among leather and wool industry workers. Many experts in biological warfare consider anthrax a perfect biological weapon due to its ability to survive and remain virulent as a spore under conditions that destroy most pathogens. It has also proved to be a very effective agent for bioterrorism, causing 22 cases of anthrax disease and 5 deaths in the fall of 2001 when circulated through the U.S. postal system in contaminated letters.[25] Depending upon the route of exposure, anthrax disease occurs in one of three clinical forms: inhalational, cutaneous, or gastrointestinal.

INHALATIONAL ANTHRAX

Inhalational anthrax is the most lethal form of anthrax disease and results from inhaling the spores. This form of the disease is extremely rare, and a single case necessitates notification of public health and law enforcement authorities for investigation. Prior to the inhalational anthrax cases of 2001, no cases had occurred in the United States for more than 20 years.[22] Once anthrax spores are inhaled, there is an incubation period lasting from several days to several weeks. The spores germinate into vegetative bacilli and release a toxin. This results in a two-stage illness including a prodromal phase and a fulminant phase.

The prodromal phase lasts from a few hours to a few days. It includes nonspecific, flulike symptoms including fever, malaise, shortness of breath, nonproductive cough, and nausea. This stage of the disease could easily be confused with influenza. However, inhalational anthrax does not normally include runny nose or sore throat, whereas many influenza-like illnesses have these symptoms. In addition, influenza does not normally include shortness of breath, vomiting, and mediastinal pain. These are common symptoms of inhalational anthrax. This prodromal period is sometimes followed by a brief improvement before progressing to the next phase of illness.

The second phase of illness is the fulminant stage. This includes the development of high-grade bacteremia characterized by fever, respiratory distress, profuse sweating, cyanosis, and shock. Patients displaying these symptoms usually progress to death within several days.

If an outbreak is known or suspected, initial diagnosis of inhalational anthrax should be made using the signs and symptoms described. This is a very challenging diagnosis. A widened mediastinum on a chest x-ray (Fig. 5-2) is considered highly suspect for inhalational anthrax. However, this clue may or may not be present at the initial patient evaluation or may be the result of another respiratory condition. Confirmation testing may be accomplished using blood cultures and polymerase chain reaction (PCR) of blood or pleural fluid. Additional immunohistochemical tests are available at the CDC or through some regional laboratories that serve as a part of the CDC's Laboratory Response Network.

CUTANEOUS ANTHRAX

The most common form of anthrax disease is cutaneous anthrax. It is a local infection resulting from skin exposure to anthrax spores. It is more likely to appear on regularly exposed areas of the body such as the head, neck, hands, and arms (Fig. 5-3). Areas of compromised skin, such as cuts, abrasions, or chronic dermatological conditions, are at greater risk and more prone to infection than exposed areas of intact skin. Once the spores become embedded in the skin, they begin to germinate and release a toxin. This causes an edema that progresses to form an ulcer within several days. The ulcer develops into a

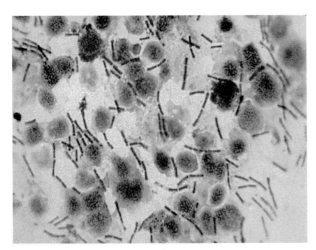

Fig. 5-1
Photomicrograph of *Bacillus anthracis*.

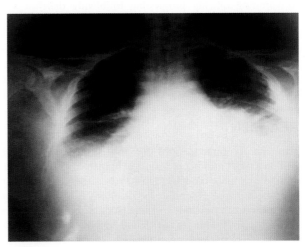

Fig. 5-2
Chest x-ray 22 hours before death showing widened mediastinum due to inhalational anthrax.

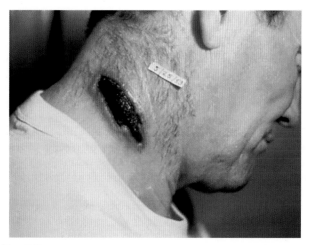

Fig. 5-3
Cutaneous anthrax lesion on the neck.

depressed, painless lesion called an *eschar*. It may be mistaken for a spider bite with one important difference: The anthrax eschar remains painless, but a spider bite causes severe pain. The eschar has a black, leathery appearance for a week or two and then loosens and falls off.

Although cutaneous anthrax is the most common form of occupational anthrax disease, it may also result from intentional release of spores. Half (11) of the 22 cases resulting from the 2001 anthrax letters were cutaneous anthrax; none of these cases were fatal.[22] However, if left untreated, cutaneous anthrax can cause a systemic disease with up to 20% mortality. If treated, cutaneous anthrax mortality is very rare (<1%).[24]

GASTROINTESTINAL ANTHRAX

There is also a gastrointestinal form of anthrax that is caused by ingestion of *Bacillus anthracis*. Ingestion may occur by consuming contaminated meat products and can be very difficult to diagnose. Initial presentation may include nausea and vomiting quickly progressing to bloody diarrhea and sepsis. Gastrointestinal anthrax can lead to the same sort of sepsis as cutaneous and inhalational anthrax and may be fatal. Although an intentional release of anthrax may cause gastrointestinal anthrax, the spore form of anthrax is far less likely to generate gastrointestinal cases; it is more likely to result from ingestion of vegetative bacilli from poorly cooked, infected meat.[24]

TREATMENT

Treatment recommendations for inhalational anthrax are based on a small number of historical human cases and limited testing in animal models (Table 5-2). Antibiotic therapy should be initiated as soon as the diagnosis is suspected. The 2001 anthrax cases included 11 inhalational anthrax cases. Six patients survived due to the rapid initiation of multiple antibiotic therapies and aggressive supportive care.[7]

If an epidemiological or criminal investigation identifies populations at risk, postexposure prophylaxis should be provided to all persons who might have been exposed (Table

Table 5-2
Anthrax Treatment Recommendations

Adult Treatment

IV ciprofloxacin (400 mg every 12 hrs) or IV doxycycline (100 mg every 12 hrs)
plus
one or two other antibiotics (including rifampin, vancomycin, penicillin, ampicillin, chloramphenicol, imipenem, clindamycin, or clarithromycin).
Other fluoroquinolones have demonstrated in vitro activity but studies are limited.

Child Treatment

IV ciprofloxacin (10 mg/kg dose every 12 hrs; max 400 mg dose)
or
IV doxycycline (>45 kg: 100 mg every 12 hrs) (≤45 kg: 2.2 mg/kg every 12 hrs)
plus
one or two other antibiotics (as for adults).

For confirmed cases, treatment should be continued for 60 days.
Maintenance therapy should be altered based upon clinical response and susceptibilities.
Upon improvement, a change to one or two oral agents can be considered.
Localized cutaneous anthrax should be treated with oral ciprofloxacin or doxycycline at equivalent doses.

Source: Inglesby T et al: *JAMA* 287:2236-2252, 2002.

5-3). It is critical that antibiotics be administered as soon as possible after exposure, before the symptoms appear. This offers the best chance for preventing or surviving anthrax disease. Patient contacts (family, friends, health care providers) who were not originally exposed to the release do not require prophylaxis.

PROTECTIVE MEASURES

A safe and effective anthrax vaccine does exist. It is a licensed, cell-free vaccine manufactured by BioPort (Lansing, Mich), the only U.S. manufacturer. Use of this vaccine has been restricted to military personnel. However, it is considered an investigational new drug (IND) for mass prophylaxis during public health emergencies. The Advisory Committee on Immunization Practices (ACIP) recommends using anthrax vaccine in combination with a prophylactic antimicrobial regimen to reduce the recommended time of antibiotic therapy from 60 days to 30 days. This includes a three-dose vaccine regimen (0, 2, 4 weeks) in combination with 30 days of antimicrobial prophylaxis.[7] Following the mailed anthrax incidents of 2001, more than 10,000 people were placed on a 60-day regimen of antimicrobial therapy. However, adherence to the full 60-day antibiotic regimen was low. Only about 42% of the persons on this prophylactic therapy were able to complete it.[31] Combining anthrax vaccinations with antimicrobial prophylaxis reduces the course of protective therapy and may facilitate complete prophylaxis for all persons at risk.

Standard precautions are adequate for all forms of anthrax disease. The only risk to health care providers is direct contact with a cutaneous lesion or exposure to body substances during invasive procedures such as surgery or autopsy. In addition, laboratory personnel should be notified of known or suspected anthrax specimens and ensure safe processing is accomplished. Biosafety level 2 is required for handling clinical specimens of anthrax.[17]

Patient decontamination is warranted only in the immediate aftermath of a known release. Decontamination simply consists of removing clothing and then showering with soap and water; bleach is not necessary. Instruments used for invasive procedures on patients with known or suspected anthrax are sterilized with a sporicidal agent such as hypochlorite (bleach).[2] If a covert release is successfully accomplished, patients seen days or weeks later will not pose a risk to health care providers and do not require decontamination.

The primary risk of infection occurs during the initial release of anthrax spores. Depending upon environmental conditions, the spores normally settle within several hours. Although the spores can survive many years in the soil, cases caused by secondary aerosolization are less likely but still possible. Environmental decontamination of surfaces following an aerosol release is a complicated and costly process. The decision to attempt this activity must be made by environmental experts.

SMALLPOX

Smallpox is a disease caused by the variola virus, a member of the orthopox virus family. This disease has claimed more lives than any other disease in human history. Even though it was eradicated in the 1970s, it still managed to kill more people in the last century than influenza, HIV, and all the casualties of all the wars combined. Smallpox was vulnerable for eradication because the only reservoir for the virus is humans and we have an effective vaccine. The World Health Organization sponsored an aggressive campaign over several years using quarantine and vaccination to bring the disease under control. By the 1970s, they had isolated the last remaining smallpox cases and in one of the greatest accomplishments in human history, smallpox was declared eradicated by 1980. Today, a single confirmed case would become a global health alert and suspected as an act of terrorism or war.

Although the natural disease has been eradicated, smallpox remains a threat as a bioterrorism agent. Following the eradication effort, laboratories around the world were asked to destroy their samples of the variola virus that causes smallpox. Only two laboratories were permitted to retain samples. One lab was in Moscow and one was at the CDC in Atlanta. There are suspicions that laboratories around the world, particularly in Iraq, Iran, and Libya, did not destroy their variola samples. In addition, defecting scientists from the former Soviet Union have alleged the existence of an immense Soviet initiative during the 1980s to create smallpox weapons. The former deputy director of the Soviet biological weapons program confirmed those suspicions when he defected in 1992.[1] This virus likely is in the hands of rogue nations or terrorists, and it may be only a matter of time before we must battle it again.

FORMS OF SMALLPOX

There are two forms of smallpox, each caused by one of two closely related variola viruses. *Variola major* is the organism that causes classic smallpox epidemics (Fig. 5-4). It is the virus most likely to be used as a weapon. In the last smallpox epidemics that occurred throughout Asia, case fatality rates of approximately 30% were observed in unvaccinated populations. *Variola minor* is far less common and far less lethal, with a case fatality rate of less than 1%.[16]

Table 5-3
Anthrax Postexposure Prophylaxis (PEP) Recommendations

Oral antibiotic therapy should be provided for at least 60 days.

Adult PEP

Ciprofloxacin (500 mg every 12 hrs)
Doxycycline: an alternative for adults if strain is susceptible (100 mg every 12 hrs)

Child PEP

Ciprofloxacin (15 mg/kg every 12 hrs; max 500 mg)
Amoxicillin: an alternative for susceptible strains in either adults or children after at least 14 days of ciprofloxacin or doxycycline have been received and is preferred for women who are or might become pregnant

(Adults or children ≥20 kg: 500 mg every 8 hrs)
(Children <20 kg: 80 mg/kg/day orally in three divided doses every 8 hrs)

Source: Inglesby T et al: *JAMA* 287:2236-2252, 2002.

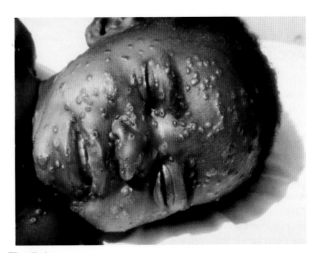

Fig. 5-4
Child with smallpox.

DIAGNOSIS AND TREATMENT

During a confirmed smallpox outbreak, diagnosis should be made based on clinical presentation alone. The greatest challenge is in the diagnosis of an index case. The most similar patient presentation is chickenpox. Smallpox lesions begin in the mouth and throat and then spread to the face and extremities. They concentrate centrifugally on the face, arms, and legs. In addition, the lesions appear on the palms and soles. Across the body, the lesions are uniform and in the same stage of development (vesicles, pustules, or scabs). In contrast, chickenpox concentrates centrally, not centrifugally. The chickenpox lesions are not seen on the palms or the soles and are not uniform in appearance. The lesions are typically in various stages of development, with pustules erupting next to scabs. An orthopox virus is quickly confirmed by electron microscopy of lesion fluid, but variola specifically can only be confirmed by rapid PCR tests at reference laboratories.

PROTECTIVE MEASURES

Smallpox is contagious person to person and usually spreads through respiratory droplets or through direct contact with infected persons or contaminated materials. Although secondary transmission typically occurs in 3 or 4 susceptible contacts per case, 20 or more secondary cases can arise from a primary case when the primary patient has a severe cough or a severe form of smallpox disease.[37] Those at highest risk include household contacts and health care providers. In a health care setting, airborne and contact precautions must be instituted. The patient should be in a negative pressure room, and personnel and visitors must wear proper respiratory protection (e,g., N-95 mask), gown, and gloves for each patient contact. (See Table 5-8.)

Any suspected cases must be immediately isolated until diagnosis is confirmed. Confirmed cases must remain isolated until all scabs separate, usually about 3 weeks. Home isolation is acceptable and may be preferred during an epidemic because of the high risk of nosocomial spread. Any confirmed contacts of smallpox cases should be quickly identified and vaccinated. They should also be monitored twice daily for 17 days following exposure. A fever higher than 38° C (101° F) may be signaling the onset of smallpox, and they should be quickly isolated.[16]

VACCINATION

Only vaccinated persons wearing appropriate personal protective equipment should be permitted to take suspect smallpox specimens. Laboratory specimens collected from suspected or confirmed smallpox cases should be placed in sealed tubes with lids taped closed and stored in a watertight container. Chain of custody must be coordinated with local law enforcement, and the specimens must be sent to specially equipped biosafety level 4 laboratories.[19]

Smallpox vaccine does not contain variola virus. It contains an attenuated strain of vaccinia virus, a close relative of variola. The original vaccine was derived from calf lymph and is no longer produced; however, remaining supplies of the old vaccine are still in use for vaccination of local smallpox response teams. A new smallpox vaccine is currently in development.

The old vaccine conferred excellent immunity for most people in all age groups when a primary "take" resulted in a scab. This is achieved with the bifurcated needle technique (Fig. 5-5). A single dose of vaccine is suspended between the tines of the bifurcated needle when it is dipped into the vaccine vial. The needle is then used to make perpendicular pricks into an area about 5 mm in diameter. Three punctures are recommended for primary vaccination and 15 punctures for revaccination. If there is no trace of blood visible after vaccination, an additional three insertions should be made by using the same bifurcated needle without reinserting the needle into the vaccine vial.[6] This technique should result in a small vaccinia skin infection. If the vaccination is successful, a small papule appears within several days. The infection peaks within two weeks, and the resulting scab separates in about three weeks (Fig. 5-6). Vaccinees should strictly follow inoculation site care and management recommendations provided after vaccination to reduce risk of inadvertent inoculation of close contacts or self.

By 1972 routine childhood smallpox vaccination was discontinued, and by 1980 no smallpox vaccine was available to the public. In the absence of a confirmed smallpox outbreak, vaccination is now indicated only for laboratory personnel who work directly with orthopox viruses and for selected response team members in each region of the country.[6]

Although there is currently an adequate supply of smallpox vaccine for everyone in the United States, no vaccination is recommended for the public unless it is in response to a confirmed outbreak. This is due to the serious risk of complications that accompanies the smallpox vaccine. Potential complications include encephalitis, progressive vaccinia, eczema vaccinatum, generalized vaccinia, and autoinoculation infections of the face, mouth, or genitalia. Most side effects can be successfully managed with vaccinia immune globulin (VIG). However, the availability of VIG is limited.[19] To reduce the likelihood of these complications, screening is required for

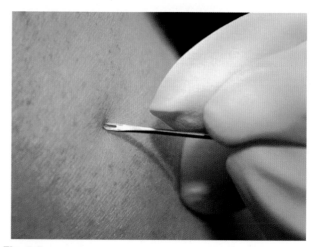

Fig. 5-5
Centers for Disease Control clinician demonstrates the use of a bifurcated needle during the 2002 Smallpox Vaccinator Workshop.

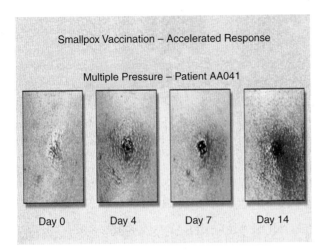

Fig. 5-6
Photographs of vaccination site "takes" that were taken at different intervals over a 2-week period.

persons with certain skin conditions, immunosuppression, and related risk factors listed in Box 5-2.

Vaccination may also be effective in preventing some morbidity and significantly reducing mortality if given within 4 days of exposure.[15] Exposure is defined as suspected inhalation of viral particles from an initial bioterrorism release, household or face-to-face contact with a confirmed smallpox case, or direct contact with contaminated materials or laboratory specimens of confirmed smallpox cases. Cidofovir, an antiviral drug with substantial renal toxicity, may also improve outcomes if given within 1 to 2 days after exposure.[20] However, there is no definitive evidence to suggest that cidofovir is more effective therapy than vaccine alone. During an outbreak, prophylactic vaccination priority must be given to all household members or close contacts, confirmed smallpox patients, exposed patients, health care workers, laboratory workers, and mortuary employees caring for deceased smallpox patients.

Smallpox infection results from inhalation or direct contact between virus particles and mucous membranes. There is normally an asymptomatic incubation period of 12 to 14 days after exposure. During this period, the virus is carried to the regional lymph nodes, causing viremia. A prodromal period follows that includes a high fever, malaise, prostration, vomiting, headache, and backache. Infected white blood cells invade the oral mucosa first, causing lesions in the mouth and throat. Infection quickly spreads to the skin on the face and extremities, causing the characteristic rash. It progresses to vesicles, pustules, and scabs over 1 to 2 weeks, and the scabs normally separate around the third week, leaving scars or pockmarks. Complications from smallpox include encephalitis, secondary bacterial infections, conjunctivitis, and blindness. Death from smallpox usually results from viremia.

There are three variants of smallpox disease. Each type is identified by the presentation of the rash. Classical smallpox is most common and accounts for more than 90% of cases.[19] The other two types of smallpox—malignant and hemorrhagic—do not appear as typical smallpox and are very difficult to diagnose. Malignant cases have an atypical velvety rash, which never matures into pustules and is associated with high mortality. Hemorrhagic smallpox is manifested by a more diffuse erythematous rash leading to petechiae and hemorrhages; it is often misdiagnosed as meningococcemia. It is uniformly fatal.

The variola virus is not stable or persistent in the environment. Following an aerosol release, the virus will be inactivated naturally within 24 hours, or slightly longer under the right conditions. Following a covert release, the buildings and materials in the path of the release do not need decontamination. The index cases would be identified following an incubation period of about two weeks. No environmental issues would be anticipated that long after a release.[19] In a health care setting, standard hospital-grade disinfectants such as quaternary ammonia are effective in killing the virus and should be used for horizontal surfaces of patient rooms or home care settings. Although it is less desirable because it can damage equipment and furniture, hypochlorite (bleach) is an acceptable alternative. Patient linens should be autoclaved or washed in hot water with bleach, and infectious waste should be placed in biohazard bags and autoclaved before incineration.

PLAGUE

Plague is a term often used to describe lethal outbreaks of infectious disease in general. However, plague is a specific disease caused by the gram-negative bacillus *Yersinia pestis*. Plague has an infamous history killing millions of people in pandemic outbreaks occurring around the world throughout recent centuries. Because plague still occurs naturally in many parts of the world, it is important to understand the baseline occurrence of naturally occurring plague. If human cases are identified in a nonendemic area, in persons without risk factors, or in the absence of confirmed rodent cases, an intentional release of *Y. pestis* as a biological weapon should be suspected. Following exposure to aerosolized plague, symptoms begin within 1 to 6 days.[21] There are three forms of plague disease: pneumonic, bubonic, and septicemic. Early symptoms for all forms of plague disease include fever, chills, myalgia, weakness, elevated white blood cell count (WBC), and headaches. Each of the three forms of plague poses different challenges and unique symptoms.

PNEUMONIC PLAGUE

Pneumonic plague is the least common but most severe form of plague. This form of the disease results from the inhalation of infectious particles either from an intentional release or from an infected person. Although it can occur secondary to bubonic plague, it also causes primary disease if it is released in an act of bioterrorism. This is the most likely form of plague disease that would result from an aerosolized biological weapon.

The mortality rate for pneumonic plague is 57%.[12] Patients with pneumonic plague initially present with dizziness, chest discomfort, and a productive cough with blood-tinged sputum. A chest x-ray may show patchy or consolidated bronchopneumonia. The pneumonia may begin in a focused portion of the lung, extend to the full lung, and then progress bilaterally as disease spreads. By the second day of the illness, the symptoms may worsen significantly. Symptoms include tachypnea, chest pain, coughing, and sputum increase, and they may include dyspnea, hemoptysis, cardiopulmonary insufficiency, and circulatory collapse.

BUBONIC PLAGUE

Bubonic plague is the most common form of plague disease. It is spread by handling contaminated infected animals or through the bite of an infected flea. Although this form of plague is less likely to be the result of bioterrorism, it is possible to intentionally spread bubonic plague through an intentional release of infected fleas. The mortality rate for this form of the disease is approximately 13%.[12]

Patients with bubonic plague present with swollen, tender, and painful buboes (enlarged lymph nodes) (Fig. 5-7). These symptoms typically occur within 24 hours of the onset of early symptoms and are generally located near the area of inoculation. Most frequently they occur in the inguinal or

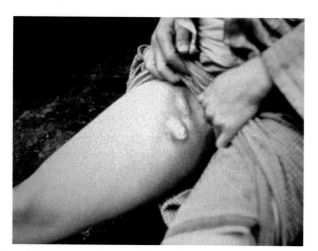

Fig. 5-7
This plague patient displays a swollen, ruptured inguinal lymph node, or bubo.

femoral lymph node region. Buboes may erupt on their own or require incision and drainage. Other possible symptoms include bladder distention, apathy, confusion, fright, agitation, oliguria, anuria, tachycardia, hypotension, and leukocytosis.

SEPTICEMIC PLAGUE

Septicemic plague is the least common form of the disease. It is a systemic infection caused by direct inoculation of *Y. pestis* into the blood stream or secondarily from untreated bubonic disease. The mortality rate for septicemic plague is approximately 22%.[12] Patients with septicemic plague initially present with nausea, vomiting, and diarrhea. Skin lesions, gangrene, and necrosis often develop later in the disease process.

DIAGNOSIS AND TREATMENT

Rapid diagnosis is essential to reduce plague mortality. In the absence of appropriate antibiotic therapy, plague illness can progress rapidly and cause death within several days. Presumptive diagnosis is accomplished with a Gram or Wayson bipolar-staining smear using lymph node aspirates, sputum, or cerebrospinal fluid (CSF). Although these tests are very reliable, they are only available at reference laboratories. Definitive diagnosis is accomplished using sputum or bubo cultures or IgM and IgG antibody testing. In addition, antibiotic resistance patterns must be quickly evaluated to identify effective treatment. Rapid diagnosis and appropriate antimicrobial therapy are the keys to effective response to a plague outbreak. Once known or suspected cases of pneumonic plague occur, assume all patients presenting with fever or cough, or tachypnea in infants, are positive and treat appropriately (Table 5-4). The antibiotic selection is based on the results of susceptibility testing, the age and condition of the patient, and the aim of the therapy. The aim may include treatment of active disease or prophylactic treatment for suspected exposures (Table 5-5).

PROTECTIVE MEASURES

There was a killed whole-cell vaccine for use against bubonic plague. Production of this vaccine has been discontinued. It consisted of a three-dose series followed by 6-month boosters and was previously used by a small number of specialized researchers. This vaccine was not effective at preventing pneumonic plague and offered little protection for most bioterrorism scenarios. New vaccines are in development to reduce the risk of pneumonic plague that could result from an act of bioterrorism, but no plague vaccine is currently available to the public.

Infection control for bubonic and septicemic forms of plague disease consists of standard precautions. However, if a bubo is draining, contact precautions should also be used until draining stops. Pneumonic plague requires droplet isolation until the patient has received at least 48 hours of appropriate antibiotic therapy. Clinical improvement of the patient's symptoms should be observed and sensitivity of the strain should be verified before removing an infected patient from isolation. For all forms of plague disease, aerosol-generating surgical procedures should be avoided, including autopsy. If

Table 5-4
Plague Treatment Recommendations

Adult Treatment (including nonpregnant, nonlactating, and immunocompromised patients)

Preferred	Alternatives
Streptomycin (1g IM twice daily) *or* Gentamicin (5 mg/kg IM or IV once daily) or (2 mg/kg loading dose followed by 1.7 mg/kg IM or IV 3 times daily)	Doxycycline (100 mg IV twice daily) or (200 mg IV once daily) *or* Ciprofloxacin (400 mg IV twice daily) *or* Chloramphenicol (25 mg/kg IV 4 times daily)

Child Treatment (including immunocompromised patients)

Preferred	Alternatives
Streptomycin (15 mg/kg IM twice daily; maximum daily dose, 2 g) *or* Gentamicin (2.5 mg/kg IM or IV 3 times daily)	Doxycycline (≥45 kg adult dose) (<45 kg 2.2 mg/kg IV 4 times daily) *or* Ciprofloxacin (15 mg/kg IV twice daily) *or* Chloramphenicol (25 mg/kg IV 4 times daily)

Preferred choices include Streptomycin or Gentamicin. Alternatives include Doxycycline, Ciprofloxacin, and Chloramphenicol. Preferred choice for pregnant women is Gentamicin. One antimicrobial agent should be used. Therapy should continue for 10 days. Oral therapy should be substituted when patient condition improves.

Source: Inglesby T et al: *JAMA* 283:2281-2290, 2000.

Table 5-5
Plague Postexposure Prophylaxis (PEP) Recommendations

Adult PEP (including pregnant and nursing women)

Preferred	Alternative
Doxycycline (100 mg orally twice daily) *or* Ciprofloxacin (500 mg orally twice daily)	Chloramphenicol (25 mg/kg orally 4 times daily)

Child PEP

Preferred	Alternative
Doxycycline (≥45 kg adult dose) (<45 kg 2.2 mg/kg orally twice daily) *or* Ciprofloxacin (20 mg/kg orally twice daily, not to exceed 1 g/d)	Chloramphenicol (25 mg/kg orally 4 times daily, not to exceed 4 g/d, not for children <2 yrs)

PEP should continue for 7 days. Asymptomatic household, hospital, or other close contacts (within 2 m) of pneumonic plague patients should receive postexposure prophylaxis. Close contacts refusing prophylaxis should be watched carefully for 7 days after exposure for signs of fever or cough. Treat immediately if symptoms occur.

Source: Inglesby T et al: *JAMA* 287:2236-2252, 2002.

required, these procedures should be accomplished in a negative pressure room. The wearing of an N-95 respirator is also required for these procedures. Only standard cleaning of patient rooms and handling of linens are necessary. Laboratory biosafety level 2 precautions are typically adequate. However, if centrifuging, grinding, or vigorous shaking of samples are anticipated, biosafety level 3 precautions are needed.

Y. pestis can remain viable for only 1 hour as an aerosol and dies quickly in sunlight, or heat or outside of the host. Environmental decontamination following aerosol release of plague is unnecessary. Standard hospital-approved disinfectants are adequate for cleaning patient rooms.

All cases of plague should be reported to the local public health authorities and the World Health Organization (WHO). If an intentional release is suspected, local law enforcement must be notified as well as the nearest field office of the Federal Bureau of Investigation (FBI).

TULAREMIA

Francisella tularensis is a hardy, highly infectious organism. Exposure to as few as 10 organisms can result in tularemia, also known as "rabbit fever" or "deer fly fever."[30] This disease is almost always rural and has occurred naturally in every state in the United States except Hawaii (Fig. 5-8). The areas that have observed the most tularemia cases include rural Missouri and Arkansas. It is important to understand the typical exposure pathways as well as the normal geographical patterns of tularemia in order to recognize unusual circumstances or patterns that may indicate an act of bioterrorism. If human cases are identified in a nonendemic area, in urban areas, or in persons without risk factors, an intentional release of *F. tularensis* as a biological weapon should be suspected.

A person may acquire tularemia in a variety of ways. The route of exposure determines the resulting form of disease. It is normally transmitted through handling infected small mammals such as rabbits or rodents. Another common route of disease transmission to humans is through the bites of ticks, deer flies, or mosquitoes that have fed on infected animals. These routes of exposure may result in ulceroglandular tularemia, a form of the disease characterized by skin ulcers and swelling of the lymph nodes, or glandular tularemia that is characterized by swelling of the lymph nodes without skin ulcers. If an infected animal is eaten after being inadequately cooked or if contaminated food or water is otherwise ingested, the resulting disease may be oropharyngeal tularemia, which is characterized by swelling of the lymph nodes and pharyngitis. It is also possible to directly inoculate the eye, resulting in oculoglandular tularemia, which is characterized by conjunctivitis and swelling of the lymph nodes.

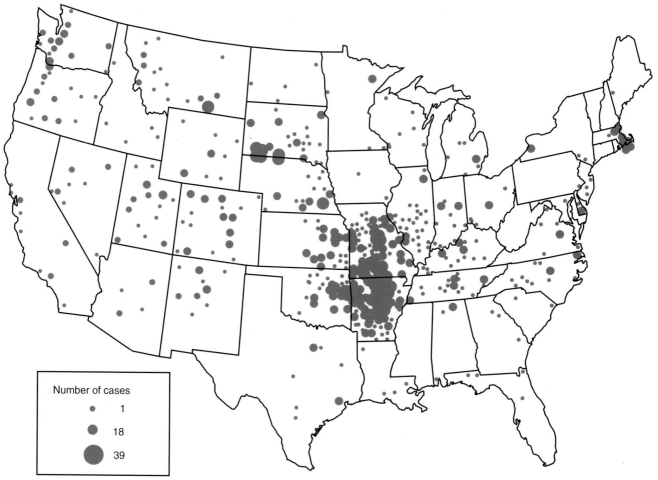

Fig. 5-8
Reported cases of tularemia in the United States, 1990-2000. Based on 1347 patients reporting county of residence in lower continental United States. (Alaska reported 10 cases, 1990-2000.) Circle size is proportional to number of cases ranging 1-39.

TYPES OF TULAREMIA

All four forms of tularemia disease described, ulceroglandular, glandular, oropharyngeal, and oculoglandular, have a very low mortality rate (<2%) and are the most common forms of tularemia disease.[14] There are other forms of this disease that may signal a bioterrorism attack. Although any form of the disease may progress to typhoidal and pneumonic forms of tularemia, these more severe forms of tularemia disease are the most likely to result from an aerosol release.

DIAGNOSIS AND TREATMENT

Inhalation of *F. tularensis* typically causes flulike symptoms after a 2- to 5-day incubation period. However, the onset of symptoms can occur within 1 day or as long as 14 days after exposure. The clinical presentation may include the rapid onset of fever, chills, myalgia, weakness, and headaches. In addition, these symptoms may progress to a nonproductive cough, sore throat, and inflammation of the bronchi, lungs, and lymph nodes. Unfortunately, there are currently no reliable

rapid diagnostic tests for tularemia. Therefore the initial identification of an intentional tularemia outbreak will rely upon presumptive diagnosis based on the described clinical presentation.

If an unusually high number of previously healthy individuals present with these symptoms, particularly in nonrural regions with low incidence of naturally occurring tularemia, the index of suspicion should be high. If inhalational tularemia is suspected, respiratory secretions should be acquired along with blood samples for confirmatory testing. Several tests may be used, including direct fluorescent antibody assays and immunohistochemical stains.[14]

Once known or suspected cases of pneumonic tularemia occur, assume all patients presenting with flulike symptoms are infected and treat appropriately (Table 5-6). The antibiotic selection is based on the results of susceptibility testing, the age and condition of the patient, and the aim of the therapy. The aim may include treatment of active disease or prophylactic treatment for suspected exposures (Table 5-7).

Table 5-6
Tularemia Treatment Recommendations

Adult Treatment (including nonpregnant, nonlactating, and immunocompromised patients)

Preferred	Alternatives
Streptomycin (1g IM twice daily) *or* Gentamicin (5 mg/kg IM or IV once daily)	Doxycycline (100 mg IV twice daily) *or* Ciprofloxacin (400 mg IV twice daily) *or* Chloramphenicol (15 mg/kg IV 4 times daily)

Child Treatment (including immunocompromised patients)

Preferred	Alternatives
Streptomycin (15 mg/kg IM twice daily; maximum daily dose, 2 g) *or* Gentamicin (2.5 mg/kg IM or IV 3 times daily)	Doxycycline (≥45 kg adult dose) (<45 kg 2.2 mg/kg IV more 2 times daily after 2.2 mg/kg IV *or* Chloramphenicol (15 mg/kg IV 4 times daily) *or* Ciprofloxacin (15 mg/kg IV twice daily; not to exceed 1 g/d in children)

Preferred choices include Streptomycin or Gentamicin.
Alternatives include Doxycycline, Ciprofloxacin, and Chloramphenicol.
Preferred choice for pregnant women is Gentamicin.
One antimicrobial agent should be used. Therapy should continue for 10 days (14 to 21 days using doxycycline or chloramphenicol).
Oral therapy should be substituted when patient condition improves.

Source: Dennis DT et al: *JAMA* 285:2763-2773, 2001.

PROTECTIVE MEASURES

A vaccine does exist for tularemia. However, it is under review by the Food and Drug Administration and is currently not available to the public.

Even though *F. tularensis* is highly infectious for anyone directly exposed to the organism, it is not spread from person to person. Standard precautions are adequate to protect health care workers and limit the risk of nosocomial infections. Aerosol-generating surgical procedures should be avoided for tularemia patients, including autopsies. Otherwise, corpses may be handled using standard precautions. Only standard cleaning of patient rooms and handling of linens are necessary. Laboratory biosafety level 2 precautions are adequate for routine procedures. However, culture examinations require the use of a biological safety cabinet. If centrifuging, grinding, or vigorous shaking of samples are anticipated, biosafety level 3 precautions are needed.

F. tularensis is capable of surviving for long periods of time in stable, cool, moist environments. However, it is unlikely that this organism could survive for a long period of time in an aerosol release and would also be unlikely to re-aerosolize. Therefore environmental decontamination following aerosol

Table 5-7
Tularemia Postexposure Prophylaxis (PEP) Recommendations

Adult PEP (including pregnant and nursing women)

Doxycycline (100 mg orally twice daily)
or
Ciprofloxacin (500 mg orally twice daily)

Child PEP

Doxycycline (≥45 kg adult dose) (<45 kg 2.2 mg/kg orally twice daily)
or
Ciprofloxacin (15 mg/kg orally twice daily, not to exceed 1 g/d)
PEP should continue for 14 days.
Preferred choice for pregnant women during mass PEP is ciprofloxacin.

Source: Dennis DT et al: *JAMA* 285:2763-2773, 2001.

release of tularemia is unnecessary. Persons suspected of being contaminated by an aerosol release should wash body surfaces and clothing with soap and water.

All cases of tularemia should be reported to the local public health authorities. If an intentional release is suspected, local law enforcement must be notified as well as the nearest field office of the FBI.

BOTULISM

Clostridium botulinum is the only toxin listed as one of the six Category A biological agents by the CDC. The other five are replicating bacterial or viral agents. It earned a place near the top of the threat list due to its widespread availability and potency. In fact, botulinum toxin is the most potent toxic substance known.[18] Exposure to this toxin causes a severe paralytic illness. There are cases of botulism occurring regularly in the United States due to improper food handling and canning. Across the country, fewer than 200 cases naturally occur each year.[11] There are four types of botulism disease: foodborne, intestinal, wound, and inhalational.

TYPES OF BOTULISM

Foodborne botulism is the most frequently occurring form of the disease and results from ingesting foods that have been contaminated with *C. botulinum* and therefore contain the resulting toxin. Although it is possible that food may serve as an intentional delivery method for botulinum, the toxin is not stable enough to survive for an extended period of time in a large volume of food. Despite its high toxicity, botulinum is also easily destroyed in food through normal cooking. If this method of delivery is selected for a bioterrorism attack, it would likely be limited to a small-scale attack. Regardless of the size or source of an outbreak, any case of botulism is considered a public health emergency because the food source may still be available to the public and cause additional cases.

Intestinal botulism occurs when *C. botulinum* spores are ingested, resulting in intestinal colonization. The germinating spores release the toxin and cause illness. This form of the disease typically occurs in infants (Fig. 5-9). However in children or adults, when an infected wound is not observed and a specific food source cannot be identified, it is typically attributed to this intestinal colonization.

Wound botulism occurs when *C. botulinum* infects the site of a wound, multiplies, and releases the toxin, causing illness. All three forms of the disease described occur naturally. However, the fourth type of disease, inhalational botulism, does not occur naturally and is the most likely form expected from an aerosol release of botulinum toxin.

The onset of botulism following exposure depends upon the quantity and duration of the exposure. Incubation for foodborne botulism ranges from 6 hours to 10 days.[32] There is a paucity of data on progression of disease following inhalation of botulinum, making it impossible to predict precisely how differently inhalational cases may progress. Initial symptoms include double or blurred vision and dryness of the mouth. Those symptoms may be the extent of the illness for a small exposure. The larger exposures may include progression of symptoms to include slurred speech, difficulty swallowing, and descending peripheral muscle weakness. Severe disease may involve the respiratory muscles, leading to ventilatory failure and death.

DIAGNOSIS AND TREATMENT

Presumptive diagnosis is based on the symptoms described. The diagnosis may be confirmed through specialized tests that are only available at reference laboratories and take several days to complete. Botulism may be mistaken for Guillain-Barré syndrome, myasthenia gravis, or a disease of the central nervous system, but it differs from other paralytic conditions in the conspicuous cranial nerve palsies, symmetry, and absence of sensory nerve damage.[3]

Treatment for botulism includes rapid administration of antitoxin and supportive care including aggressive respiratory monitoring and support. These essential therapies pose tremendous challenges to an effective public health response. The need for ventilators may quickly exceed the critical care capacity of the affected community. In addition, the efficacy of the antitoxin therapy depends upon how early it is initiated in the course of illness.[34] Therefore the local response must include well-trained providers with a high index of suspicion and a logistical system to rapidly deliver antitoxin where it is needed. This therapy cannot be used prophylactically for exposed persons who are not yet displaying symptoms. Persons who suspect exposure must be monitored for the onset of initial symptoms prior to administration of antitoxin. There is also no vaccine currently available for the public.

PROTECTIVE MEASURES

Because botulinum is a toxin and not an infectious organism, person-to-person transmission will not occur and only standard precautions are needed. Exposed skin and clothing may be cleaned with soap and water.

VIRAL HEMORRHAGIC FEVERS

Viral hemorrhagic fevers (VHFs) are caused by one of a number of viruses from the arenavirus, filovirus, bunyavirus, or flavivirus families. Included in these viral families are the organisms that cause diseases such as Ebola, Marburg, Rift Valley, and Lassa fevers (Fig. 5-10). These RNA viruses depend upon various animal and insect hosts for survival, and naturally occurring disease is somewhat restricted to the areas of their primary hosts. People are not the natural reservoirs for VHF viruses but are sometimes accidentally exposed and

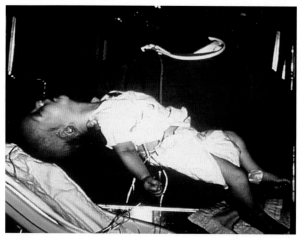

Fig. 5-9
Six-week-old infant with botulism that is evident as a marked loss of muscle tone, especially in the region of the head and neck.

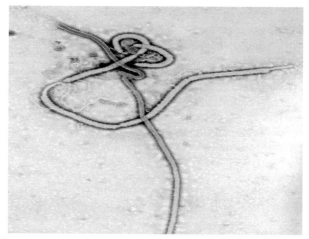

Fig. 5-10
Transmission electron micrograph of the Ebola virus.

infected by coming into contact with an infected animal host or through the bite of an arthropod vector. Outbreaks of these diseases are usually isolated and unpredictable. The clinical feature that these VHF viruses have in common is that they all cause microvascular damage leading to various hemorrhagic presentations.

DIAGNOSIS AND TREATMENT

VHFs rank high on the list of biological agent threats due to the infectiousness of these pathogens at very low doses as an aerosol. Animal studies have sufficiently demonstrated the risk of infection posed by aerosolization of these pathogens.[23,33] Following a VHF aerosol release, an incubation period takes from 2 to 21 days depending upon the pathogen used. Those exposed would normally have a flulike prodromal illness of less than 1 week, including symptoms such as high fever, headache, malaise, myalgias, nausea, and bloody diarrhea. Severe cases may then show signs of bleeding from orifices, under the skin, and in internal organs and progress to shock and multiorgan failure.

Diagnosis is initially based on the clinical criteria and requires a high index of suspicion. Immediate reporting of suspicious cases is vital for an effective response. Treatment must begin before receiving confirmatory lab testing results.[4] In fact, VHF testing capabilities are limited and may not be available to confirm diagnosis. Treatment options of VHFs are also very limited and consist primarily of supportive care with close monitoring of blood pressure, maintenance of fluid balance and circulatory volume, and ventilatory support as needed. Although Ribavirin may offer some benefit for certain kinds of VHFs, there currently are no FDA-approved antiviral drugs for treatment of these diseases. The case fatality rate can be very high. In fact, one recent Ebola outbreak had a case fatality rate of approximately 90%.[26]

PROTECTIVE MEASURES

Given the inordinate risk posed by these organisms to health care workers, strict adherence to infection control precautions is essential. These recommendations include patient isolation in a negative pressure room, strict hand hygiene, and use of double gloves, impermeable gown, face shield, eye protection, and leg and shoe coverings. In addition, HEPA respiratory protection should be worn by anyone entering the patient's room.[4] The risk to prehospital contacts may be somewhat lower because the patients will likely be in the earlier stages of disease and less infectious.

Laboratory specimens must be handled in a biological safety cabinet following biosafety level 3 practices, and virus cultivation requires a level 4 laboratory. Cleaning of environmental surfaces visibly contaminated with body fluids may be accomplished using standard EPA-registered hospital disinfectants or a 1:100 dilution of household bleach.[13]

CHAPTER SUMMARY

In recent years, infection control has become a higher priority across the continuum of health care delivery in the United States. Despite strides made in the reduction of nosocomial

infections and the protection of first responders and health care workers, most infection-control programs still lack the managerial support and worker compliance needed to be fully effective.

With regard to bioterrorism preparedness, it is not possible to overstate the importance of basic infection-control procedures. The key aspect of biological weapons that instills terror is the potential for acquiring and passing infection. Those responding to an attack will either be part of the problem by contributing to the spread of the disease or part of the solution by complying with basic infection-control procedures. The basic principles of hand washing, standard precautions, and use of personal protective equipment must be enhanced for our daily routines and not simply studied for preparedness. Table 5-8 gives more details on bioterrorism-related infection-control recommendations.

ADDITIONAL INFORMATION

For more information on bioterrorism preparedness, please refer to the following websites:

ACADEMIC SITES

Center for the Study of Bioterrorism, Saint Louis University
http://bioterrorism.slu.edu/
Center for Civilian Biodefense Strategies, Johns Hopkins University
http://www.hopkins-biodefense.org/
Center for Infectious Disease Research and Policy, University of Minnesota
http://www.cidrap.umn.edu/cidrap/

PROFESSIONAL ORGANIZATION SITES

Association for Professionals in Infection Control and Epidemiology, Bioterrorism Resource Page
http://www.apic.org/bioterror/default.cfm
Infectious Diseases Society of America, Bioterrorism Resource Page
http://www.idsociety.org/BT/ToC.htm
American College of Emergency Physicians, Bioterrorism Resource Page
http://www.acep.org/1,4634,0.html

GOVERNMENT SITES

Centers for Disease Control and Prevention, Public Health Emergency Preparedness and Response Program
http://www.bt.cdc.gov/
Department of Homeland Security
http://www.ready.gov/
U.S. Army Medical Research Institute of Infectious Diseases
http://www.usamriid.army.mil/

Table 5-8
Sample Patient Management Guidelines for Bioterrorism-Related Illnesses

IMPORTANT PHONE NUMBERS (fill in your local numbers in the spaces provided)

Infectious Diseases: _____-_____

Infection Control: _____-_____

Emergency Dept.: _____-_____

USAMRIID: 301-619-2833

CDC Emergency Response Office: 770-488-7100

	Anthrax	Brucellosis	Cholera	Glanders	Bubonic Plague	Pneumonic Plague	Tularemia	Q Fever	Smallpox	Venez. Equine Encephalitis	Viral Encephalitis	Viral Hemorrhagic Fever	Botulism	Ricin	T-2 Mycotoxins	Staph. Enterotoxin B
	Bacterial Agents								Viruses				Biological Agents			
Isolation Precautions																
Standard precautions for all aspects of patient care	X	X	X	X	X	X	X	X	X	X	X	X	X	X	X	X
Contact precautions (gown and gloves; wash hands after each patient encounter)			X‡	X*	X*				X			X			X*	
Airborne precautions (negative pressure room; N-95 masks for all individuals entering the room)									X			X†				
Droplet precautions (surgical mask)						X						X†				
Patient Placement																
No restrictions	X	X	X	X			X	X		X	X		X	X	X	X
Cohort like patients when private room is unavailable			X‡	X*	X	X			X			X			X*	
Private room			X‡	X*	X*	X			X			X			X*	
Negative pressure room									X			X†				
Door closed at all times									X			X†				
Patient Transport																
No restrictions	X	X	X	X	X		X	X		X	X		X	X	X	X
Limit movement to essential medical purposes only			X‡	X*	X*	X			X			X			X*	
Place mask on patient to minimize dispersal of droplets						X			X			X†				
Cleaning and Disinfection																
Routine cleaning of room with hospital-approved disinfectant	X	X	X	X	X	X	X	X	X	X	X		X	X	X	X
Disinfect surfaces with 10% bleach solution or phenolic disinfectant												X				
Dedicated equipment (disinfect prior to leaving room)			X‡	X*	X*				X			X			X*	
Linen management as with all other patients	X	X	X	X	X	X	X	X	X	X	X	X	X	X	X	X
Linens autoclaved before laundering or wash in hot water with bleach added												X				
Postmortem Care																
Standard precautions	X	X	X	X	X	X	X	X	X	X	X	X	X	X	X	X
Droplet precautions (surgical mask)						X										
Contact precautions (gown and gloves)				X*	X*				X			X			X*	
Avoid autopsy or use airborne precautions and HEPA filter						X			X			X†				
Routine terminal cleaning of room with hospital-approved disinfectant	X	X	X	X	X	X	X	X	X	X	X		X	X	X	X
Disinfect surfaces with 10% bleach solution or phenolic disinfectant												X				
Minimal handling of body; seal body in leak-proof material												X				
Cremate body whenever possible									X							

Table 5-8–cont'd
Sample Patient Management Guidelines for Bioterrorism-Related Illnesses

IMPORTANT PHONE NUMBERS (fill in your local numbers in the spaces provided)	Bacterial Agents									Viruses				Biological Agents		
	Anthrax	Brucellosis	Cholera	Glanders	Bubonic Plague	Pneumonic Plague	Tularemia	Q Fever	Smallpox	Venez. Equine Encephalitis	Viral Encephalitis	Viral Hemorrhagic Fever	Botulism	Ricin	T-2 Mycotoxins	Staph. Enterotoxin B
Infectious Diseases: _____-_____																
Infection Control: _____-_____																
Emergency Dept.: _____-_____																
USAMRIID: 301-619-2833																
CDC Emergency Response Office: 770-488-7100																
Discontinuation of Isolation																
48 hours of appropriate antibiotic and clinical improvement						X										
Until all scabs separate									X							
Until skin decontamination is completed (1 hour contact time)															X	
Duration of illness			X‡	X*	X*							X				

Source: Saint Louis University, Center for the Study of Bioterrorism and Emerging Infections, October 2001. Adapted with permission from an original table designed by LTC Suzanne E. Johnson, RN, MSN, CIC, Walter Reed Army Medical Center.

Standard precautions prevent direct contact with all body fluids (including blood), secretions, excretions, nonintact skin (including rashes), and mucous membranes. Standard precautions routinely practiced by healthcare providers include splash/spray and gowns to protect skin and clothing during procedures.

USAMRIID, United States Army Medical Research Institute of Infectious Diseases.

*Contact precautions needed only if the patient has skin involvement (bubonic plague: draining bubo) or until decontamination of skin is complete (T2 Mycotoxins).

†A surgical mask and eye protection should be worn if you come within 3 feet of the patient. Airborne precautions are needed if the patient has cough, vomiting, diarrhea, or hemorrhage.

‡Contact precautions needed only if the patient is diapered or incontinent.

REFERENCES

1. Alibek K: *Biohazard,* New York, 1999, Random House.
2. American Public Health Association: Anthrax. In Benson AS, editor. *Control of communicable diseases manual,* Washington, DC, 1995, American Public Health Association.
3. Arnon SS et al: Botulinum toxin as a biological weapon: medical and public health management, *JAMA* 285:1059-1070, 2001.
4. Borio L et al: Hemorrhagic fever viruses as biological weapons: medical and public health management, *JAMA* 287:2391-2405, 2002.
5. Bush LM et al: Index case of fatal inhalational anthrax due to bioterrorism in the United States, *N Engl J Med* 345:1607-1610, 2001.
6. Centers for Disease Control and Prevention: Recommendations for using smallpox vaccine in a pre-event vaccination program: supplemental recommendations of the Advisory Committee on Immunization Practices (ACIP) and the Healthcare Infection Control Practices Advisory Committee (HICPAC), *MMWR Morb Mortal Wkly Rep* 52:1-16, 2003, http://www.cdc.gov/mmwr/preview/mmwrhtml/m2d226.htm, retrieved September 28, 2004.
7. Centers for Disease Control and Prevention: Notice to readers: use of anthrax vaccine in response to terrorism: supplemental recommendations of the Advisory Committee on Immunization Practices, *MMWR Morb Mortal Wkly Rep* 51:1024-1026, 2002, http://www.cdc.gov/mmwr/preview/mmwrhtml/mm5145a4.htm, retrieved September 28, 2004.
8. Centers for Disease Control and Prevention: Clinical issues in the prophylaxis, diagnosis, and treatment of anthrax, conference summary 2001, *Emerg Infec Dis* 8:222-225, 2002, http://www.cdc.gov/ncidod/eid/vol8no2/01-0521.htm, retrieved September 28, 2004.
9. Centers for Disease Control and Prevention: Tularemia—United States, 1990-2000, *MMWR Morb Mortal Wkly Rep* 51:182-184, 2002, http://www.cdc.gov/mmwr/preview/mmwrhtml/mm5109a1.htm, retrieved September 28, 2004.
10. Centers for Disease Control and Prevention: Biological and chemical terrorism: strategic plan for preparedness and response, recommendations of the CDC Strategic Planning Workgroup, *MMWR Morb Mortal Wkly Rep* 49(RR-4):1-14, 2000, http://www.cdc.gov/mmwr/preview/mmwrhtml/rr4904a1.htm, retrieved September 28, 2004.
11. Centers for Disease Control and Prevention: *Botulism in the United States 1899-1996: handbook for epidemiologists, clinicians, and laboratory workers,* Atlanta, 1998, Centers for Disease Control and Prevention, http://www.cdc.gov/ncidod/dbmd/diseaseinfo/botulism.pdf, retrieved September 28, 2004.
12. Centers for Disease Control and Prevention: Fatal human plague—Arizona and Colorado, 1996, *MMWR Morb Mortal Wkly Rep* 46:617-620, 1997, http://www.cdc.gov/mmwr/preview/mmwrhtml/00048352.htm, retrieved September 28, 2004.
13. Centers for Disease Control and Prevention: Notice to readers update: management of patients with suspected viral hemorrhagic fever—United States, *MMWR Morb Mortal Wkly Rep* 44:475-479, 1995, http://www.cdc.gov/mmwr/preview/mmwrhtml/00038033.htm, retrieved September 28, 2004.
14. Dennis DT et al: Tularemia as a biological weapon: medical and public health management, *JAMA* 285:2763-2773, 2001.

15. Dixon CW: *Smallpox*, London, 1962, J & A Churchill.
16. Fenner F et al: *Smallpox and its eradication*, Geneva, 1988, World Health Organization, http://www.who.int/emc/diseases/smallpox/Smallpoxeradication.html, retrieved September 28, 2004.
17. Franz DR et al: Clinical recognition and management of patients exposed to biological warfare agents, *JAMA* 278:399-411, 1997.
18. Gill MD: Bacterial toxins: a table of lethal amounts, *Microbiol Rev* 46:86-94, 1982.
19. Henderson DA et al: Smallpox as a biological weapon: medical and public health management, *JAMA* 281:1735-1745, 1999.
20. Huggins JW et al: Potential antiviral therapeutics for smallpox, monkeypox, and other orthopoxvirus infections. Presented at the WHO Advisory Committee on Variola Virus Research, Geneva, December 3-6, 2001.
21. Inglesby T et al: Plague as a biological weapon: medical and public health management, *JAMA* 283:2281-2290, 2000.
22. Inglesby T et al: Anthrax as a biological weapon, 2002: updated recommendations for management, *JAMA* 287:2236-2252, 2002.
23. Johnson E et al: Lethal experimental infections of rhesus monkeys by aerosolized Ebola virus, *Int J Exp Pathol* 76:227-236, 1995.
24. Lew D: Bacillus anthracis. In Mandell GL, Bennett JE, Dolin R, editors: *Principles and practice of infectious disease*, New York, 1995, Churchill Livingstone.
25. Mina B et al: Fatal inhalational anthrax with unknown source of exposure in a 61-year-old woman in New York City, *JAMA* 287:858-862, 2002.
26. Muyembe-Tamfum JJ et al: Ebola outbreak in Kikwit, Democratic Republic of the Congo: discovery and control measures, *J Infect Dis* 179(suppl 1):S259-S262, 1999.
27. Pavlin JA: Epidemiology of bioterrorism, *Emerg Infec Dis* 5:528-530, 1999.
28. Pavlin JA et al: Innovative surveillance methods for monitoring dangerous pathogens. In Knobler SL, Mahmoud AF, Pray LA, editors: *Biological threats and terrorism: assessing the science and response capabilities,* Washington, DC, 2002, National Academy Press.
29. Rotz LD et al: Public health assessment of potential biological terrorism agents, *Emerg Infec Dis* 8:225-230, 2002.
30. Saslaw S et al: Tularemia vaccine study, I: intracutaneous challenge, *Arch Intern Med* 107:121-133, 1961.
31. Shepard CW et al: Antimicrobial postexposure prophylaxis for anthrax: adverse events and adherence, *Emerg Infect Dis* 8:1124-1132, 2002.
32. St. Louis ME et al: Botulism from chopped garlic: delayed recognition of a major outbreak, *Ann Intern Med* 108:363-368, 1988.
33. Stephenson EH, Larson EW, Dominik JW: Effect of environmental factors on aerosol-induced Lassa virus infection, *J Med Virol* 14:295-303, 1984.
34. Tackett CO et al: Equine antitoxin use and other factors that predict outcome in type A foodborne botulism, *Am J Med* 76:794-798, 1984.
35. Thacker SB: Historical development. In Teutsch SM, Churchill RE, editors: *Principles and practice of public health surveillance*, New York, 1994, Oxford University Press.
36. Torok TJ et al: A large community outbreak of salmonellosis caused by intentional contamination of restaurant salad bars, *JAMA* 278:389-395, 1997.
37. Wehrle PF et al: An airborne outbreak of smallpox in a German hospital and its significance with respect to other recent outbreaks in Europe, *Bull World Health Organ* 43:669-679, 1970.

Chemical Weapons

CHRIS MAILLIARD

CHAPTER OBJECTIVES

At the conclusion of this chapter the student will be able to:

- Understand the history of chemical warfare and how it provides important lessons for protecting ourselves and treating our patients.
- Identify chemicals first responders should be concerned about.
- Identify the four classes of chemical warfare agents.
- Describe the characteristics, signs and symptoms, and mechanism of action of the chemicals discussed in this chapter.
- Triage and treat patients affected by a chemical agent.
- Describe the indicators of a possible chemical release.
- Identify the factors that can influence the release of a chemical agent.

CASE STUDY

On March 20, 1995, the Aum Shinrikyo cult released a nerve agent in the Tokyo subway system at the height of the morning rush hour. The nerve agent was an impure version of sarin, which the terrorists placed into plastic bags that they pierced with the pointed tip of an umbrella. The attack was planned very precisely and involved four cars on three different trains. All three trains were scheduled to arrive under the Ministry of Government offices at about the same time. The scope of the incident rapidly grew to involve thousands of injured people at 15 underground stations. In all, more than 5500 people were exposed; 3227 patients went to the 41 hospitals in the Tokyo area, 550 by ambulance. More than 100 first responders had to be treated for chemical exposure.

How would your agency respond to an incident of this magnitude?

What resources are available in your area to help with this type of incident?

What are your priorities in this type of incident, and how would you perform triage?

HISTORY OF CHEMICAL AGENTS

Whether or not gas will be employed in the future is a matter of conjecture, but the effect is so deadly to the unprepared that we can never afford to neglect the question.

General John J. Pershing, 1919

When General Pershing assessed the future of chemical weapons shortly after World War I, he was speaking about the gases used during that war, chlorine and mustard. His words hold just as true today, however, as they did then. Today the threat is not only to the armies on the battlefield but also to the firefighters, emergency medical technicians (EMTs), paramedics, police officers, and other first responders in cities and towns around the country. The threat may even be greater to these first responders because of one simple fact: lack of training and experience with this type of weapon.

Chemical weapons pose such a huge threat to first responders that many proactive fire departments, Emergency Medical Services (EMS) agencies, and hospitals have already outfitted their personnel with the proper personnel protective equipment and antidotes. Since September 11, 2001, and the anthrax attacks that followed in October 2001, the number of agencies that began to look at this threat proliferated. Some

agencies still have taken only minimal precautions to deal with chemical weapons. Some agencies still believe that if a chemical agent were released, the first group of responders on the scene will be killed. This is not only unnecessary but also completely preventable. They might believe that a chemical agent will never be released in their town, or they can't justify spending the money on equipment and training that may never be used. This is unacceptable.

When the topic of chemical warfare agents comes up, what comes to mind? Sarin? VX? Maybe mustard? What about chlorine, anhydrous ammonia, and cyanide? This is where a "normal" hazardous materials call and chemical warfare can collide. These three chemicals all exist in industry and are transported on our roads and railways daily. All three of these chemicals can be powerful weapons in the hands of a person or group with goal-oriented behavior. (Two, chlorine and cyanide, have already been weaponized and used.) Should our response to incidents like these change because they could be terrorist acts?

This chapter discusses the history of chemical warfare agents, including current threats and threat assessments. It provides you with the most current information on the four classifications of agents—blood agents, choking (pulmonary) agents, nerve agents, and vesicants—and it provides reference material to help you understand these deadly agents. Because there are only isolated uses of chemical agents as acts of terrorism, when we begin to discuss the history of chemical weapons we must look at the military uses.

MILITARY USE OF CHEMICAL AGENTS

In the never-ending search to find new and more efficient ways to kill and strike fear into their enemies, militaries from around the world began to look at using chemicals as one way to achieve this goal. Throughout history there are accounts of armies improvising with fire, coal, sulfur, and other materials directed at the enemy in an effort to achieve a tactical advantage. One of the first documented accounts of this occurred in 423 BC, when the army of Sparta used "beam smoke" (composition unknown) to overwhelm an Athenian-held fort.

In 1855 Sir Lyon Playfair of Britain suggested using cyanide in shells aimed at Russian soldiers during the Crimean War. His idea was rejected by command, stating that it was an inhumane form of warfare. Sir Lyon responded, "There's no sense to this objection. It is considered a legitimate mode of warfare to fill shells with molten metal that scatters upon the enemy and produces the most frightful modes of death. Why a poisonous vapor that would kill men without suffering is to be considered illegitimate is incomprehensible to me. However, no doubt in time chemistry will be used to lessen the sufferings of combatants." During the nineteenth century there were several other attempts at using chemicals against enemies; for example, the French dipped their bayonets into cyanide during the Franco-Prussian War.

On April 22, 1915, outside the town of Ypres, Belgium, the age of modern chemical warfare was ushered in (Fig. 6-1). It was here on the stalled Western Front of World War I that German soldiers opened 6000 canisters of chlorine into an east wind, releasing approximately 150 tons of the toxic gas on

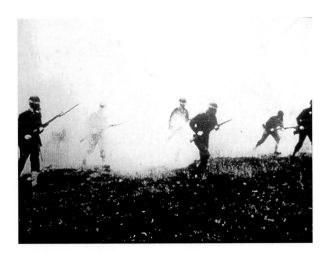

Fig. 6-1
Chlorine used on the World War I battlefield.

**Factors Influencing the   Box 6-1
Effectiveness of Chemical
Agents**

Many factors can influence the effectiveness of chemical agents. These include the amount of agent that is released, size of the target population, topographical features of the target site, and the persistence of the agent. The following environmental features are also important and should be noted when responding to a chemical agent incident.

Winds allow chemical agents to disperse rapidly in certain topographical areas. Lack of winds can cause higher concentrations of chemical agents in one area.

High temperatures can decrease the persistence of some agents, and cold can increase the persistence of other agents.

Rain can dispose of some agents, dilute some agents, and promote hydrolysis in some agents. Most agents can still be used effectively in the rain.

unsuspecting Allied soldiers. This attack most likely caused no more than 800 deaths, but the psychological toll it played on the Allied troops was devastating. The 15,000 Allied troops that retreated during the attack had the unfortunate experience of observing the effect that chemical weapons can have on the battlefield.

In the months and years that followed, both sides were busy creating new chemical weapons and new ways to protect their soldiers. Because chlorine attacks only the respiratory system, work concentrated on developing masks to prevent inhalation injury. However, during World War I several other agents were weaponized and used at least once, including phosgene, diphosgene, chloropicrin, and cyanide.

In July 1917 the Germans again escalated the concept of chemical warfare with the release of the blister agent mustard. The attack occurred again in the town of Ypres, and it caused massive casualties. Mustard was found to be a very effective weapon not because it killed so many but because of the long time it incapacitated soldiers. This in effect took all those soldiers out of action and further depleted resources to care for the injured.

Mustard also presented the soldiers with a new problem: a persistent, dermal active agent. The military uses a 24-hour time frame to rate persistence. If a chemical will evaporate or break down in the environment within 24 hours it is considered to be nonpersistent. If the agent will evaporate slowly and continue to be active beyond 24 hours it is considered persistent. Some authorities reduce this time limit to 12 hours. Weather conditions also affect the agent's persistence (Box 6-1).

Because mustard is a persistent agent, it did not evaporate quickly, causing a large amount of contamination not only to the air but also to equipment. This new agent also mandated the development of a protective suit to further keep the troops safe, as well as a way to decontaminate personnel and equipment.

Following World War I, Col. Edward Vedder of the U.S. Army Medical Corps became the first commander of the research facility that eventually became the United States Army Medical Research Institute of Chemical Defense. In 1925 he wrote a textbook about managing chemical weapons casualties, *The Medical Aspects of Chemical Warfare*. His classes opened with a picture of a soldier whose face was partially destroyed by a bullet; Col. Vedder asked which was more humane, this soldier's injury, or a quick death by cyanide?

At the start of World War II, countries on both sides thought this war would use massive amounts of chemical weapons. As it turned out, this was not the case. The Allies had committed to a non–first-strike policy on the use of chemical weapons; however, the Allies planned to use chemical weapons if they were the targets of a chemical attack. The Germans, for unknown reasons, did not initiate any chemical attacks. One possible reason is that Hitler himself was a victim of mustard in World War I and therefore averse to using chemical weapons.

It wasn't until the end of World War II that the true scope of the German chemical weapons program was realized. Sometime in the late 1930s, a German chemist, Gerhard Schrader, synthesized tabun (GA), an extremely toxic organophosphorus compound. Two years later Dr. Schrader developed sarin (GB), a similar but even more toxic agent. These two agents became the first of a new group of chemical weapons to be known as nerve agents.

After World War II, countries continued to develop and stockpile chemical munitions. Egypt used mustard against the North Yemen troops in support of South Yemen in the Yemen War between 1963 and 1967. When the United States entered the Vietnam War, the new type of warfare demanded a way to clear the jungle. The U.S. military used herbicides (Agent Orange, the best known, was named for the orange stripe on the 55-gallon drum that contained it) to defoliate the jungle terrain. In 1975 the United States ratified the Geneva Convention but with the exception that defoliants and riot-control agents did not apply.

In the 1980s Iraq used chemical weapons against Iran. Iraq also used chemical agents against the Kurds in northern Iraq.

These included mustard and an unknown agent with a rapid onset, most likely sarin or cyanide. The threat of Iraq using chemical weapons continued with the invasion of Kuwait in 1990. The allied coalition was heavily prepared to battle in a chemical warfare environment. This threat never materialized during the 100-hour ground war, but during the United Nations inspections after the cease-fire in 1991 large stockpiles of nerve agents and mustard were found in a town near Baghdad.

The United States' chemical weapons stockpile includes nerve agents (GB and VX) and vesicants (mustard [H and HD]). These weapons are being incinerated on Johnston Atoll, a group of islands 850 miles southwest of Hawaii. This facility was the original chemical disposal facility and has been in operation for several years. Several other depots around the United States storing chemical weapons are being converted to chemical disposal facilities. These facilities are located in Aberdeen, Maryland (mustard); Anniston, Alabama (mustard, VX, GB); Blue Grass, Kentucky (mustard, VX, GB); Newport, Idaho (VX); Pine Bluff, Arkansas (mustard, VX, GB); Pueblo, Colorado (mustard); Tooele, Utah (mustard, VX, GB); and Umatilla, Oregon (mustard, VX, GB).

TERRORIST USE OF CHEMICAL AGENTS

Today the threat of a country or terrorist group using chemical weapons as a way to achieve their goals is as real as ever. The Soviet Union, which had the world's largest development, testing, and production facilities in the 1980s, now has poor control over these facilities. The ability of a rogue nation or group to acquire these weapons is remarkably easy.

Nonwartime uses of chemical agents are fortunately very few. One well-known attack was the release of sarin in the Tokyo subway system by the Aum Shinrikyo sect (Fig. 6-2). Because the Tokyo attack was the only release of a chemical agent on a civilian population, it is difficult to predict the casualties and response that would come from an attack in the United States. There have been other threats and plots of chemical release in the United States, but these have never

materialized. One such scenario that almost played out in Dallas in March 1997 involved a plot, by a couple who belonged to an offshoot of the Ku Klux Klan, to detonate several large hydrogen sulfide tanks at a storage facility. This was to be a diversion so they could rob banks and armored cars on the other side of the city.

CURRENT THREAT AND THREAT ASSESSMENT

Following the attacks on Washington and New York in September 2001, the threat of any type of attack is high. Whether an aggressor chooses to use chemical agents as the weapon remains to be seen. The Federal Bureau of Investigation (FBI) is the lead agency for investigating and analyzing information on domestic threats. The FBI has researched the major chemicals that could be used as weapons. They work with state and local officials to determine what agents should be considered possible weapons of mass destruction. This process is called *threat assessment.* The FBI breaks down threat assessment into four levels: strategic, area-specific, weapon and device, and tactical.

The *strategic threat assessment* studies persons or groups that have made threats or actual attacks against a target. The FBI looks for three criteria that the person or group must have to carry out the attack. These are:
- Behavioral resolve: The terrorists must actually carry out the plan when the time comes.
- Technical feasibility: The terrorists must know what they are doing. If a person sets a vial of liquid in front of a bank teller and tells her "This is the deadly nerve agent sarum" (rather than sarin), this person has lost credibility as a terrorist.
- Operational practicality: The operation must work as planned. For example, a 55-gallon drum of cyanide dumped into a large city's water supply will probably not even show up in a test.

The FBI looks at many *area-specific* events as possible targets for a terrorist group. A few of these include the Olympics, meetings of the World Trade Organization, and presidential inaugurations. If the event has a high profile or if the organizers have received a credible threat, the government may pre-position federal agents to protect the event.

At the *weapon and device* level the FBI looks at the scientific and technological aspects of chemical agents to determine if they can be used as weapons. The three criteria are the difficulty of acquiring the product, the difficulty of making it into an effective weapon, and the product's stability and ease of use. Once this assessment is made, the FBI gives more weight to agents that have been used as weapons in the past.

The *tactical* level of threat assessment deals with an event that has just happened. This would be an event similar to the Tokyo attack. The federal response to this type of event starts with the local responders. If there has been a threat against a business, for example, the first responders should contact the local FBI office, which will notify the FBI WMD Operations Team. This WMD Operations Team will assess the threat using all available information, including past threats, any

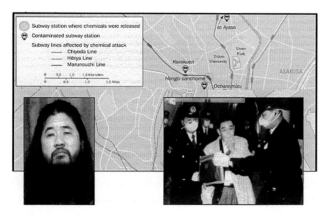

Fig. 6-2
The Tokyo subway attack exposed more than 5000 victims.

current threat, and what the first responders witnessed on the scene. The FBI will then determine if the threat is credible or not (Box 6-2).

RESPONSE TO A CHEMICAL AGENT RELEASE

When firefighters, paramedics, police, and others are responding to a release of any chemical agent—whether the release is accidental or an act of terrorism—several tasks must be accomplished to mitigate the incident. Personnel safety is the first priority in this response. If the responders become victims, they are now part of the problem instead of being part of the solution (Box 6-3).

In the event of a chemical release, many affected people may not be sick enough to stay at the scene. These victims most likely will dispatch themselves to a local hospital or clinic. Staff at medical facilities must be able to treat these people without becoming contaminated themselves. Many hospitals have decontamination rooms near the entrance to the emergency department. However, many of these rooms have become just another storage area. Emergency department staff must be able to use the proper PPE and understand how to properly decontaminate patients arriving at the emergency department. Because the local fire, EMS, and police departments will be at the scene of the incident, the staff at the hospital may not be able to rely on these local resources, and therefore they must be self-sufficient.

BLOOD AGENTS

Blood agents are usually absorbed into the body by breathing. Once in the body and blood stream they cause lethal damage at the cellular level by acting on the enzyme cytochrome

oxidase. The blood agents include the two cyanides: hydrogen cyanide (AC) and cyanogen chloride (CK). The United States maintained a small number of cyanide munitions during World War II. Japan allegedly used cyanide against China before and during World War II, and Iraq may have used cyanide against the Kurds in the 1980s.

CYANIDES

Cyanide is widely used, manufactured, and transported in the United States. More than 300,000 tons of cyanide are produced annually (Fig. 6-3). It is used in printing, agriculture, and photography as well as in the manufacture of paper and plastics. It is also a combustion product of burning synthetic

---

The FBI List of Top Ten Chemical Agents   **Box 6-2**

The FBI has identified the following 10 agents as most likely to be used in a chemical attack:
1. Ammonia
2. Arsine
3. Chlorine
4. Cyanide
5. Hydrogen sulfide
6. Methyl isocyanate
7. Phosgene
8. Phosphine
9. Sulfur dioxide
10. Fluorine

How many of these chemicals do you have in your community? How accessible are they? How close do they get to major residential and business centers? How are they transported? Remember, chemical weapons are not just sarin, mustard, and VX.

Responding to the Scene of a Chemical Release Incident   **Box 6-3**

The following is a list of functions that must be performed at all incidents:
1. Size up the scene. This allows incoming crews to know where to go and what to do.
2. Control the scene and establish a perimeter. This must happen quickly to prevent potential patients from leaving the scene and to keep unauthorized people and potential victims out.
3. Identify the product. Gather as much information about the scene as possible to help in identifying the product.
4. Examine the scene before entry. Determine the appropriate personal protective equipment and other equipment that should be used. Obtain baseline vital signs on all entry team personnel.
5. Establish a decontamination area. This must be done before personnel enter the area.
6. Plan the entry, including air monitoring, patient removal, and reconnaissance.
7. Enter the hot zone and carry out assigned tasks.
8. Contain or neutralize the release. Try to accomplish this early.
9. Decontaminate patients, victims, and the response team. Complete decontamination must be ensured if air monitors are not available.
10. Triage patients. It is easiest to perform this after decontamination has been completed.
11. Treat patients. Treatment can be performed concurrently with decontamination if necessary and if the proper equipment is available.
12. Consult with local hospitals and experts for up-to-date information.
13. Transport patients to the most appropriate hospital.
14. Examine the responders after entry. Assess entry team members and place them into rehab as necessary.
15. Collect evidence. Responders may be used to help with this process.
16. Clean up. Turn property over to responsible party for delegation of cleanup.
17. Perform debriefing and write after-action reports.

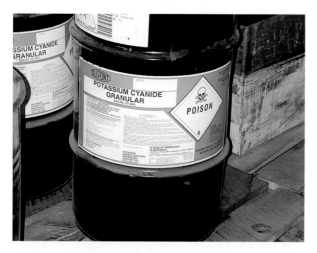

Fig. 6-3
Cyanide is a widely used and readily available product.

Table 6-1
Comparison of Hydrogen Cyanide and Cyanogen Chloride

Characteristic	Hydrogen Cyanide (AC)	Cyanogen Chloride (CK)
Vapor density (68° F)	0.99	2.1
Vapor pressure (mm Hg)	740	1000
Persistence	<1 hour	Nonpersistent
LCt_{50} (mg-min/m^3)	2500	11,000
LD_{50} (mg on skin)	100 mg/kg	N/A
NAERG Guide No.	131, 117, 154	125
NAERG ID No.	1614, 1613, 1051	1589

NAERG, North American Emergency Response Guidebook.

materials such as carpet, furniture, and upholstery. Rail cars with 30,000-gallon tanks of cyanide represent potential transportation and terrorist threats.

Characteristics. At room temperature, hydrogen cyanide is a colorless liquid. Hydrogen cyanide is predominantly absorbed through inhalation, but gaseous, liquid, and crystallized cyanide can also be taken up through the skin. Hydrogen cyanide is difficult to use in warfare because it is highly volatile and nonpersistent. If hydrogen cyanide is released in an open area, high concentrations are hard to obtain, although if it is released in a confined area, high and lethal doses can easily be obtained. Hydrogen cyanide has a faint odor that is similar to that of bitter almonds (although not all people can smell this). Cyanide is the least toxic of the "lethal" chemical agents.

Hydrogen cyanide belongs to a group of agents known as the CN group. The CN compounds hydrolyze slowly in water, allowing for a gradual loss of toxicity. CN compounds are also readily oxidized by strong oxidants. Hydrogen cyanide has an attraction for oxygen and is flammable. Along with its attraction for oxygen, CN compounds, AC included, also have a strong attraction for metal ions (a reason for its lethal effects).

After it is absorbed, cyanogen chloride breaks down to eventually produce hydrogen cyanide. Therefore almost everything about cyanogen chloride is the same as for hydrogen cyanide except that it, like other cyanogen halides, produces an added irritant effect to persons who are exposed to it. Cyanogen chloride, like hydrogen cyanide, is colorless, highly volatile, soluble in water, and nonpersistent. See Table 6-1 for a comparison of hydrogen cyanide and cyanogen chloride.

Mechanism of Action. Hydrogen cyanide is so lethal because it readily binds with metal-containing enzymes, such as those in the cytochrome oxidase enzyme system, an enzyme system that is essential for oxidative processes within the cell. When a cyanide ion binds with such an enzyme, cellular respiration is stopped because the cells can no longer produce ATP and process the oxygen that they receive. When cellular respiration ceases, bodily functions no longer receive the necessary oxygen and nutrients needed to survive, and they therefore shut down. Overall the cause of death due to hydrogen cyanide exposure is suffocation.

Cyanogen chloride has the same mechanism of action as hydrogen cyanide does except that cyanogen chloride irritates the mucus membranes and eyes. It also causes burning sensations in the throat and lungs, and over the entire upper respiratory tract, of an exposed individual.

Signs and Symptoms. The symptoms of cyanide exposure vary depending on several factors, including the total dose of the poison, the route of poisoning, and the exposure time. In the initial stages of cyanide poisoning, several things occur. Initially the victim becomes restless and the respiratory rate increases. Other early symptoms are similar to those of hypoxia and include giddiness, headaches, heart palpitations, and respiratory difficulty. As poisoning progresses, vomiting, convulsions, respiratory failure, and coma are most likely to occur. In cases of high concentrations an increase in respiration occurs within seconds of exposure, followed by 20 to 30 seconds of convulsions and cardiac arrest within 1 minute.

Detection. Cyanide poisoning is detected by an M256A1 kit and colorimetric tubes.

Decontamination. Decontamination is usually not necessary unless clothing is wet. In that case, remove the patient's clothing and decontaminate the patient with water, hypochlorite, or a mild soap such as baby shampoo.

Triage. Immediate: Patient is apneic, but pulses are present within minutes of exposure.
Delayed: Patient is recovering from effects after therapy.
Minor: Patient has mild effects; poisoning is not life threatening.
Dead or dying: Patient is pulseless and apneic.

Treatment. Patients who do not die immediately following exposure to hydrogen cyanide must be treated rapidly. The patient must first be removed to a fresh-air environment. Airway and circulatory system management are vital in the early stages of treatment. The antidotes for cyanide exposure include amyl nitrite, sodium nitrite, and sodium thiosulfate. These drugs are packaged together in a kit called the Pasadena Cyanide Antidote Kit (formerly known as the

Lilly Kit) (Fig. 6-4) (Box 6-4). It is important to remember when treating a cyanide exposure that the antidotes themselves are poisonous and can cause damage to the body; therefore be sure you are dealing with a cyanide exposure. Generally, a victim who has had inhalation exposure and survives long enough to reach medical care will need little treatment.

PULMONARY AGENTS

Pulmonary agents are the chemicals first responders should fear the most. These chemicals are easy to obtain, and they usually do not require any manufacturing process to turn them into weapons (Fig. 6-5). These agents (also referred to as choking agents or pulmonary irritants) primarily attack the

lungs and lung tissue after inhalation and are characterized by pronounced irritation of the upper and lower respiratory tract. The three agents addressed in this chapter (phosgene, chlorine, and ammonia) are all on the FBI's top ten list of agents most likely to be used as chemical weapons of mass destruction. See Table 6-2 for a comparison of phosgene, chlorine, and anhydrous ammonia.

PHOSGENE (CG)

Phosgene is a chemical widely used today in the manufacture of dyes, coal tar, pesticides, and pharmaceuticals. It was widely used as a weapon in World War I until mustard was introduced on the battlefield. The Bhopal, India, disaster of 1984 at the Union Carbide plant involved the release of 50,000 pounds of methylisocyanate. This chemical is composed of phosgene and methylamine. The chemical affected 150,000 people; 10,000 were severely injured and 3300 were killed. The effects of the release were thought to be due to a combination of isocyanate and phosgene.

Characteristics. Phosgene is a colorless gas with an odor of new-mown hay. Phosgene is a highly volatile nonpersistent

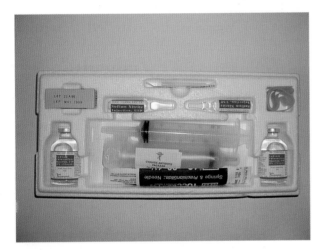

Fig. 6-4
The cyanide antidote kit can be used to treat cyanide toxicity.

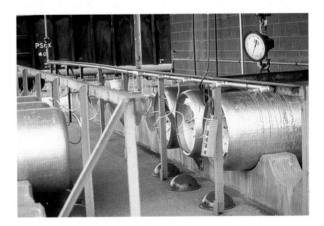

Fig. 6-5
Chlorine is used at a number of industrial facilities.

Cyanide Antidote Kit	Box 6-4

Adult Dose

Amyl nitrite: Place one ampoule in front of nose and mouth, or in bag valve mask, for 15 seconds; remove for 15 seconds. Repeat.
Sodium nitrite: 300 mg (10 ml of 3% solution) IV over 2 minutes.
Sodium thiosulfate: 12.5 g (50 ml of 25% solution) slow IV push.

Pediatric Dose

Pediatric doses must be calculated based on hemoglobin concentration, body surface area, or body weight. Body weight dose is:
Amyl nitrite: Place one ampoule in front of nose and mouth, or in bag valve mask, for 15 seconds; remove for 15 seconds. Repeat.
Sodium nitrite: Child <25 kg 10 mg/kg (0.33 ml/kg of 3% solution) IV over 2 minutes. Do not exceed 10 ml or 300 mg.
Sodium thiosulfate: Child <25 kg 1.65 ml/kg of the 25% solution slow IV push. Do not exceed 12.5 g.

Table 6-2			
Comparison of Phosgene, Chlorine, and Anhydrous Ammonia			
Characteristic	**Phosgene**	**Chlorine**	**Anhydrous Ammonia**
Vapor density (68° F)	3.41	2.47	0.62
Vapor pressure (mm Hg)	22.6	100.2	94
LCt_{50} (mg-min/m^3)	3200	6000	—
LC_{50} (ppm)	800	293 over 1 hour	2000 over 4 hours
NAERG Guide No.	125	124	125
NAERG ID No.	1076	1017	1005

NAERG, North American Emergency Response Guidebook.

agent. The vapor density of phosgene (3.4) allows it to stay in the air and low-lying places for long periods of time. Phosgene is a gas at temperatures greater than 47° F. It reacts rapidly in water and is quickly hydrolyzed into hydrochloric acid and carbon dioxide. Phosgene is easy to produce but is unstable in storage and therefore must be kept refrigerated.

Mechanism of Action. Phosgene is an inhalation or vapor hazard. It dissolves slowly in water to form carbon dioxide and hydrochloric acid (HCl). In contact with the upper airways, the hydrochloric acid causes a transient irritation of the eyes, nose, sinuses, and throat. It can also irritate the upper airway and bronchi, causing a dry cough.

Phosgene penetrates slowly into the airways due to its poor water solubility. There is a symptom-free period of up to 48 hours. Over the first several hours, the carbonyl group of the phosgene attacks the surface of the alveolar capillaries. Eventually, serum leaks from the capillaries into the alveoli. The fluid fills the tissues, causing severe hypoxia and apnea. As the fluid leaks into the alveoli, massive amounts of fluid (up to 1 liter per hour) pour out of the circulation. The patient develops a severe noncardiogenic pulmonary edema and hypovolemic shock.

Signs and Symptoms. Directly after a person is exposed, symptoms include coughing, choking, a feeling of pressure on the chest, nausea, vomiting, and headache. After the initial symptoms there is a period, lasting from 2 to 24 hours, when the exposed person appears free from any abnormalities. The patient then develops signs and symptoms of pulmonary edema. As time wears on and the edema progresses, general discomfort and dyspnea increase and frothy sputum develops. The patient may then develop signs of hypovolemic or cardiogenic shock. If the patient can rest and survive until the danger of the pulmonary edema has passed, the patient has a greater chance for recovery.

Detection. Phosgene is detected by photoionization detector (PID) and colorimetric tubes.

Decontamination. Decontamination for vapor exposure is with fresh air; decontamination for liquid exposure is with water and a mild soap.

Triage. Immediate: Patient has severe dyspnea with pulmonary edema.
Delayed: Patient has dyspnea without objective signs and should be monitored closely.
Minor: Patient is asymptomatic with known exposure.
Dead or dying: Patient has pulmonary edema, cyanosis, and hypotension.

Treatment. Removing the patient to a fresh-air environment and providing supportive airway and circulatory system management is generally all that is required. The effects of an acute exposure to some of these agents may not be seen immediately but rather over several hours. Exposed patients should be medically evaluated and if necessary kept hospitalized for continued evaluation.

CHLORINE

Chlorine is a very common chemical used widely in industry. It is used in the production of chlorinated inorganic and organic chemicals and in the manufacture of solvents and plastics. It is also used as a bleaching or cleaning agent and in water treatment facilities for purifying drinking water. Chlorine was the first chemical used in modern warfare when the Germans released it against the Allies in 1915.

Characteristics. Chlorine is a greenish-yellow gas or amber liquid (under pressure) with a pungent odor. Chlorine has a vapor density of 2.5 and is highly volatile and nonpersistent. Chlorine is also a strong oxidizer and very corrosive.

Mechanism of Action. Chlorine is an inhalation or vapor hazard and is water soluble. When chlorine gas is inhaled, it combines with water and produces hydrochloric acid and free oxygen radicals. The free oxygen radicals oxidize cell walls and destroy tissue. Destruction of the alveoli results in noncardiogenic pulmonary edema, which is the primary cause of death from exposure to chlorine.

Signs and Symptoms. Lance Sergeant Elmer Cotton described the effects of chlorine gas in World War I:

> It produces a flooding of the lungs—it is an equivalent death to drowning, only on dry land. The effects are these—a splitting headache and terrific thirst (to drink water is instant death), a knife edge of pain in the lungs and the coughing up of a greenish froth off the stomach and the lungs, ending finally in insensibility and death. The color of the skin from white turns a greenish black and yellow, the tongue protrudes and the eyes assume a glassy stare. It is a fiendish death to die.[1]

This is a first-hand account of how the signs and symptoms of chlorine may appear. The primary signs and symptoms from exposure to chlorine include eye and airway irritation, dyspnea, chest tightness, headache, vomiting, and delayed-onset pulmonary edema.

Detection. Chlorine is detected by colorimetric tubes, specific gas monitors, and odor.

Decontamination. Decontamination for vapor exposure is with fresh air; decontamination for liquid exposure is with water and a mild soap. Vapor exposure may warrant water decontamination if the patient has any skin irritation or burns.

Triage. Immediate: Patient has severe dyspnea with pulmonary edema.
Delayed: Patient has dyspnea without objective signs and should be monitored closely.
Minor: Patient is asymptomatic with known exposure.
Dead or dying: Patient has pulmonary edema, cyanosis, and hypotension.

Treatment. Removing the patient to a fresh-air environment, giving oxygen, and providing supportive airway and circulatory system management is generally all that is required. The effects of an acute exposure to chlorine may not be seen immediately but rather over several hours. Exposed patients should be medically evaluated and if necessary kept in the hospital for continued evaluation.

ANHYDROUS AMMONIA

Anhydrous ammonia is used in both agriculture as a fertilizer and in industrial facilities as a refrigerant for cooling and freezing. It is used commonly in meat, poultry, and fish processing facilities, dairy and ice cream plants, cold storage warehouses, and other food processing facilities.

Characteristics. Anhydrous ammonia is a colorless gas in lower concentrations. In higher concentrations it can form a white cloud. Ammonia has a low odor threshold of 20 parts per million (ppm), and 2000 ppm is the LC_{50}. Ammonia has a vapor density of 0.62, causing it to disperse in the atmosphere if released outdoors. It is a volatile, nonpersistent agent. Anhydrous ammonia is transported as a liquid under pressure.

Mechanism of Action. Anhydrous ammonia reacts with water in tissue to form the strong alkali ammonium hydroxide. Ammonium hydroxide can cause severe alkaline chemical burns to skin, eyes, and especially the respiratory system. Mild exposures primarily affect the upper respiratory tract, while more severe exposures tend to affect the entire respiratory system. Ammonium hydroxide can break down tissue, which liberates water, thus perpetuating the conversion of ammonia to ammonium hydroxide. In the respiratory tract, this process causes the destruction of cilia and opens the mucosal barrier to infection. Liquid anhydrous ammonia can freeze skin on contact.

Signs and Symptoms. Common symptoms and signs include eye and airway irritation, severe general pain, dyspnea, chest tightness, laryngeal edema, and pulmonary edema. Anhydrous ammonia can cause partial-thickness and full-thickness burns or frostbite, or both, when in contact with the skin.

Detection. Anhydrous ammonia is detected by PID, colorimetric tubes, and odor.

Decontamination. Decontamination for vapor exposure is with fresh air; decontamination for liquid exposure is with copious amounts of water and a mild soap. Vapor exposure may warrant water decontamination if the patient has any skin irritation or burns.

Triage. Immediate: Patient has severe dyspnea with pulmonary edema.
Delayed: Patient has dyspnea without objective signs and needs to be monitored closely.
Minor: Patient is asymptomatic with known exposure.
Dead or dying: Patient has pulmonary edema, cyanosis, and hypotension.

Treatment. Removing the patient to a fresh-air environment and giving oxygen and providing supportive airway and circulatory system management is generally all that is required. The effects of an acute exposure to ammonia may not be seen immediately but rather over several hours. Exposed patients should be medically evaluated and if necessary kept in the hospital for continued evaluation.

VESICANTS

Vesicants (also known as blister agents or mustard agents) are named for the most obvious injury they inflict on a person. These agents burn and blister the skin or any other part of the body they contact (Fig. 6-6). They also severely damage the skin and eyes as well as the lungs, gastrointestinal tract, and other internal organs (Fig. 6-7).

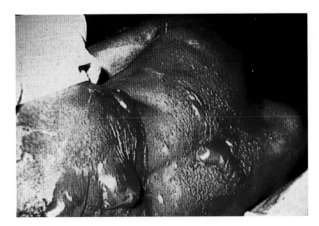

Fig. 6-6
Blister formation secondary to mustard agent exposure.

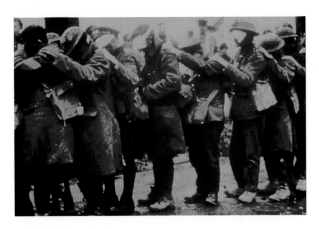

Fig. 6-7
During World War I many patients were temporarily blinded by mustard agent exposure.

Blister agents are most commonly used on the battlefield to force enemy troops to use personal protective equipment during battle, thereby decreasing the soldiers' effectiveness. These agents contaminate almost everything with which they come into contact.

The agents discussed here are sulfur mustard, nitrogen mustard, lewisite, and phosgene oxime. The effects of these four agents are very similar in mechanism of action, signs and symptoms, and treatment. Sulfur mustard is the best known and most used of the vesicants, and the information here will focus primarily on this agent. See Table 6-3 for a comparison of mustard, lewisite, and phosgene oxime.

SULFUR MUSTARD (H) AND DISTILLED MUSTARD (HD)

Sulfur mustard was first synthesized in the early 1800s, and it has been a major military threat since its introduction to warfare during World War I. During the war, mustard produced the largest number of chemical casualties despite its late initial use. Mustard has been used in wars throughout the 1900s:

Table 6-3

Comparison of Mustard, Lewisite, and Phosgene Oxime

Characteristic	Mustard (HD, HN)	Lewisite (L)	Phosgene Oxime (CX)
Vapor density (68° F)	5.4-7.1*	7.1	3.9
Vapor pressure (mm Hg)	0.072-0.29*	0.39	11.2 (77° F)
Persistence	Hours to days	Hours to days	Nonpersistent
LCt_{50} (mg-min/m³)	1500 (Inhalation) 10,000 (Skin)	1200	3200
LD_{50} (mg on skin)	100 mg/kg	40 mg/kg	N/A
NAERG Guide No.	153	153	154
NAERG ID No.	2810	2810	2811

NAERG, North American Emergency Response Guidebook.
*These are the low-end and high-end numbers for H, HD, and the three nitrogen mustard agents. Each has slightly different properties. Vapor density also depends on the purity of the agent.

Italy used it against Abyssinia in the 1930s, Egypt used it against Yemen in the 1960s, and Iraq used it against the Kurds in the 1980s. Mustard is still considered a major military threat from former Warsaw Pact and third world countries.

Characteristics. In its pure state, mustard is colorless and almost odorless. (There may be an odor of mustard, garlic, or rotten onions.) At room temperature, mustard is a liquid with a low volatility. These agents can be thickened with a polymer to create a persistent threat. At warmer temperatures, blister agents become nonpersistent but they have a higher concentration of vapor, which increases the respiratory threat. Under temperate conditions, mustard evaporates slowly and is primarily a liquid hazard, but its vapor hazard increases with increasing temperature. At 100° F or higher, it is a definite vapor hazard. Mustard freezes at 57° F, and because a solid is difficult to disperse, mustard is often mixed with substances that have a lower freezing point. Sulfur mustard (H) can contain up to 30% impurities (mostly sulfur). Distilled mustard (HD) is almost pure.

Mechanism of Action. Mustard can easily and rapidly penetrate most fabrics (except those of protective clothing) and reach the skin. Penetration through the skin is rapid, with an increase in penetration in areas of high heat, moisture, and thin skin. During World War I, 42% of the mustard victims had damage to the scrotum, in contrast to only 4% with damage to the more exposed hands. Other important modes of exposure include ocular, respiratory, and ingestion.

When a person is exposed to mustard, approximately 10% of the agent binds with the skin and the remaining 90% is absorbed into the body. It spreads to all major organs, but because of the dilution factor of mustard, systemic symptoms are only seen with very high doses. Systemic problems include damage to the bone marrow similar to that caused by radiation exposure. Once mustard fixes to tissue, the molecule is no longer intact, so blisters that develop from exposure pose no risk to responders.

Mustard must first dissolve in an aqueous solution such as sweat or extracellular fluid. Although mustard molecules dissolve

slowly in such solutions, once they dissolve they rapidly (seconds to minutes) rearrange to form extremely reactive cyclic ethylene sulfonium ions that immediately bind to intracellular and extracellular enzymes, proteins, and other cellular components. Mustard has many biological actions, but the exact mechanism by which it produces tissue injury is not known. Mustard also possesses mild cholinergic activity, which may be responsible for effects such as early GI symptoms and miosis.

Signs and Symptoms. Signs and symptoms of mustard exposure can begin 2 to 48 hours after exposure, but by then the damage has already been done. Signs and symptoms include erythema and blisters on skin; irritation, conjunctivitis, and corneal opacity and damage in the eyes; mild upper respiratory signs or marked airway damage; and gastrointestinal effects. No immediate pain is felt from exposure to mustard agents.

Detection. Mustard is detected by APD 2000 (advanced portable detector) or CAM (chemical agent monitor) handheld devices, PID, colorimetric tubes, M256A1 chemical agent detector kit, M-8 paper, or M-9 tape.

Decontamination. Decontamination of these agents is critical. Washing with 0.5% household bleach is a standard military decontamination technique. Washing with a mild soap such as baby shampoo is an effective alternative. Scrubbing and hot water should be avoided, as both enhance the absorption of the agent.

Triage. Immediate: Patient has moderate to severe respiratory signs and symptoms.
Delayed: Patient has skin lesions over up to 50% of body surface area and mild to moderate respiratory effects.
Minor: Patient has skin lesions over less than 5% of body surface area; lesions are not in vital areas.
Dead or dying: Severe respiratory effects developed within 4 to 6 hours after exposure. Lesions cover more than 50% of body surface area with limited resources.

Treatment. There is no antidote for the mustard agents. Symptomatic management of lesions and supportive airway management is usually all that is required. Only a small portion of patients will have long-term effects.

NITROGEN MUSTARD (HN-1, HN-2, AND HN-3)

All of the nitrogen mustards are dark, oily liquids. These mustards are much more dangerous than sulfur mustard. The most toxic and most volatile of the three nitrogen mustard compounds is HN-2, but HN-3 is more stable and therefore used more often. Except that it is more dangerous than sulfur mustard, everything else about the nitrogen mustards is the same as for sulfur mustard.

LEWISITE (L)

Lewisite is a dark, oily liquid with a slight odor of geraniums. Lewisite is a quick-acting blistering agent that causes immediate intense pain as well as more pronounced blistering than most blistering agents. Once inside the body it causes systemic destruction. Another major difference between this and other mustards is that it causes low blood pressure, lung swelling, and bowel troubles. An exposure to a high concentration of lewisite can kill in 10 minutes, whereas a low exposure can cause symptoms to occur in 30 minutes. Lewisite is the only vesicant that has a known antidote, British anti-lewisite (BAL; dimercaprol). Lewisite is most often mixed with other chemical weapon agents to produce an extreme effect on a victim.

PHOSGENE OXIME (CX)

Phosgene oxime is a mustard produced in both liquid and solid forms. The only difference between phosgene and the other mustards is that its typical mustard agent effects occur immediately after exposure.

NERVE AGENTS

The nerve agents are probably the best-known type of chemical agent. They are the most toxic of the chemical agents, but they are also the hardest to acquire or manufacture. Nerve agents are chemically related to organophosphate pesticides, but they are several times more deadly. The G agents were originally developed just before and during World War II by German industry. These include GA (tabun), GB (sarin), GD, (soman), and GF. The only true V agent known is VX. This agent was developed in the United Kingdom. The only other possible V agent is one developed by the former Soviet Union, which has characteristics similar to those of VX.

Characteristics. In their pure states nerve agents are colorless liquids; when impure they tend to be yellowish. Some of these agents may have a fruity odor, but this is a very unreliable sign. The G agents tend to be nonpersistent, volatile agents, whereas VX is a very persistent nonvolatile agent (it evaporates at about the same rate as motor oil). The vapor hazard increases significantly when the agent is exposed to high temperatures or is aerosolized.

Mechanism of Action. Nerve agents are very potent organophosphorus compounds that directly affect the enzyme acetylcholinesterase, and their effects are caused by the resulting excess acetylcholine. Acetylcholine is the primary chemical neurotransmitter in the parasympathetic nervous system. This excess acetylcholine is due to the nerve agent's inhibiting the enzyme acetylcholinesterase. After a nerve agent inhibits the tissue enzyme, the enzyme cannot hydrolyze acetylcholine; acetylcholine thus accumulates and continues to stimulate the affected organ or muscle (Fig. 6-8). The systems most commonly affected include the skeletal muscles, smooth muscles, exocrine glands, and some nerves in both the central nervous system and the ganglia. Once the enzyme has been inhibited, the effect cannot be reversed without the proper medication (pralidoxime [2-PAM]).

Signs and Symptoms. The signs and symptoms for all nerve agents are very similar; the only difference is in the onset of signs and symptoms. The onset can vary greatly depending on several factors including weather, geography, and whether the release was indoors or outdoors. The most important factor is whether the victim was exposed to a vapor or a liquid. Vapor exposure can lead to signs and symptoms in just a few seconds to a couple of minutes, whereas an exposure to a liquid agent may take several minutes to several hours.

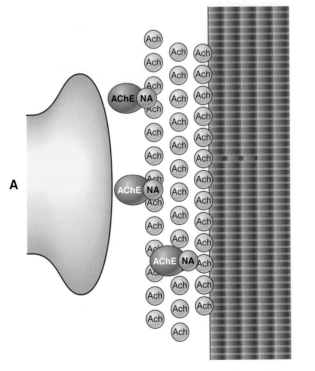
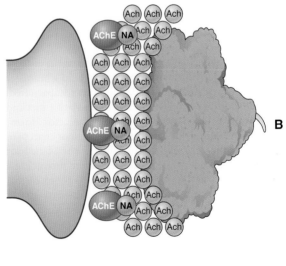

Fig. 6-8
A, Effects of nerve agent toxicity at smooth muscle receptor sites. **B,** Effects of nerve agent toxicity at organ receptor site.

The specific signs and symptoms include muscle twitching, miosis, headache, rhinorrhea, salivation, and dyspnea in the mild cases. A patient with a severe exposure may show all these symptoms and develop severe difficulty breathing, generalized muscle twitching, weakness or paralysis, seizures, loss of bladder and bowel control, and loss of consciousness. The classic SLUDGE (salivation, lacrimation, urination, defecation, gastrointestinal pain, and emesis) syndrome may be seen.

Detection. Nerve agents are detected by APD 2000 or CAM handheld devices, PID, colorimetric tubes, M256A1 kit, M-8 paper, and M-9 tape.

Decontamination. Decontamination of these patients is critical. Washing with 0.5% household bleach is a standard military decontamination technique. The use of mild soap or baby shampoo is an effective alternative.

Triage. Immediate: Patient is unconscious, seizing, or postictal and has breathing difficulty or is apneic with immediate therapy available (Mark 1 kit, diazepam [Valium], and airway). Patient has severe symptoms with respirations, no loss of consciousness, and has not seized.

Delayed: Patient is recovering from exposure and has already received treatment.

Minor: Patient is walking wounded.

Dead or dying: No pulse or blood pressure can be obtained.

Treatment. There are two specific antidotes for nerve agent exposure, atropine and 2-PAM. Atropine is an acetylcholine blocking agent; it takes the place of the acetylcholine at the receptor sites. This corrects bradycardia and dries out secretions produced by overstimulation of organs. Atropine does not correct respiratory muscle weakness so the patient will likely need respiratory support. The second medication, 2-PAM (pralidoxime chloride), disengages the agent from the enzyme, thereby returning normal function to the acetylcholinesterase. These two drugs are paired in the Mark 1 nerve agent antidote kit (Fig. 6-9). The Mark I kit is a two-part auto-injector that contains 2 mg atropine and 600 mg pralidoxime chloride.

The current military procedure for nerve agent exposure is as follows: If you have been exposed to a nerve agent and are experiencing mild signs and symptoms, you should administer a Mark 1 kit to yourself. If a responder becomes incapacitated, the responder's buddy should administer three Mark 1 kits and 10 mg diazepam (also available in auto-injector form) (Fig. 6-10). The Mark 1 kits and the auto-injector diazepam are for adult patients only. The manufacturer of the Mark 1 kit (Meridian Medical, Columbia, Md) will soon be producing a pediatric version of the kit. Consult your local protocols for the pediatric doses of atropine and 2-PAM. Aggressive airway management and supportive care should also be started when necessary.

In some cases atropine should be given 2 to 5 mg every 15 to 30 minutes for the adult patient until secretions are dry and ventilation can be accomplished with ease. 2-PAM can also be given intravenously at 1 to 2 g in 100 ml normal saline for the adult patient.

The success of 2-PAM treatment depends on the aging process of the agent used. Aging is the time the nerve

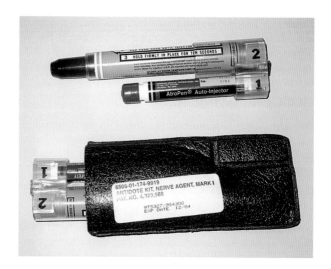

Fig. 6-9
The Mark 1 kit contains atropine and pralidoxime chloride.

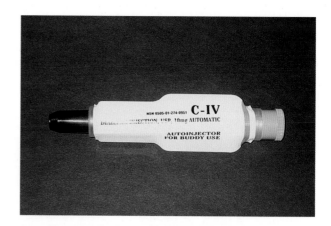

Fig. 6-10
Auto-injectors of diazepam (Valium) are available for the treatment of nerve agent exposure.

agent–acetylcholinesterase bond takes to mature. When the bond ages, then the acetylcholinesterase is deactivated. Once the enzyme is deactivated the body will have to regenerate it over an extended period of time. This time varies by agent: soman ages in 2 minutes, sarin ages in 4 to 6 hours, and VX ages in 1 hour. See Table 6-4 for a comparison of tabun, sarin, soman, and VX.

CHAPTER SUMMARY

Response to a chemical release, either accidental or intentional, can be chaotic, especially if you are dealing with hundreds of patients. Knowing the basics of chemical agents, how to manage them, and how to protect yourself and colleagues is a vital first step to ensuring a successful outcome.

Table 6-4
Comparison of Tabun, Sarin, Soman, and VX

Characteristic	Tabun (GA)	Sarin (GB)	Soman (GD)	VX
Vapor density (68° F)	5.6	4.86	6.3	9.2
Vapor pressure (mm Hg)	0.037	2.1	0.4	0.0007
Persistence	Nonpersistent	Nonpersistent	Nonpersistent	Persistent
LCt_{50} (mg-min/m^3)	400	100	70	100
LD_{50} (mg on skin)	1000	1700	50	10
NAERG Guide No.	153	153	153	153
NAERG ID No.	2810	2810	2810	2810

NAERG, North American Emergency Response Guidebook.

REFERENCE

1. Gibert M: *First World War,* 1994, London, Weidenfeld and Nicolson.

BIBLIOGRAPHY

Currance P, Bronstein A: *Emergency care for hazardous materials exposure,* ed 2, St Louis, 1994, Mosby.
Federal Emergency Management Agency: *Chemical Stockpile Emergency Preparedness Program, frequently asked questions,* http://www.fema.gov/rrr/csepp2.shtm, retrieved September 15, 2004.
Medical Research Institute of Chemical Defense: *Medical management of chemical casualties handbook,* ed 3, Aberdeen Proving Ground, Md, 1999, United States Army, http://www.vnh.org/CHEMCASU/titlepg.html, retrieved September 15, 2004.
Scripp R: *FBI chemical/biological threat assessment lecture,* FBI/WMD countermeasures unit, Atlanta, April 2002, National Disaster Medical System conference.

Siddell FR, Patrick WC, Dashiell TR: *Jane's chem-bio handbook,* Coulsdon, UK, 1998, Jane's Information Group.
U.S. Army Solider and Chemical Biological Command: *Homeland defense,* http://www.ecbc.army.mil/hld/index.htm, retrieved October 18, 2004.
U.S. Department of Health and Human Services: *The Metropolitan Medical Response System field operations guide,* Washington, DC, 1998, U.S. Department of Health and Human Services.
U.S. Department of Transportation: *2000 Emergency response guidebook,* Washington, DC, 2000, United States Department of Transportation.
Valley National Gases: *BOC gases, material safety data sheets,* June 1996, http://www.vngas.com/msds.cfm, retrieved August 15, 2003.
Vedder EB: *The medical aspects of chemical warfare,* Baltimore, 1925, Williams and Wilkins.

CASE STUDY

The local sports team has just won the national championship. At a local hospital, the emergency department (ED) staff are still congratulating each other when the charge nurse sees live news footage of large crowds burning cars and breaking windows downtown, just a few blocks away, and the police deploying tear gas. Affected people are seen streaming out of the area.

What is the likelihood that patients will self-refer to the ED?

What preparations should be taken to prepare for these patients?

What physical security precautions should be taken?

What personal protective equipment is required?

What can be done to reduce contamination of the ED?

What are the health risks from riot agents?

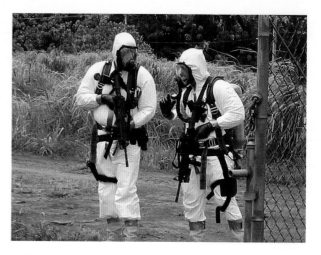

Fig. 7-1
Law enforcement personnel using personal protective equipment.

Law enforcement uses several types of riot agents, each with a different chemical composition and mechanism of action. This chapter reviews the agents by name, type, mechanism of action, delivery system, decontamination, and treatment.

The classic law enforcement riot agents are O-chloro-benzylidene malononitrile (CN) and chloroacetophenone (CS). The CN and CN designators are arbitrary NATO code names for the chemicals, having nothing to do with their chemical composition. The newer and increasingly common police riot agent is oleoresin capsicum (OC, pepper spray). Also gaining wide acceptance is an OC-CS mix. These agents are discussed in detail later in this chapter. Now in deployment are newer agents, such as pepper foam and malodorants. This chapter will give you insight into the new agents being fielded.

PERSONAL PROTECTIVE EQUIPMENT

All riot agents are relatively benign. They are said to have a high safety factor. They cause symptoms at a low level of exposure; lethal affects only result from an extremely high level of exposure. Hospital personnel should not need PPE, because they should not be working in an agent-saturated environment.

Prehospital providers are likely to have to respond into an area with high levels of riot agents. Emergency medical personnel are encouraged to learn what agents and delivery systems your area agencies use. Plan accordingly and coordinate with local law enforcement. Services should acquire appropriate PPE, such as gas masks (Fig. 7-1).

Borrowing PPE from the police department will not be easy and should not be counted on unless it is determined in advance that the PPE will be available. Loan agreements must

also be written into policy and PPE must be available 24 hours a day. In all cases proper fit testing and training should be conducted before using any protective equipment.

SELF-REFERRED PATIENTS

OFF-GASSING

Hospital personnel should expect self-referred, chemically exposed patients. Off-gassing from exposed patients will almost certainly fill the air in the waiting areas with riot agents, will expose uncontaminated waiting patients, and depending on airflows could allow riot agents to enter the emergency department (ED). While off-gassing from a single patient might not be enough to affect the ED, cumulative off-gassing from several patients can put enough agent in the air to cause persons in the waiting areas to develop symptoms from the agent.

SECONDARY EXPOSURE

Secondary exposure to riot agents should not be harmful to healthy staff members and patients. Secondary exposure may theoretically aggravate patients' preexisting or underlying respiratory problems, but in practice this is exceedingly rare.[1] If staffing allows, basic decontamination should be performed before patients reach triage and waiting areas.

PREPLANNING FOR THE EVENT

PREPARING THE HOSPITAL

Police most often deploy chemical agents against unruly crowds. These circumstances usually force a great number of persons out of the area, while relatively few are arrested. This means the great majority will be exposed but not arrested and will be therefore free to roam. Plans should be made for an alternate waiting area for chemically exposed patients.

It is imperative that the ED be part of the warning list when the police believe there is an impending civil unrest event with the potential for deployment of chemical agents. Hospital security should prepare so that when they become aware that police have deployed chemical agents they can restrict hospital access to a designated entrance. This is advantageous for reasons of limiting cross-contamination as well as controlling access by patients who could be agitated and angry. Assaults on hospital staff are a growing issue, and access control is a key to reducing the threat from this type of incident.

DECONTAMINATION

REMOVAL OF CLOTHING

The most basic and effective form of decontamination for riot agents is the removal of clothing. The great majority of chemical contaminants are held in the patient's clothes. Removing the clothes and closing them in a plastic bag isolates most of the potential contaminants.

Security can have plastic bags outside, so at least outer garments (e.g., jackets, sweaters) can be removed and bagged to reduce the amount of off-gassing inside the hospital. Once inside, patients can be changed into scrubs or disposable paper suits and the remainder of their clothes placed into plastic bags to reduce cross-contamination.

OVERVIEW OF CHEMICAL AGENTS

CN AND CS

GENERAL

CN (O-chlorobenzylidene malononitrile) and CS (chloroacetophenone) are lab-created compounds and are not derived from natural substances. These agents were originally developed for the military and then used by law enforcement. Their names are the NATO code designators and have no relation to their chemical structure.

CS and CN are listed as a group because the symptoms, delivery systems, decontamination, and treatment are the same. The primary difference is that CS is generally more potent. Both have relatively short action times, and the severity of symptoms decreases rapidly with time.

HISTORY

CN and CS were initially developed for use by the military; they were designed to disperse crowds and reduce the effectiveness of opposing troops. Starting in the 1950s, law enforcement started deploying military-specification CN and CS to disperse crowds. Over time, manufacturers began packing tear gas into containers designed to be carried on police officers' belts (Fig. 7-2).

MECHANISM OF ACTION

CN and CS are both chemical irritants. They do not cause any permanent physical damage, but they irritate the mucous membranes (and to a much smaller, but still intense, degree, the skin) on contact. Both have questionable effectiveness on

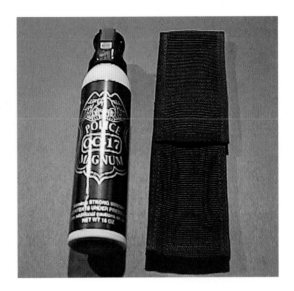

Fig. 7-2
O-chlorobenzylidene malononitrile (CN) container.

intoxicated or emotionally disturbed persons, as they only cause pain and have limited direct physiological effects (as compared to OC, which acts as an inflammatory regardless of whether the subject can feel pain or not).

DELIVERY SYSTEMS

CN and CS are commonly distributed in several forms: powder, spray, pyrotechnic dispensers, and heat-based dispensers.

Powder is CN and CS in their native form. CN and CS are fine crystalline powder, and in some riot applications they may be used in this form. The powder will lie on surfaces until disturbed, then rise into the air. This delivery system is typically seen in riots using grenades with a small explosive charge to disperse the powder (Fig. 7-3).

In sprays, crystals of agent are suspended in a liquid under pressure or dissolved in a solution. This can be sprayed from a container, which can vary in size from a can small enough to hang on a keyring to backpack-sized dispensers.

Pyrotechnic dispensers are designed to burst from a pyrotechnic charge, reducing the CS or CN to microcrystals and dispersing them over a given area. Pyrotechnic dispensers pose a risk of injury from the explosive charge used to disperse the agent.

Heat-based dispensers are designed to heat the CN or CS crystals and release a chemical smoke. Unlike the crystal-liquid suspension, chemical smoke completely disperses through a given space and is difficult to protect against with improvised masks. Chemical smoke tends to penetrate deep into the lungs. Smoke canisters get extremely hot from the incendiary used to heat the chemical agent, so burns from unintentional contact with the canister are common. The device could also ignite secondary fires.

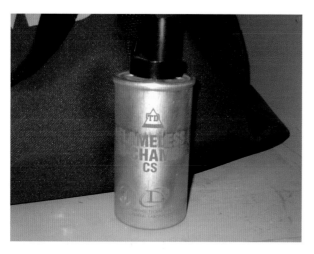

Fig. 7-3
Riot control grenades.

Severe rhinorrhea (running nose)
Lacrimation (watering eyes)
Mild blepharospasm (involuntary closing of eyes)
Pain in the exposed mucosa (eyes, nose, mouth)
Corneal abrasions if agent has been sprayed in the eyes
Moderate dyspnea (shortness of breath)
Painful breathing (particularly from smoke form)
Irritation to exposed skin (usually minor)
Mild bronchospasm and wheezing in victims with preexisting respiratory conditions

SIGNS AND SYMPTOMS

CN and CS cause essentially the same symptoms, although CS effects are generally more severe (Box 7-1). CN and CS are notorious for causing unpredictable reactions in the exposed party. Some persons are severely affected, and others seem immune. The primary sign is mucous membrane irritation by the chemical agent. This affects the eyes, eyelids, conjunctiva, nose, lips, and mouth.

DECONTAMINATION

CN and CS in crystal form tend to cling to clothing, skin, and hair, and during large-scale deployments they are often visible on the patient. In smoke form they are usually not visible. Removing as much clothing as practical is the single most effective decontamination action one can take.

For CN or CS in *smoke form,* remove clothing and allow residual agent to off-gas. Water may be used but is of questionable value (other than psychological).

For CN or CS in *crystal form,* in most cases the best treatment is moving air across the contaminated area, allowing the agent to blow away.[2] In cases of visible gross contamination, water is useful for removing large amounts of agent, but ultimately the remaining agent will not be removed until the water dries and the agent can blow away.

Use copious amounts of plain water for removing *gross* contamination only. Make sure the water flows away from the face. The hair is, after clothes, the next most effective reservoir for contamination. Use particular care that water does not run from the hair to the eyes, and dry the hair after use of water for decontamination. Use of water on clothing does *not* remove the contaminant, it merely holds it to the clothes until the water dries; then the agent is released into the air again.

Special Note on Decontaminating Law Enforcement Personnel. Law enforcement treatment during riots or civil disturbances is usually geared toward getting personnel back to duty. If possible, avoid using water on their clothing. Visible agent can be physically removed from the clothing. If the officer's head is decontaminated, use the same precautions as above. Pay particular attention to the hair and decontaminate repeatedly to remove as much agent as possible. The officer's helmet will cause sweat on the head, which will tend to carry agent back into the eyes.

TREATMENT

Eyes. Apply plain water or saline directly to the eyes, being careful to allow the water to run away from the eyes. A nasal cannula can be connected to IV tubing and placed over the bridge of the nose to provide a constant stream of fluid into the eyes, rather than having a staff member stand and pour fluid into the eyes (Fig. 7-4). Consider the use of Morgan therapeutic irrigation lenses. For continued pain, evaluate the patient for the presence of corneal abrasions.

Nasal Mucosa. Time is the best remedy. Mucous production will carry contaminants away from the mucosa and out of the nose, and is the most effective treatment. Do not attempt to lavage or irrigate the nose or allow the patient to blow the nose, as this will result in increased pain and irritation.

Mouth. Patients may rinse the mouth with water to remove the agent, but the taste of the agent will dwell in the mouth for an extended period of time (usually a day).

Treat respiratory symptoms as necessary. Dyspnea or painful respiration (chest pain on breathing) are generally caused by deep inhalation of agent, and in otherwise healthy persons it is not a danger to the patient.[3] Screen the patient for underlying conditions that may be aggravated by chemical agent. There is no way to decontaminate the respiratory system. Breathing will blow off some contaminant. Use of oxygen will reduce tidal volume, and with it discomfort, but may increase time to normalcy.

To treat intact skin with mild symptoms, water may be used. Flush broken skin with copious amounts of water.

Special Note on PPE. For EMS personnel, a HEPA mask will protect the airways from crystal CS and CN; goggles (without vents) will protect the eyes. A HEPA mask will not protect against CS or CN in smoke form.

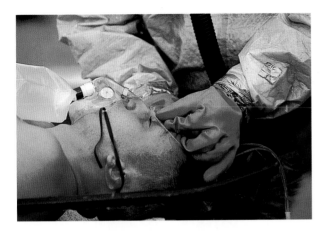

Fig. 7-4
A nasal cannula can be used for eye irrigation.

OLEORESIN CAPSICUM

GENERAL

OC is an organic compound derived from concentrated peppers. OC is different from CN and CS in that it is much more potent, has a much longer duration of action, and has actual physical effects.

HISTORY

OC is one of the few police-specific agents and is a relatively new addition to the law enforcement arsenal. OC was developed as a response to complaints about the limited effectiveness of CN and CS against aggressive offenders (Fig. 7-5).

OC is still in development, and new forms, such as OC-CS mixes and pepper foam, are being introduced. Whereas CN and CS started as crowd control weapons and evolved into forms carried by individual officers, OC evolved exactly the opposite way.

MECHANISM OF ACTION

OC is both an irritant (many times more powerful than CN or CS) and an inflammatory. OC causes pain through an enzymatic action at the nerve endings, short circuiting the heat receptor and causing the perception of pain while no actual damage is being done. OC also causes inflammation whether the subject feels pain or not. From a law enforcement perspective, this is a dramatic improvement over CN and CS, which were ineffective against persons who did not feel pain.

DELIVERY SYSTEMS

OC is delivered in many ways, but in all cases OC is an extract of pepper. Grenades use a small explosive charge to distribute the OC in liquid or powder form. In a spray, OC extract is suspended in a liquid under pressure and sprayed from a container, which can be as small as a keyring-sized can or as large as a backpack-sized dispenser. OC can be delivered in a water-based foam that is sprayed directly onto the target. The foam "melts" to a liquid and runs down the target. Pepperballs

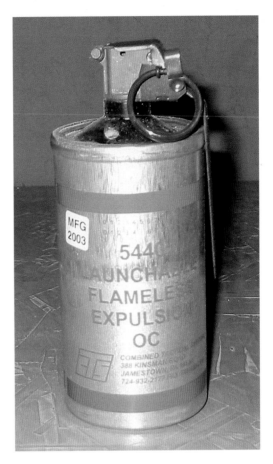

Fig. 7-5
Oleoresin capsicum (OC) spray.

are small plastic balls (roughly marble sized) filled with OC powder that are fired from a paintball gun and break open on impact.

SIGNS AND SYMPTOMS

In most cases, OC causes very severe (but not life-threatening) symptoms (Box 7-2). As with any agent, however, some persons are severely affected whereas others seem immune. The primary symptom is direct and severe irritation of the mucosa by the agent. This affects the eyes, eyelids, conjunctiva, nose, lips, and mouth.

DECONTAMINATION

OC is a very pernicious agent and tends to cross-contaminate items and objects. Touching your eye after touching a contaminated item will serve as a valuable learning experience. Treat a very contaminated patient the same as one who is very bloody. Place a barrier between the patient and the stretcher or seat. OC tends to cling to clothing, skin, and hair, and during large-scale deployments it is often visible on the patient.

Clothing. As with all chemical agents, the vast majority of the contaminant is retained by the clothes. Removing as much clothing as practical is the single most effective decontamination

Common Signs and Symptoms of OC   Box 7-2

Profound rhinorrhea (running nose)
Lacrimation (watering eyes)
Severe blepharospasm (involuntary closing of eyes)
Extreme pain in exposed mucosa (eyes, nose, mouth)
Direct spray to the eyes may cause corneal abrasions
Dyspnea (shortness of breath)
Painful breathing (particularly from smoke form)
Pain to exposed skin (usually minor)
Visible discoloration of the skin may be seen due to vasodilation and dyes added to the agent
Patients with preexisting respiratory conditions may experience mild bronchospasm and wheezing

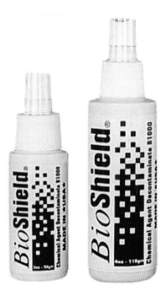

Fig. 7-6
BioShield Decontamination Wash for oleoresin capsicum exposure.

act one can perform. This is particularly true with pepper foam, which "melts" into the target and severely contaminates clothing.

Several decontamination solutions are available. Evidence suggests milk (of any type) is also an effective solution due to the antagonistic relationship between lactic acid and the active enzyme in OC.

EMS Personnel. For EMS personnel, a HEPA mask protects the airways, although you will still smell the powerful agent odor. Goggles (without vents) protect the eyes. Some type of head cover (skullcap, surgical cap) is recommended to prevent contamination of the hair.

In most cases, the best treatment is moving air across the contaminated area, allowing the agent to blow away. In cases of visible gross contamination, water is useful for removing large amounts of agent, but ultimately the remaining agent will not be removed until the water dries and the agent can blow away. In high-humidity environments, the application of water may actually increase decontamination time due to the long drying time, but in hot, very high humidity environments where the patient will continue to sweat and will never really dry off, the use of water is an acceptable intervention.[4] If water is used as a decontamination agent, blot the skin dry (do not rub) and discard the object used to dry the skin. For field use, decontamination towelettes or sprays are useful (Fig. 7-6). They also reduce contaminated runoff, which in turn reduces the chance of cross-contamination.

Use copious amounts of plain water for removing *gross* contamination only. Make sure the water flows away from the face. The hair is the next most common reservoir for contamination (after clothes). Use particular care that water does not run from the hair to the eyes, and dry the hair after using water for decontamination. Use of water on clothing does *not* remove the contaminant, it merely holds it to the clothes until the water dries; then the agent is released into the air again.

Special Note on Decontaminating Law Enforcement Personnel. Law enforcement treatment is usually geared toward getting personnel back onto the line. Avoid, if possible, the use of water on their clothing. Visible agent can be physically removed from the clothing.

If the officer's head is decontaminated, use the same precautions as for patients. Pay particular attention to the hair and decontaminate repeatedly to remove as much agent as possible. The officer's helmet will cause sweat on the head, which will tend to carry agent back into the eyes. Take particular care not to let runoff run down the body, because the neck, underarms, genitalia, and perineum are quite sensitive to OC.

TREATMENT

Decontaminate the patient as described.

For the eyes, plain water and time are the best treatment. Saline will cause increased pain; apply plain water directly to the eyes, being careful to allow the water to run away from the eyes. For continued pain, evaluate the patient for the presence of corneal abrasions.

For nasal mucosa, time is the best therapy. Mucous production will carry contaminants away from the mucosa and out of the nose and is the most effective treatment. Do not attempt to irrigate or lavage the nose or allow the patient to blow the nose, as this will result in increased pain and irritation.

For the mouth, water and time will help. Patients may rinse their mouth with water to remove the agent, but the taste of the agent will dwell in the mouth for an extended period of time (usually 1 day).

For the respiratory system, treat the symptoms. Dyspnea and painful respiration (chest pain on breathing) are generally caused by deep inhalation of agent, and in otherwise healthy persons it is not a danger to the patient.[5] Screen the patient for underlying conditions, which may be aggravated by chemical agents. After severe OC exposure, oxygen may reduce the common anxiety from air hunger. There is no way to decontaminate the respiratory system. Breathing will blow off some contaminant.

Symptoms in intact skin are usually mild; water is not recommended as it will likely increase the time to relieve symptoms. Broken skin, however, must be flushed with copious amounts of water.

MALODORANTS (STINK BOMBS)

Malodorants are a new class of riot agents. Whereas CN, CS, and OC were designed to use pain to cause people to vacate a given area, malodorants simply make a place or person smell so bad that people do not want to be around. Malodorants have no direct physical effects, but some people may present with somatic effects from the remarkably intense odor.

HISTORY

Malodorants have great promise as riot agents in overcoming some of the inherent limitations of CN, CS, and OC. CN and CS are not sufficiently powerful to displace intensely motivated protesters or rioters, which led to the introduction of OC as a riot agent. OC's disadvantage is that its inflammatory action and blepharospasm can result in a large crowd of effectively blind, dyspneic people who may be incapable of leaving the area. Malodorants have nearly the dispersal power of OC, without taking away people's ability to navigate.

MECHANISM OF ACTION

Malodorants are an artificial mixture of compounds designed to smell as bad as possible. The compound is one that does not cause olfactory fatigue, so the odor stays at the same intensity regardless of length of exposure. The exact nature of the compound and its components are still a trade secret.

DELIVERY SYSTEMS

Malodorant is delivered in different ways, but it is a liquid in all forms. Grenades use a small explosive charge to aerosolize and distribute the liquid. Spray is still in development. Stinkballs are small plastic balls (roughly marble sized) filled with malodorant liquid that are fired from paintball guns and break open on impact.

SIGNS AND SYMPTOMS

Malodorants have no direct physical effects other than the odor, but the profoundly obnoxious odor can (and is intended to) result in somatic effects such as nausea, vomiting, dyspnea, and vertigo.

DECONTAMINATION

As yet, there is no specific decontamination agent for malodorants. Standard cleaning methods (soap, water) should be used. As with all chemical agents, the vast majority of contaminants are retained by the clothes. Removing as much clothing as practical is the single most effective decontamination action one can take.

Special Note on Decontaminating Law Enforcement Personnel. Law enforcement treatment is usually geared toward getting personnel back onto the line. If possible, avoid using water on their clothing because it will trap contaminants in the clothing. Air is the best current way to remove malodorants unless the clothing can be washed.

TREATMENT

Decontaminate the patient and treat any somatic symptoms. Treat any strikes by stinkballs on sensitive areas (eyes, mouth, genitalia) as you would any other low-velocity trauma.

CHAPTER SUMMARY

Riot agents are relatively harmless under normal conditions, but during large-scale deployments they can cause significant challenges to an emergency department. The hospital's preparation will determine the level to which the event affects the hospital's response. Contamination of the ED's air will significantly reduce the effectiveness of the staff and may cause pain and discomfort. Proper design of a response plan will minimize the risks from both the agent and potentially hostile patients.

REFERENCES

1. Medical Research Institute of Chemical Defense: *Medical management of chemical casualties handbook*, ed 3, Aberdeen Proving Ground, Md, 1999, United States Army, http://www.vnh.org/CHEMCASU/titlepg.html, retrieved September 17, 2004.
2. U.S. Departments of the Army, Navy, and Air Force: *NATO handbook on the medical aspects of NBC defensive operations*, Washington, DC, 1996, Departments of the Army, Navy, and Air Force, http://www.vnh.org/MedAspNBCDef/toc.htm, retrieved September 17, 2004.
3. Fraunfelder FT: Is CS gas dangerous? Current evidence suggests not but unanswered questions remain [editorial], *BMJ* 320: 458-459, 2000.
4. Colon A: Personal experience in high-humidity environments.
5. Onnen J: *IACP report: oleoresin capsicum*, Alexandria, Va, International Association of Chiefs of Police, June 1993.

Incident Management Systems

Gary Christman

CHAPTER OBJECTIVES

At the conclusion of this chapter the student will be able to:

- Describe the origin of the incident command system.
- Explain the concepts of the incident command system.
- Identify the positions of the incident command system.
- Describe the role of emergency medical services in the incident command system.
- Explain the task force and strike team concept.
- Explain the unified command concept and unity of command.

CASE STUDY

An explosive device with a radiological component (dirty bomb) has been detonated at a large metropolitan fair. There are numerous casualties. Federal, state, and local government agencies are all responding to the scene. A safe and efficient response mandates that all of these agencies communicate and operate under an effective command structure.

Who is in charge at this type of incident?

How can all of these agencies coordinate their activities?

What type of incident management system is needed?

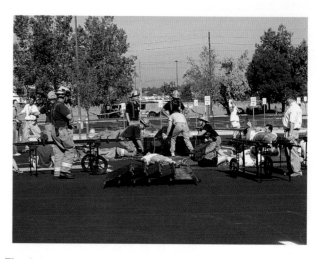

Fig. 8-1
The complexities of a mass casualty incident mandate the use of an incident management system.

BACKGROUND

The National Incident Management System (NIMS) is a major part of all types of responses both small and large. It allows for the control and safety of responders as well as information and logistical resources involved in a major response. The part of the National Incident Management System that manages on-scene responder focus and safety is the Incident Command System (ICS). The system has been proved to be the best system for emergency response.

The Emergency Medical System (EMS) will play a major role in the response to a weapons of mass destruction (WMD) incident and all incidents involving mass casualties. The incident command system lends consistency and efficiency to the operations. Using the incident command system or unified command system will help save the lives of both first responders and civilians.

ORIGIN

All incidents involving mass casualties or potential mass casualties must be organized under a system that can support operations of many agencies with the single focus of managing the incident in a safe and efficient manner (Fig. 8-1). The incident command system was first used in California in the early 1970s during a series of severe wildfires. The operational group, including local, state, and federal agencies, decided that they needed a system that could control a large operation involving many agencies.

This system, the Fire Fighting Resources of California Organized for Potential Emergencies (FIRESCOPE), was the original incident command system. FIRESCOPE found many areas that needed to be organized. The system looked at a number of issues within the operation of an incident, including span of control, terminology, resource management, planning, documentation, and communications.

The incident command system was recognized, adopted, and endorsed by the National Fire Academy, the International Associations of Chiefs of Police, and the American Public Works Association. The system was also recognized by the hospital system, which adopted the Hospital Emergency Incident Command System (HEICS). The basic structure of the ICS makes up the foundation of the new National Incident Management System (NIMS).

LAWS PERTAINING TO INCIDENT COMMAND

On March 6, 1990, the Occupational Safety and Health Administration (OSHA) made into law the Hazardous Waste Operations and Emergency Response (HAZWOPER) standard. This standard provided a protection package for employees involved in cleaning up hazardous waste or in emergency response to hazardous materials incidents. This regulation is OSHA rule 29 CFR 1910.120. Part of this standard mandates the use of a recognized incident command management system by all agencies responding to or participating in an incident involving hazardous material.

Knowing that not all employees in all states are covered by the OSHA rule, the EPA passed a parallel standard (40 CFR 311) that covered all employees no matter where or for whom they worked. The EPA standard extended the coverage to volunteers and government workers who are not covered by OSHA rules. These two standards made it mandatory for all agencies, the EMS, and hospitals to use a recognized incident command system when responding to an incident involving hazardous materials. Most WMD incidents will involve the use of hazardous materials.

ORGANIZATION

The incident command system mimics the general business practice used by most corporations and small companies. The structure can expand and contract depending on the incident. The one constant position is that of *incident commander*. The first person on the scene will be the incident commander until that person is replaced by a higher ranking or more knowledgeable, qualified person. The incident commander takes on all responsibilities of the incident until he or she delegates responsibilities to others, creating the other ICS positions (Fig. 8-2).

The incident command system has five major functional areas that span the needs encountered when responding to an incident. These areas are incident command, operations, planning, logistics, and finance and administration. Each section, if needed, will expand to control several areas depending on the needs and conditions of the incident (Fig. 8-3). The five

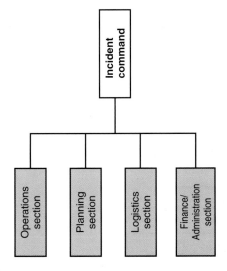

Fig. 8-2
The incident commander has the ultimate responsibility for managing the incident.

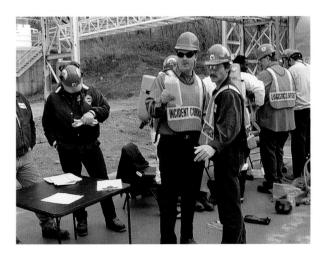

Fig. 8-3
Five major functional areas (sections) of the incident command system.

functions do not have to be used unless the incident is large enough and warrants them.

INCIDENT COMMANDER

The incident commander has the overall responsibility for the response to the incident. All response decisions and communications pass through the incident commander or someone she or he designates. The incident commander is responsible for making the decision to fill the other four functional area positions and positions below them. The incident commander performs the duties for any functional area whose positions are not filled.

The incident commander position can comprise more than one person representing more than one agency. This concept is known as *unified command* and is covered later in this chapter.

Some staff positions report directly to the incident commander. These include the safety officer, the public information officer, and the liaison officer.

The safety officer is responsible for all safety concerns at the incident. The safety officer must stop or modify any unsafe acts, then immediately report those changes to the incident commander. At complex incidents a safety sector may be used (Fig. 8-4).

The public information officer is responsible for developing and presenting information to the news media. This is a vital concern and must not be overlooked. The news media can be of major assistance in getting information to the public. This can help alleviate public fears and provide information on topics such as evacuation.

The liaison officer serves as a filter for the people wishing to speak to the incident commander. The liaison officer must have immediate access to the incident commander and can allow critical information to be given to the incident commander.

OPERATIONS

The operations section chief leads the operations section. The operations section chief is responsible for all tactical operations at the scene of the incident. This section is established by the

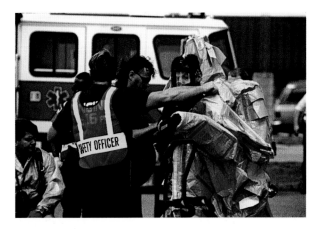

Fig. 8-4
Safety officer at a weapons of mass destruction incident.

incident commander as needed based on the size and complexity of the incident and the number of responders.

The operations section chief is responsible for a number of tasks at the scene of the incident, including helping to develop the incident operations plan, requesting resources, communicating with subordinate sectors, supervising the staging areas and personnel operating under the operations section, keeping the incident commander updated on the incident, and developing the objectives for the incident.

The operations section can have several subordinate sectors depending on the incident. The agencies could include police, fire, EMS, public works, and any other agencies with tactical responsibility (Fig. 8-5). Depending on the incident, the operations section may be divided into divisions and the divisions into working groups.

Divisions. The operations section is broken into divisions when the incident covers a large geographical area or crosses over borders or jurisdictions. Divisions split responders into separate areas, such as north and south divisions or parking lot and inside venue divisions. Each division will have a division leader who reports to the operations section chief. When multiple divisions are set up they must be given independent names to prevent confusion. Once the divisions are organized, working groups will be set up in each division.

Sectors. A lot of discussion has taken place concerning the names used for the working groups established under divisions of the operations section. *Branches, groups, sectors,* and *units* are the terms used to identify these working groups. *Sector* seems to be the most often used so that is the term we will use here.

A sector is an organizational level for a specified function. Sectors can be established temporarily or for the duration of the incident. Each sector handles a specific tactical function of the operation. In a mass casualty incident, divisions may be broken into triage and treatment sectors. Each sector will have an officer to oversee it.

Working under the operations section but independently of the divisions will be the other sectors that are needed to handle a mass casualty incident. These may include a transportation sector and a communications sector for medical operations. Communications will play a large role in assuring both internal and external communication. Transportation could be broken down into different groups depending on the needs of the incident. Transportation concerns must be controlled by one sector leader so patients do not overwhelm one location and can receive proper treatment. This will be necessary to control patient flow to hospitals and Disaster Medical Assistance Teams (DMATs). Different transport sectors that could be used include air transportation units and

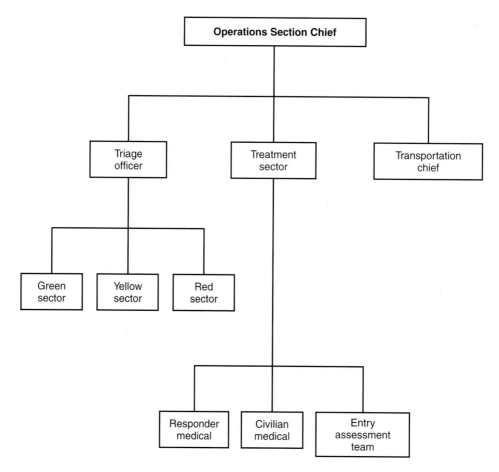

Fig. 8-5
Example of medical sectors at a WMD incident.

ground transportation units. Keep in mind when using air transportation you will need a safety officer, communications, and fire suppression and rescue to operate this sector properly.

Task Forces. Task forces are teams made up of several different agencies with common communications and a team leader. Task forces may include security, hot zone extraction, decontamination, medical treatment, and communications. This concept allows for a group of different resources to be immediately available for assignment and operation.

Strike Teams. The response to a WMD incident will require major EMS involvement. Strike teams are like resources assigned to carry out specific tasks. It may be necessary to make up teams of EMS responders to handle specific duties. These could include evacuation, special weapons and tactics (SWAT), hazardous materials response, inoculation for biological weapons, and support of area hospitals and clinics (Fig. 8-6).

PLANNING

Planning will be responsible for collecting data from the operations section. Once the information is collected it will be evaluated and disseminated as needed to manage the incident. Planning writes the operations plan for the incident. The planning section will have to work closely with the other sections to make sure they have the resources and finances to make the plan functional. Once the plan is established the planning section will have to make sure that the plan is updated according to the progress of the incident. This will also include the demobilization of all resources back to normal service when they are no longer needed.

LOGISTICS

The logistics group will be responsible for procuring all needed resources during the incident, including facilities, material, and services. The logistics function could be divided into several different sectors. Besides locating resources for the operation, they will also be dealing with donated goods. Historically, one of the largest problems facing logistics is donated goods. Well-intentioned people have been known to donate everything, including winter coats at a hurricane scene. Logistics will have to determine what can be used and what must be removed from the scene. Logistics will also have to deal with cash and check donations being dropped off and mailed to the incident.

ADMINISTRATION AND FINANCE

Administration and finance will be responsible for billing, documentation, and procurement. Documentation of the incident is extremely important for several reasons. The documentation will be used to recover funds for service, evidence in court of actions taken during the operation, and after-action program improvement.

CONCEPTS

The incident command system is set up so that everyone operates under the same concepts (Box 8-1). When you respond to an incident or bring outside agencies into your incident, working within the same system and concepts will reduce confusion and the risk of responder injury or death.

COMMON TERMINOLOGY

Common terminology must be followed throughout the incident to minimize confusion. For years emergency responders have been using 10 codes (e.g., 10-4, "acknowledge") and verbal shorthand to communicate within their agency. When this terminology is used with other agencies at an incident scene, mass confusion is the common outcome when one 10 code could mean "evacuate the scene" to one agency and "all clear" to another.

Communications must be in plain English both on the scene and on the radio to reduce the possibility of confusion between agencies. More than just first responders will be on the scene of a WMD incident. As we have seen in large responses, such as to the New York World Trade Center, many different agencies, from public works to private contractors, will be attempting to work together effectively and safely.

COMMAND POST

The command post is the location where incident operations are directed. It may be an officer's vehicle, a specially designed mobile command post, or a tent. In long-term incidents, the command post may be located in a building. There should be only one incident command post at the incident. Once the command post is established, the incident commander should stay at the command post so he or she can be easily found. The command post is usually marked with a green flag or light. In large or complex incidents an emergency operations center (EOC) may be established to support the incident commander. EOC operations are discussed in detail later (Fig. 8-7).

UNIFIED COMMAND

The unified command structure is used when there are a number of agencies that have an overall responsibility to the incident. This structure will be seen in a WMD event. Lead representatives from each involved agency will make up the unified command.

The unified command group will be making the decisions about the goals, objectives, and priorities for the response to the incident. The unified command group will change as the incident changes. The unified command can expand or contract depending on the needs of the incident.

Within a unified command there must be a leader. The agency with the current incident focus will usually take the lead of the unified command. This may change several times during the incident as the response focus changes. In a terrorist incident the lead agency for crisis management (the prevention of the incident) is usually the FBI. In the consequence-management phase (responding to the aftermath of the incident) the local incident commander is usually the FEMA commander (Fig. 8-8).

The unified command concept should not be confused with unity of command. Unity of command means that responders report to only one supervisor. If responders receive conflicting orders from a second command-level person, they should refer that person to their supervisor for clarification.

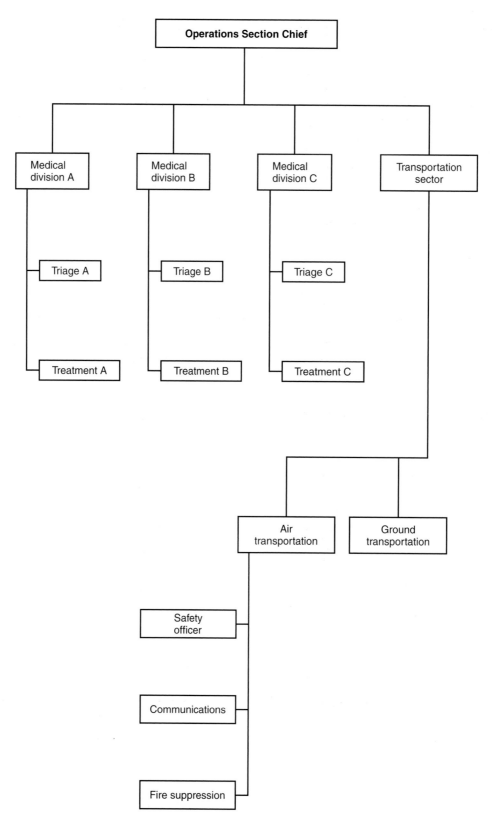

Fig. 8-6
Example of medical strike teams at a WMD incident.

Incident Command System Concepts — Box 8-1

- Common terminology
- Command post
- Unified command
- Consolidated response plan
- Span of control
- Integrated communication
- Staging areas

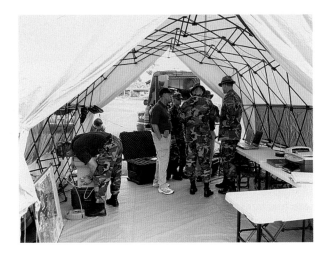

Fig. 8-7
Incident command post.

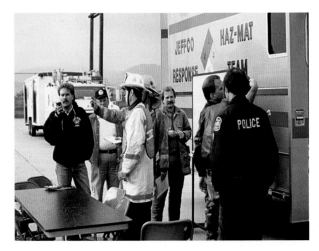

Fig. 8-8
In complex incidents a unified command system is usually established.

CONSOLIDATED RESPONSE PLAN

A plan is necessary when responding to any type of emergency. This will be especially true when facing the complexities of a WMD incident. In emergency work, plans for responding to incidents within our jurisdictions are common, but developing a plan for every possible incident is not feasible. A general plan showing who will be responsible for different aspects of an incident is adequate for a small incident that only involves responders from the same jurisdiction.

When responding to a large-scale incident or a WMD incident you must have a specific response plan that is updated whenever the incident changes. These plans will cover a number of different aspects of the response, including shift change, resource management, action, and demobilization. The plan will be governed by the incident and will grow as the response progresses.

SPAN OF CONTROL

Accountability is a priority in the response to any emergency. It is especially important in a WMD incident. Responders at these incidents must understand and follow a manageable span of control. The span of control recommended by the ICS is three to seven responders per supervisor with the optimum number of five. This makes the accountability of responders easier and keeps supervisors from being overwhelmed by a large number of responders.

INTEGRATED COMMUNICATIONS

Communication problems have been the downfall of many emergency responses. Communication has a high priority in any response, large or small. It is imperative to establish a communications sector and a plan stating how communications will take place. The communications sector will need to establish standard operating procedures for radio traffic using plain English. A number of personnel will be using communications devices that they are not familiar with.

Radios most often come to mind when we think of emergency response communications. In a WMD incident or any large incident involving a number of agencies, radios may represent only a small part of the communication devices. Different communication devices including phones, satellite communications, Internet, and intranet may be needed. A complex communications setup will require a qualified person in a full-time position to handle the communications function.

With a number of different agencies on the scene, communicating with all agencies with one or two frequencies will be impossible. Multiple frequencies and unified command will help to solve this problem. New communication devices that allow multiple frequencies and systems to communicate with each other are becoming more common and will be a major asset when responding to large incidents.

STAGING AREAS

Many resources will be required to manage a WMD incident. The ICS must be able to manage the resources. The resources will be needed at different times and possibly at different locations. If every piece of equipment arrived at the same time and location the result would be chaos. Only those resources that are needed immediately should be at the emergency site.

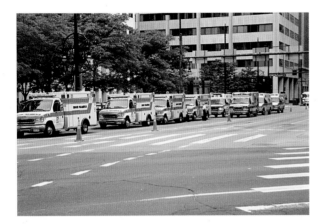

Fig. 8-9
Because of the resources required at a weapons of mass destruction incident, numerous staging areas may be necessary.

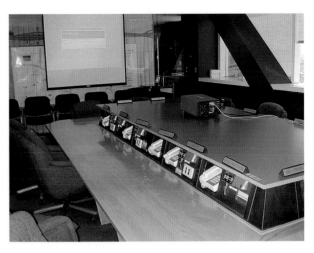

Fig. 8-10
Emergency operations centers are established to support the incident commander and field operations.

Other resources should be directed to a staging area where they can stay until they are needed (Fig. 8-9). Depending on the incident there may be more than one staging area. Staging areas are usually established at a site remote from the command post. Considerations in establishing staging areas include:
• A safe area with proximity to the emergency site
• Easy access in and out
• Parking areas for equipment
• Storage space for supplies
• Temperature-controlled space for personnel, if possible
• Security control with checks for possible secondary devices

The staging areas are under the control of a staging area manager who reports to the operations section chief. The staging area manager should establish a check-in and distribution procedure. Communications among the staging officer, operations officer, and incident commander must be maintained at all times. The operations section chief should be kept informed about what resources are available.

EMERGENCY OPERATIONS CENTERS

Most jurisdictions have established emergency operations centers (EOCs) as part of their emergency response to major incidents. The EOC is where senior response officials, department heads, and government officers and officials gather to coordinate the response to an emergency (Fig. 8-10).

Multiple EOCs could be operating during a WMD incident. The local, county, and state EOCs may all be in operation. Federal assets may establish a regional operations center or a joint operations center to bring key personnel together. The individual response agencies may also establish operations centers to support their teams.

The establishment of EOCs does not reduce the importance of the ICS or limit the responsibilities of the incident commander. The two systems must work together and complement each other. The EOCs are established to support the ICS with guidance, information, and resources and supplies that are not available to the incident commander. Some functions are better handled away from the command post. For instance providing food and shelter for responders is better managed by an EOC than by the incident commander.

CHAPTER SUMMARY

The incident command system is required by law for any agency responding to a hazardous materials incident. An incident involving weapons of mass destruction is one of the most complex hazardous materials incidents possible. Many agencies, including federal, state, and local governments as well as contractors, will be responding. An incident management system is necessary for an effective and safe response. The system has been proven to work and will save the lives of both responders and citizens.

BIBLIOGRAPHY

Department of Justice: *Incident command for weapons of mass destruction* (training course), Anniston, Ala, Center for Domestic Preparedness, 2002.

FEMA: *Hospital emergency incident command system* (training course), Fort McClellan, Ala, Noble Training Center, year unknown.

FEMA Emergency Management Institute: *Advanced incident command system*, course no. G196, Emmitsburg, Md, 2003-2004.

FEMA Emergency Management Institute: *Incident command system: law enforcement*, course no. G190, Emmitsburg, Md, 2003-2004.

FEMA Emergency Management Institute: *Intermediate incident command system*, course no. G195, Emmitsburg, Md, 2003-2004.

FEMA Emergency Management Institute: *Incident command system/emergency operations center interface workshop*, course no. G191, Emmitsburg, Md, 2003-2004.

Chapter **9**

Field Management of a Weapons of Mass Destruction Incident

PHIL CURRANCE

CHAPTER OBJECTIVES

At the conclusion of this chapter the student will be able to:

- Discuss the importance of preplanning in safely and effectively responding to weapons of mass destruction (WMD) incidents.
- Describe proper EMS response procedures for a WMD incident.
- Identify the control zones that should be established at a WMD incident and discuss EMS activities in each zone.
- Discuss patient triage and movement at a WMD incident.
- Discuss patient decontamination procedures.
- Discuss the types of personal protective equipment (PPE) that will be needed.
- Identify responder medical support procedures.
- Identify the need for evidence preservation.
- Identify special EMS resources and equipment that will be needed at a WMD incident.
- Discuss special patient transportation concerns.
- Describe actions that will be necessary after the incident is concluded.

CASE STUDY

An unknown chemical agent has been released into the ventilation system at a county court building. Numerous patients have made their way from the building but there are many others unconscious inside the building. Many different response agencies including police department, fire department, local EMS, state National Guard units, and county health department personnel are at the scene.

Who is in charge?

What items should have been addressed during preplanning?

How should the scene be controlled?

What should be done about people in surrounding buildings?

What on-scene activities are EMS responders responsible for?

What activities will be required at the conclusion of the incident?

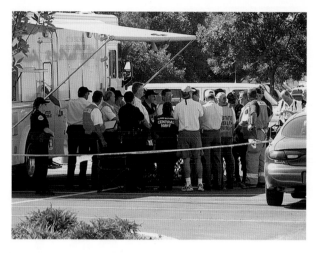

Fig. 9-1
Many agencies will be represented at a WMD incident.

EMERGENCY RESPONSE PLAN

One of the most important tools to help ensure the safety of personnel is an emergency response plan. Every agency with emergency response responsibilities should have an emergency response plan. This plan should be developed, rehearsed, modified as necessary, and rehearsed again. It should establish the response agency's actions when faced with a major emergency. At a minimum the plan should include:

- Assessment of local hazards and potential targets
- Preemergency planning and coordination with outside agencies and private parties
- Personnel roles, lines of authority, training, and communications
- Emergency recognition and response practices
- Emergency alerting and response procedures
- Safe distances and places of refuge
- Site security and control
- Evacuation routes and procedures
- Personal protective equipment and emergency equipment
- Decontamination procedures
- Emergency medical treatment
- Incident termination procedures, including postincident analysis of response and follow-up
- Reporting and tracking of responder exposure

Emergency response organizations may use the local emergency response plan or the state emergency response plan as a model to prevent duplication. If the local or state plan is used, it still must be modified to be specific to the emergency response organization.

A comprehensive response plan must address the potential hazards and targets in the area. Industrial chemicals that are used, stored, or transported through the area in large quantities should be identified. The many regulations covering chemicals and hazardous materials can assist in developing this assessment. One is the 1986 EPA Superfund Amendment and Reauthorization Act (SARA). This law established a list of

OVERVIEW

Response to an incident involving weapons of mass destruction is on every responder's mind. It is essential to be prepared when facing these incidents. Weapons of mass destruction can include explosives, chemical agents, biological agents, or radiological hazards. Secondary devices may be used to injure or kill emergency responders. It is impossible for any one agency to successfully handle one of these incidents. Many different agencies will play a part in these responses (Fig. 9-1). Preplanning and efficient scene management techniques are essential in responding to these incidents.

PREPLANNING

Preplanning is a vital part of safe and effective response to a WMD incident. Response to these incidents involves a great deal of risk to the responders. Their health and safety depend on a highly organized response. A WMD incident comprises the complexities of a crime scene, a hazardous materials release, and a mass casualty incident. It will certainly stress even the most organized response system. Many agencies will be needed to manage this scene safely and efficiently. Many aspects of this type of response must be determined far in advance of an actual emergency.

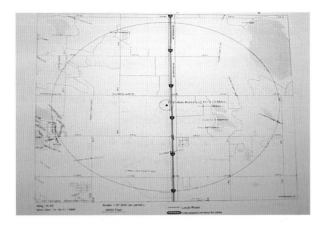

Fig. 9-2
The Risk Management Area of Concern map for an industrial facility that uses anhydrous ammonia.

Signs of a WMD Incident	Box 9-1

Clues that you may be involved in a WMD incident can include:
A response to a target hazard or target event
A recent threat
Multiple victims (especially nontrauma victims)
First responders becoming victims
Hazardous materials involved
Reports of explosions
Reports of unusual odors or vapor clouds
Reports of dissemination devices
Reports of unusual or unscheduled paint or insecticide spraying
Secondary attack or explosion

what the EPA considers extremely hazardous substances (EHSs) and mandates emergency planning and reporting if industries manufacture or store more than listed amounts.

An OSHA law, the Process Safety Management Standard (29 CFR 1910.119), will also assist in this emergency planning hazard assessment. This standard lists chemicals that could cause a catastrophic problem when released. The standard requires that facilities conduct emergency planning, failure mode analysis, and training and have process diagrams and emergency shutdown procedures. Major industrial facilities in your area may identify which chemicals they have that meet these criteria.

Similar to the OSHA Process Management Standard is the EPA's Risk Management Program. This standard is also concerned with chemicals that could cause a catastrophic problem. While the OSHA standard is concerned with worker safety, this EPA standard is focused on the safety of people living in the surrounding area (Fig. 9-2). If identified chemicals are stored in quantities greater than the specified amounts, the company must carry out emergency planning and public notification.

Additional information regarding chemicals found at local industries can be obtained from fire department inspections and reports concerning prior releases and incidents. The local police department, county sheriff, and state patrol can be excellent sources of information regarding which chemicals are routinely transported through the area.

The federal regulations can assist the responder in identifying the locations of chemical hazards in the area, but access to this information is not limited to emergency responders. Terrorists may also gain access to this information and use it for their own planning and target identification.

Potential targets include federal and local government buildings, areas of historical importance, areas where large numbers of people gather, and critical infrastructures such as water and power plants, transportation facilities, and hospitals. This information will allow the response agency to plan training, protective equipment, and resource needs. Although

it is not possible to identify all potential problems in the area, information should be gathered on as many hazards and targets as possible.

INCIDENT RECOGNITION AND SAFE APPROACH

Depending on the type of incident, the release of a weapon of mass destruction may not be apparent during the initial response. Responders should always be alert for clues to the presence of this type of incident (Box 9-1).

During hazardous materials incidents many responders are injured during the initial approach. Add to this the large scale of an intentional release and the possibility of a secondary device during a terrorist attack. The ability to respond safely and have a positive impact on the scene depends on the responder's ability to recognize the type of incident.

INCIDENT PRIORITIES

The first priority is to protect responders. Rescues from contaminated areas should not be attempted until the chemical has been identified and properly trained responders with appropriate PPE are available. This is difficult to do when it is obvious that people are in distress and need help. However, if untrained and unprotected responders enter the area to carry out a rescue, they are likely to become victims themselves and become part of the problem, not part of the solution.

The hazard area should be isolated and secured from entry by unauthorized personnel. A safe zone that is upwind, uphill, and upstream from the incident should be established. Because gases and vapors spread the fastest and go the farthest, upwind is the most important factor in selection of a safe zone. Because most vapors are heavier than air, they will accumulate in low areas. Therefore all low-lying areas should be avoided. If the incident has occurred inside a structure, avoid areas around the building's ventilation exhaust.

Isolation and evacuation distances will vary depending on agent, weather, and situation. Suggested evacuation and protective distances can be found in the *North American Emergency Response Guidebook* (NAERG), and the Chemical

Transportation Emergency Center (CHEMTREC) may be able to provide more detailed information.

Never assume that the scene is safe because the substance does not have any apparent odor or obvious color. Many agents are colorless and odorless.

INCIDENT RESPONSE

SAFE APPROACH

Response must be to a safe area away from obvious and fore-seeable dangers. Areas that are upwind, uphill, and upstream from the incident are best. Upwind is essential. Initial priorities always are to ensure that responders are in a safe area and that the incident is isolated. At the first hint that you are respond-ing to an incident involving a weapon of mass destruction, responders should stop a safe distance from the contaminated area (Fig. 9-3). The NAERG gives distance suggestions. If no other personnel are on site, EMS responders will need to establish a command post and set up an incident command system (ICS). Ensure that other emergency personnel are responding to a safe area. If an ICS is already established, EMS responders should report to the incident commander or staging area as directed.

STAGING AREAS

A staging area is a resource marshaling area that units report to while awaiting specific assignments and direction. Only resources that are needed immediately at the scene of the emergency should be on site. Different personnel and resources are needed at different times and in different locations. In addition, when they are needed, they must be available to respond in a controlled, organized, and effective manner. Above all, the safety of the responders must be ensured. The way to achieve these goals is to use staging areas.

Depending on the size and nature of the incident, one or more staging areas may be established. The staging area provides a safe location where personnel and resources may wait until needed, prevents the freelancing of incoming units, and provides accountability for the units on scene and their status. Key considerations for selecting a staging area include:

- Proximity to the incident scene
- Easy access in and out
- Parking areas and storage space
- Security for equipment and supplies

INCIDENT COMMAND SYSTEM AND RESPONDER CONTROL

Federal regulations (OSHA 29 CFR 1910.120 and EPA 40 CFR 311) mandate that emergency response to all incidents involving hazardous substances be managed under an incident command system. (See Chapter 8.) This system is designed to focus the actions of all responders on safely and efficiently mitigating the incident. All personnel responding to the incident must be able to function under an effective ICS.

The ICS is a management tool consisting of procedures for organizing personnel, facilities, equipment, and communica-tions at the scene of an emergency. Functional areas are established to address concerns of command, operations, logistics, planning, and administration.

The incident commander should designate a safety officer who is knowledgeable in the operations being implemented at the emergency response site (Fig. 9-4). This person is specifically charged with identifying and evaluating hazards and providing direction with respect to the safety of operations for the emergency at hand. When the safety officer judges activities to be immediately dangerous to life or health (IDLH) or to involve an imminently dangerous condition, he or she must have the authority to alter, suspend, or terminate those activities. The safety officer should immediately inform the incident commander of any actions needed to correct hazards at the emergency scene.

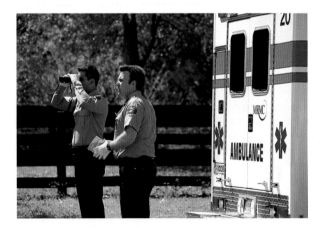

Fig. 9-3
EMS responders stopping at a safe distance at the first clue of a WMD incident.

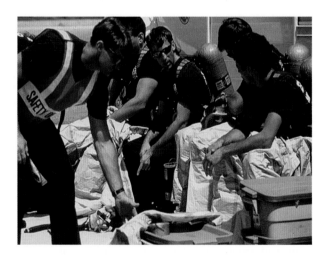

Fig. 9-4
The safety officer should have the authority to stop or modify all unsafe acts.

BYSTANDER AND VOLUNTEER MANAGEMENT

Remember that bystanders, witnesses, and well-meaning persons who stopped to assist may be exposed or contaminated. These people need to be screened for possible exposure and injuries. If contamination is possible, decontamination will be necessary. The level of decontamination will depend on the degree of contamination. Names and addresses should be noted in case future information indicates an exposure.

A frequent problem at large incidents is control of the people who show up to volunteer. Many people may suddenly descend on the emergency wishing to help. Most of these people will be genuine and sincere in their desires, but there is always the possibility that some people will be there to further their own agendas or obtain souvenirs.

In any case, volunteers must be screened and protected from harm. Most of these people will not be trained and will not have proper protective equipment. A staging area should be designated where volunteer credentials can be checked and proper assignments made. Portable ID systems can be used at the scene to credential responders and volunteers. Access control should be established to ensure that noncredentialed personnel do not gain access to restricted areas.

In some recent incidents donated equipment and supplies have become a problem. Unneeded supplies have been plentiful, and needed equipment has been hard to obtain. Logistics personnel must be able to manage donated supplies as well as those procured through normal channels. Logistics personnel should work with the public information officers to request that donations be limited to needed and usable items.

COMMUNICATIONS

Communications will be a major problem at any large emergency. Agencies from local, state, and federal agencies will all be responding. Coordinating these response agencies is vital. Major progress has been made to standardize radio frequencies so that different response agencies can communicate effectively (Fig. 9-5).

RADIO SYSTEMS

Significant technological advances such as trunking systems and 800-megahertz systems have been developed. Many larger departments are taking advantage of these developments while departments with smaller budgets are still using older technology. The result is that standardized radio frequencies and coordinated communications are mostly a thing of the past. New equipment developments also include communication mixing systems that will allow different frequencies to be able to communicate. Because these are very expensive they will not usually be available in the early hours of most incidents.

Plans must be developed to share radios and to overcome these issues. Many agencies are now using cellular or digital phones as a major part of their communication plan. These are used for emergency backup, personnel notification, hospital communication, and so on. At large incidents cellular and

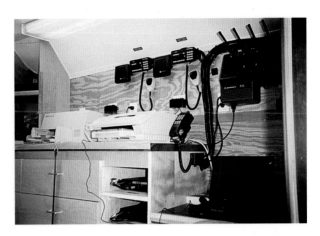

Fig. 9-5
Communication systems must be able to link various agencies at a WMD incident.

digital sites will be quickly overwhelmed, and these systems may quickly be out of service.

Another problem is using a radio while wearing personal protective equipment. Throat and ear units will make communication easier when wearing a helmet or protective equipment.

HAND SIGNALS

Writing boards and hand signals can also be used to improve communication between responders wearing PPE. Hand signals must be predetermined and practiced in training to reduce confusion and miscommunication. Typical hand signals include the following:
- Both hands over the head: Emergency help needed
- Hands gripping throat: Low air or out of air
- Thumbs up: Yes or I understand
- Thumbs down: No
- Grip partner's arm or both hands around waist: Leave area immediately

EMERGENCY COMMUNICATION

Emergency communication also should be established. An emergency signal should be designated that will warn responders to leave the hot zone immediately and be on the lookout for potential problems. Air-powered foghorns or personnel-alert sirens work well. In high-noise areas, a visual signal, such as a strobe light, may need to be added. All communication devices used in a potentially explosive atmosphere must be intrinsically safe and should be checked and maintained regularly to ensure proper operation.

COMMUNICATION WITH VICTIMS

Another communication issue is communication with victims. Communication will be necessary to advise victims where to go and what to do. The mechanics of mass casualty decontamination can be confusing, and victims will need direction. Many units are using written signs in multiple languages to communicate with victims (Fig. 9-6).

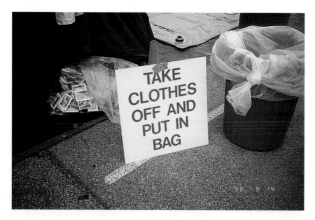

Fig. 9-6
Signs or verbal messages should be in place to guide
victims at a WMD incident.

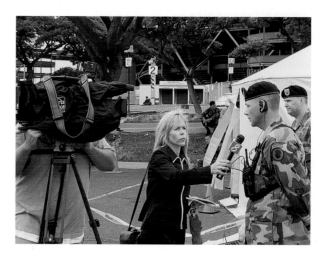

Fig. 9-7
The media should be viewed as an asset, not an
adversary.

Some units have developed cassette player–speaker units to
deliver messages in multiple languages during the decontamination process. Sporting goods suppliers have portable,
battery powered, water-resistant cassette player–speaker units
that are used as hunting game caller units. These units, coupled
with loop recording tapes, can be very effective at delivering
messages on a continuous basis. Add a portable cassette recorder
to the inventory and messages can be customized on the fly.

WORKING WITH THE MEDIA

The media will be a part of a large-scale response, especially
when terrorism is suspected. Although many responders feel
that the media are intrusive and a hindrance to their job, they
can be also be a major asset (Fig. 9-7).

The media can alert the public and provide them with
information about exposure effects and where to seek care.
Real-time medical information provided by qualified experts
through the media can help the public to differentiate between
real and somatic symptoms of the incident. People who need
medical care can be directed to the appropriate facility. This can
help distribute the population to different facilities and prevent
facility overload. Information about evacuation and protection
in place can be provided to the public through the media.

PUBLIC INFORMATION OFFICER

Plans must include media relations. Each response agency
should have a designated public information officer (PIO) with
backup personnel. Every person designated should attend PIO
training. The incident commander should designate a lead
PIO for the incident. Each agency PIO should work with the
designated incident PIO so that the public does not receive
conflicting information. The incident PIO should report directly
to the incident commander. Frequent reports should be made
to the PIO so that the most current information is available.

Designated media staging areas must be established where
media representatives' identities can be ascertained and verified.

Strict badge access must be maintained. Media briefings can be
held in the staging area. Briefings should be held at regular
scheduled intervals whether there is new information to report
or not. Reporters are under the pressure of deadlines, and if
information is not available through the PIO they will get it
somewhere else. This information may not be accurate or the
information that the incident commander wants released.

EVACUATION VERSUS PROTECTION IN PLACE

Terrorist attacks involving chemical, biological, or radiological
agents may involve a large part of the community. Mass
evacuations may complicate the response by exposing the
evacuating population to the agent or by choking off access to
emergency responders. It is often assumed that evacuation is
the best protective measure for the public. Although that is
probably true when there is time to safely move the public
from harm's way, it may be disastrous in the case of an event
involving chemical, biological, or radiological weapons. Short
warning times, the rapid spread of the toxic agent, and time
factors required to move large segments of the population
must be considered. Evacuations take time and personnel.
People must not only evacuate their homes or workplaces, they
must also evacuate the area. Mass evacuation can cause large
traffic jams. In many cases the agent may be moving much
faster than people can evacuate. Cars and buses do not provide
adequate protection against most chemical vapors, resulting in
public exposure.

In some cases a better strategy may be protection in place
(also called in-place sheltering). This concept strives to protect
the public in homes or other structures. It uses the concept
that an "air bubble" is present inside the building or can be
created by sealing the structure and limiting the air exchange
from external to internal environments.

Protection in place uses the same basic concepts and engineering strategies that allow buildings to be heated and cooled. Air exchange rates are reduced by shutting down air-handling systems and ensuring that all doors and windows remain closed. Newer, more energy-efficient structures will provide better protection. Even greater levels of protection can be afforded by sealing windows and doors with plastic and tape. This concept may be the only method available when the public could be exposed during the evacuation process. It may also be the only choice available for facilities that may be difficult or impossible to evacuate on short notice, such as schools, nursing homes, and hospitals.

The problem with protection in place is that it is a short-term protection procedure. Contamination will eventually make its way inside the structure. Usually a maximum time of 3 hours of protection in a modern structure is given as a planning guideline.

Evacuation and protection in place can be used to complement each other. There is no single protective measure that can be used in all situations. As the conditions of the event change, so must the strategies that are employed to protect the public. In all cases the incident commander must approve the decisions.

SCENE MANAGEMENT

Site security is necessary to limit scene access to properly trained and equipped response personnel. These events are news-worthy and attract a lot of attention. Bystanders and news media personnel may easily end up in the wrong area and become unwilling participants. Force protection is also necessary. Secondary devices, terrorists mixed in the patient population, and looting are all distinct possibilities. Many police departments are training and equipping their staff to operate in contaminated environments and to provide security force protection duties (Fig. 9-8).

CONTROL ZONES

Control zones should be established during an incident to reduce the chances of accidental spread of contaminants by responders. Different types of operations will occur within these zones, and the flow of personnel in and out of the zones can be controlled.

Control zones are necessary to ensure that response personnel and the public are protected against hazards, contamination is confined to the appropriate areas, and personnel can be accounted for and evacuated if necessary. Typically, three zones are established: the hot zone, warm zone, and cold zone (Fig. 9-9).

HOT ZONE

The hot, or exclusion, zone is the area in which contamination currently exists or areas that may be contaminated in a short time. Activities in this zone include scene characterization, patient rescue, and mitigation activities. Entrance into this zone will require proper training and appropriate PPE, given the identified or suspected threat (Fig. 9-10).

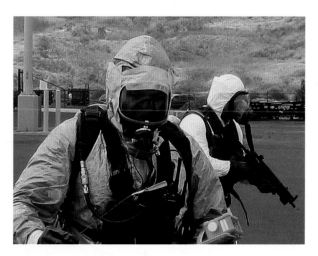

Fig. 9-8
Law enforcement personnel capable of operating in personal protective equipment will be a valuable asset at a WMD incident.

Activities in this zone must be conducted using the buddy system. This means that responders must work in teams of at least two people and that a backup team must be ready. All people exiting this area must be decontaminated. The buddy system alone may not be sufficient to ensure that help will be provided in an emergency. At all times, responders in the hot zone should be in line of sight of or have verbal communication with backup personnel in the warm or cold zone.

Because this area is contaminated, the most obvious patient management technique is rapid patient removal. EMS units do not usually operate in the hot zone, but responder involvement will depend on area needs, standard operating procedures, training, and specific incident considerations. These issues must be dealt with as a part of preplanning. Awareness Level EMS responders are restricted to the cold zone, and Operations Level responders may work in the warm zone. Because entry into the hot zone may involve direct contact with the agent, EMS responders who work in the hot zone should be trained to a technician or specialist equivalent (Box 9-2).

In multiple or mass casualty incidents, triage may be needed in the hot zone. If patients are trapped in the hot zone, they may require EMS treatment during extrication activities. Patient care activities in this area should routinely include rapid patient removal, with attention to possible spine injuries. If the patient is trapped or pinned, stabilizing care may be required (medical procedures must be carried out by qualified personnel). Airway control and isolation of the spontaneously breathing patient's airway with an escape mask will limit any further inhalation exposure. If the patient needs ventilatory support, it should be provided with a demand valve or bag-valve-mask with a chemical filter. Rapid spine immobilization should be carried out as necessary, and the patient should be removed rapidly from the area.

Because of the difficulties of assessing and treating patients while wearing PPE, patient care in this zone is extremely limited.

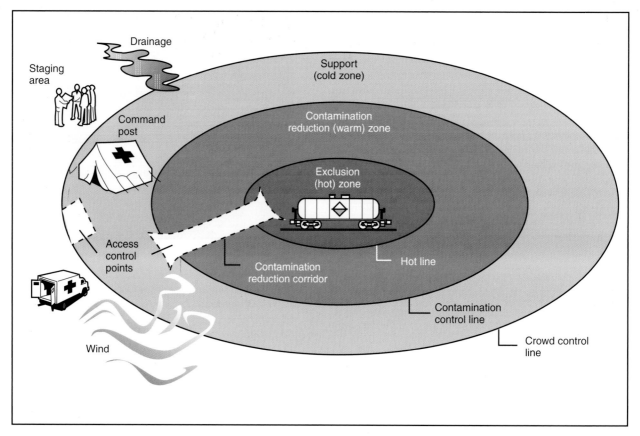

Fig. 9-9
Response zones are established to isolate the scene and protect responders.

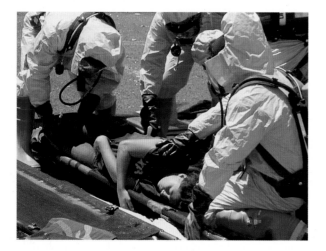

Fig. 9-10
Responders should extract victims from the hot zone as quickly as possible.

Patient Care Activities in the Hot Zone*   Box 9-2

- Medical or trauma stabilization care may be required if the patient is pinned or trapped (medical procedures must be carried out by qualified personnel). Because of the contaminated environment, invasive procedures must be kept to the absolute minimum.
- Airway control
- Isolation of spontaneously breathing patient's airway with an escape mask, SCBA, filtered bag-valve-mask, or ventilator
- Rapid patient removal, with attention to possible spinal injuries, when extrication procedures are complete

*Activities in this zone require proper preplanning, training, and personal protective equipment.

Remember that any activity, including rescue, will require proper preplanning, training, and appropriate PPE.

WARM ZONE

The warm zone, also called the contamination reduction zone (CRZ), is the transition area between the contaminated and clean areas. It is designed to reduce the probability that the clean areas will become contaminated or affected by scene hazards. This is an area of potential contamination and must be adequately controlled (Fig. 9-11).

The decontamination procedures and the distance between the hot zone and clean areas limit the physical transfer of hazardous substances into clean areas. Decontamination procedures take place in a designated area within the warm zone called the *contamination reduction corridor,* the *decon corridor,* or the *decon line.* The number of personnel allowed in this area is kept to a minimum, and they must be properly trained (Operations Level at a minimum) and wearing appropriate PPE. The level of protection in this zone usually is one level below that of the entry team but may be the same level, depending on the hazards that are present. Conversely, air-purifying respirators may be used if air-monitoring results show that the level of contamination is within their protective envelope. (Detailed PPE information can be found in Chapter 12.)

All personnel must be decontaminated before exiting this area. No eating, drinking, or smoking is allowed in this zone. In special circumstances, such as an extended warm zone established because of possible explosions, a forward haven may be established. This is a safe location established in the warm zone in which support functions may be carried out.

Similar to actions in the hot zone, EMS activities in the warm zone require special preparation. Responders with medical training should be available to manage the patients' medical needs during decontamination. EMS involvement again will depend on area needs, standard operating procedures, training (preplanning concerns), and specific incident considerations.

Patient care should be available during decontamination. Ambulatory patient self-decontamination should be supervised and assisted as necessary by properly trained personnel. In multicasualty incidents, triage for decontamination priority may be needed as patients are removed from the hot zone. Qualified personnel also should be available to provide immediate care of injured team members during decontamination.

Usual patient care activities provided in the warm zone include basic life support during decontamination. Airway, breathing, circulation, cervical-spine (c-spine) immobilization, decontamination, and evaluation for systemic toxicity (ABC²DE) should all be considered priority items. Spinal immobilization and oxygen administration should be ensured and continued. As in the hot zone, ventilatory support should be carried out with a demand valve or bag-valve-mask with chemical filter and oxygen as needed.

Invasive procedures, such as starting intravenous (IV) lines or endotracheal intubation, should be limited until complete decontamination can be ensured. Cardiopulmonary resuscitation (CPR) should be performed as necessary during decontamination. Starting or continuing CPR must be based on patient-to-responder ratios and standard triage procedures. As in the hot zone, any activity in this area will require proper preplanning, training, and appropriate PPE (Box 9-3).

COLD ZONE

The cold, or support, zone is an area under responder control but is located safely away from the emergency. All support and rehabilitation functions are located in the cold zone (Fig. 9-12).

The command post and staging area are located in this zone. The command post should be situated in a secure location, away from the danger area. A view of the incident scene is nice but not essential. Adequate communication must be available for the command post. A staging area also should be established in a safe location. Responding units can be amassed in the staging area, which should allow easy access to all sides of the incident so units can be dispatched easily as

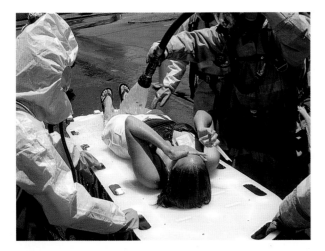

Fig. 9-11
Patient care and decontamination can occur simultaneously in the warm zone.

Patient Care Activities in the Warm Zone*   Box 9-3

- Medical care during decontamination
- ABC²DE
  - Airway
  - Breathing
  - Circulation (hemorrhage control)
  - Cervical-spine stabilization
  - Decontamination
  - Evaluate for systemic toxicity
- Oxygen administration
- Limited invasive procedures
- CPR as necessary and feasible

*Activities in this zone require proper preplanning, training, and personal protective equipment.

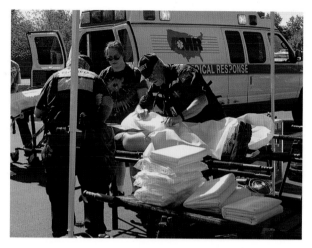

Fig. 9-12
Once the patient is decontaminated, basic and advanced life-support procedures can be carried out in the cold zone.

needed. The person in charge of the staging area must have reliable communication with the incident commander or operations officer.

At this type of incident, EMS personnel will be most active in the cold zone. Patients who have been decontaminated and are as clean as reasonably possible will be cared for in the cold zone. They should be passed to clean caregivers, on a clean backboard, to limit contamination spread. All patient-care equipment that was used in the warm zone should be considered contaminated and must remain in the warm zone. As in the other zones, responder involvement will depend on area needs, standard operating procedures, training (preplanning concerns), and incident-specific considerations (Box 9-4).

CONTROL ZONE CONFIGURATION

The control zones can be established in any configuration necessary to control the incident. For example, for an incident inside a building, the hot zone may be the building itself. A warm zone may surround the building, with the decontamination area set up immediately outside the door. The cold zone would be an area farther out but still surrounding the building.

The line separating the hot and warm zones is called the *hot line.* It should be clearly marked by cones, signs, barrier tape, or existing landmarks. The line separating the warm and cold zones is designated the *contamination control line* and also should be clearly marked. Access-control points should be established to regulate the flow of personnel into the warm and hot zones and help verify that proper procedures for entering and exiting are followed.

The entrance and exit to the hot zone should be located at the decontamination corridor. At large incidents, there may be more than one decontamination entrance and exit point. In these cases, access control must be coordinated so that all personnel can be accounted for in cases of hot zone evacuation.

Patient Care Activities in the Cold Zone*   **Box 9-4**

- Ensure that adequate decontamination has been performed
- Transfer patient from decontamination personnel to medical caregivers to limit contamination spread
- Place patient on clean backboard or stretcher
- Perform basic and advanced life support functions as required

*Activities in this zone will require proper preplanning, training, and minimal personal protective equipment.

Considerations When Establishing Control Zones   **Box 9-5**

Visual survey of the immediate environment
Determination of locations of agent and possible movement patterns
Evaluation of data from detection devices
Distances needed to prevent an explosion or fire from affecting personnel outside the hot zone
Possible areas of secondary device concealment
Distances that personnel must travel to and from the hot zone
Physical area necessary for site operations
Meteorological conditions and predictions

In addition to the primary exit, an emergency exit should be established in case personnel cannot reach the primary exit during an emergency evacuation (Box 9-5).

SAFETY PLAN

Each incident should be handled using an incident-specific safety plan. The safety of all responders and many EMS activities are directed by the safety plan. The incident-specific safety plan must be user friendly and should be a guide or checklist for mitigation of the incident. It also serves to document the response activities and serves as a briefing tool for responders. The safety plan is a dynamic document that should change as scene conditions change. Checklists can be established to assist in developing the safety plan.

PATIENT TRIAGE AND MOVEMENT

The release of a weapon of mass destruction is designed to result in mass casualties. Medical response will almost certainly be overwhelmed. Triage procedures will be necessary to effectively handle the patient population. Triage may be employed many times at MCIs. One triage may be necessary to prioritize which patients are extracted first from the hot zone. A second triage may be necessary to determine which patients should move through the decontamination line first. A third triage may

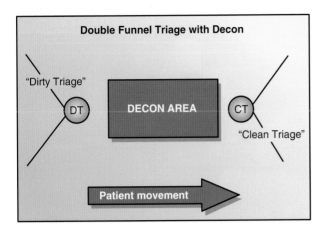

Fig. 9-13
Patients must be triaged multiple times during the extraction and decontamination process.

Simple Triage and Rapid Treatment (START)   Box 9-6

- Ambulatory victims should immediately be moved into one location. These patients should be tagged GREEN. START triage should then be performed on the nonambulatory patients.
- Assess respirations: If 30/min or less, go to perfusion assessment. If more than 30/min tag RED; if no respirations, tag BLACK.
- Assess perfusion: If capillary refill time is 2 seconds or less or you can feel a radial pulse go to mental status assessment. If no radial pulse or capillary refill time is greater than 2 seconds, tag RED. Also, control any external bleeding at this time.
- Assess mental status: If the victim can follow simple commands and is oriented to person, place, and time, tag YELLOW. If the patient does not follow commands or is unconscious, tag RED.

be needed to prioritize patient treatment and transportation after decontamination (Fig. 9-13).

Triage can be difficult under disaster conditions. Add to that the restrictions caused by personnel protective equipment and it becomes a major undertaking. Experienced personnel should be chosen to carry out triage duties. Backup personnel should be identified. Information on decontamination, patient treatment, transportation, and hospital availability is essential for making good triage decisions.

SIMPLE TRIAGE AND RAPID TREATMENT

There are many different triage systems. One of the most popular is the Simple Triage and Rapid Treatment (START) system. START was developed specifically for MCIs where a more rapid sorting of multiple victims is needed at any one time. Ambulatory victims should immediately be moved into one location. These patients should be tagged GREEN. Then START should be performed on the nonambulatory victims. There are four classifications for START (Box 9-6):
- Red: immediate
- Yellow: delayed
- Green: ambulatory (minor)
- Black: deceased (not salvageable)

Here are the three points of assessment for START:
- Assess respirations: If 30/min or less, go to perfusion assessment. If more than 30/min tag RED; if no respirations tag BLACK.
- Assess perfusion: If capillary refill time is 2 seconds or less or you can feel a radial pulse, go to mental status assessment. If no radial pulse or capillary refill time is greater than 2 seconds, tag RED. Also, control any external bleeding at this time.
- Assess mental status: If the victim can follow simple commands and is oriented to person, place, and time, tag YELLOW. If the patient does not follow commands or is unconscious, tag RED.

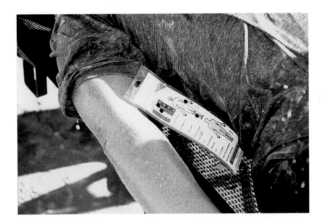

Fig. 9-14
Decontamination triage tag.

EQUIPMENT

Another concern is triage equipment. Thousands of tags may be needed at an MCI. Most agencies do not have anywhere near that number on hand. Triage colored (red, yellow, green, black and white striped) surveyor's tape can be used when standard triage tags run out. Some agencies use blue tape to signify that a patient has been decontaminated.

Paper triage tags and decontamination usually don't mix. There are waterproof triage tags that are designed especially for decontamination operations. Some are designed with a hole-punch system to minimize writing when wearing protective equipment (Fig. 9-14).

PATIENT EVACUATION

Incidents involving many nonambulatory victims will present problems with patient movement. Responders entering the hot zone will be wearing extensive protective

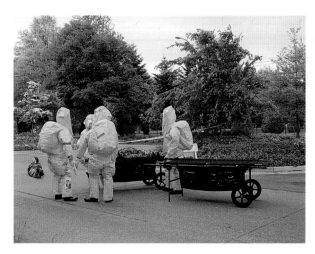

Fig. 9-15
Using stretcher carts to move patients allows responders to work more efficiently.

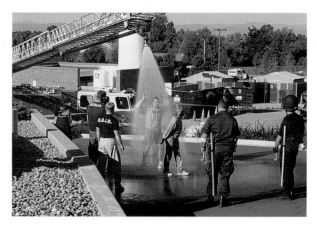

Fig. 9-16
An emergency decontamination system, or drench drill, can decontaminate a large number of people but is not without problems.

equipment. Their numbers will be limited. Responders will quickly tire trying to carry stretcher patients from the hot zone. This will severely limit the number of patients who can be successfully extracted from the hot zone. Manufacturers are inventing new products to help solve this problem. Products include units that can be dragged and wheeled carts that can carry stretchers (Fig. 9-15).

Multiple units will be necessary to move the number of patients involved in these incidents. Patient movement devices should also be available to use on the clean side of decontamination to reduce the physical stress of moving clean patients to care areas or transport.

DECONTAMINATION

Mass decontamination remains one of the significant bottlenecks at MCIs or WMD response. Some agencies are using a procedure known as the *drench drill* (Fig. 9-16). The drench drill uses fire department apparatus or hoses to decontaminate extremely large numbers of patients in a very short period of time. A simple method is to place two fire engines side by side (approximately 15 feet apart) and install fire hose fog nozzles directly on the panel discharge gates. Some departments use a nozzle on an elevated ladder or platform to create an overhead spray.

Although this procedure does move a lot of people through the decontamination process, some concerns must be addressed. Cold water is used, so hypothermia is a concern in cooler temperatures. If clothes are left on during the drench drill, contamination could be driven to the skin. This presents a problem due to lack of privacy and the patient's unwillingness to disrobe. Because of these concerns many teams are using decontamination trailers or special tents and patient roller systems or carts to increase mass casualty decontamination efficiency.

Nonambulatory patients should be moved from the contaminated area to the decontamination area. Trained and properly protected medical personnel should provide essential medical care during the decontamination process. Adequate blankets should be available to reduce the effects of hypothermia.

As in standard decontamination operations, runoff should be collected if possible. Due to the amount of runoff associated with mass decontamination operations, this may be an extremely difficult task. Patient decontamination should not be delayed to allow for runoff containment.

Some WMD decontamination teams use video cameras to photograph both ambulatory and nonambulatory patients' faces as they leave the decontamination area. The videotape is then given to local or federal law enforcement agencies to document the identities of the patients who were decontaminated. Detailed decontamination information for patients and responders can be found in Chapter 13.

PERSONAL PROTECTIVE EQUIPMENT

All responders operating in the warm and hot zones must use appropriate PPE. The exact level and type of PPE will be dictated by the type of incident and contaminant. Responders operating in the hot zone will most likely need vapor-tight, fully encapsulating suits and self-contained breathing apparatus (SCBA) (Level A) or non–vapor-tight, chemical resistant suits and SCBA (Level B) (Figs. 9-17 and 9-18). In some cases, where the contaminant and concentrations have been identified, chemical-resistant suits and an air-purifying respirator (APR) with appropriate cartridges (Level C) may be adequate (Fig. 9-19).

New tests conducted by the U.S. Army Soldier Biological and Chemical Command (SBCCOM) show that firefighter's structural firefighting clothing (turnout) and SCBA could provide protection against chemicals such as nerve agents. The study suggests that turnout (coat, pants, boots, gloves, hood,

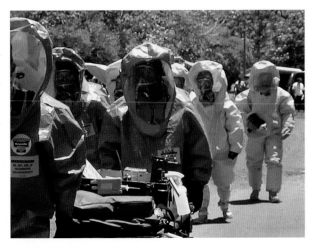

Fig. 9-17
Level A suits provide the highest degree or respiratory and skin protection.

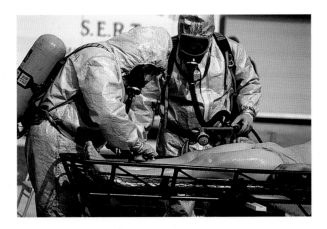

Fig. 9-18
Level B suits are used when the highest level of respiratory protection is needed but a lower level of skin protection is adequate.

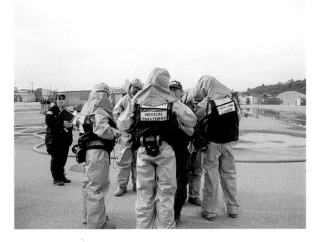

Fig. 9-19
Level C protection consists of an air-purifying respirator and chemical-resistant suit, gloves, and boots.

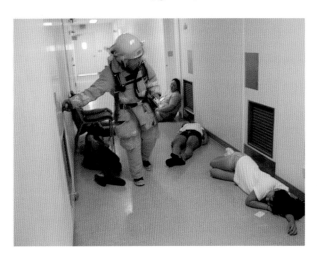

Fig. 9-20
Tests have shown that structural firefighting clothing and self-contained breathing apparatus can offer short-term protection for rescue and reconnaissance.

and helmet, and all openings sealed with tape) plus SCBA could be used in an indoor environment for a short time. If there are no viable patients in the area (suggesting a higher level of contamination), tape-sealed turnout plus SCBA can provide 3 minutes of protection for a rapid reconnaissance. If there are viable patients in the area, this gear can provide up to 30 minutes of protection for rescue operations (Fig. 9-20).

In all cases direct contact with the agent should be avoided. A separate test showed that powered air-purifying respirators (PAPRs) with appropriate cartridges provide protection against many chemical, biological, and radiological warfare agents.

Responders operating in the warm zone will need a lesser degree of protective equipment than those operating in the hot zone. Chemical suits with SCBA (Level B) or chemical suits with air-purifying respirators (Level C) will be needed based on the specifics of the incident. Chemical and air monitoring

data are needed to make an appropriate decision. In all cases decisions about selection of PPE should be made by an experienced and qualified person. Responders should never attempt to use PPE without adequate training and fit testing. More detailed information on PPE can be found in Chapter 12.

RESPONDER MEDICAL SUPPORT

EMS responders can play an integral part in the health and safety of response personnel at a WMD incident. Responders will be working for extended periods of time in protective equipment. They will be at a high risk of heat stress. Many of the agents that they will be facing are extremely toxic. If responders are exposed or injured, immediate care may save their lives. The EMS responder's assessment skills and knowledge

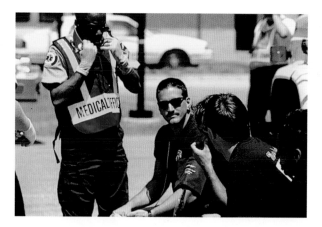

Fig. 9-21
EMS providers should be on scene to manage responders' medical needs.

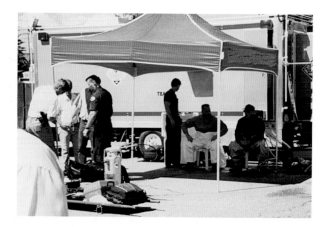

Fig. 9-22
Establishing and using a rest and rehabilitation area will help reduce heat-stress injuries.

of anatomy and physiology, coupled with an understanding of heat stress and PPE, make them the ideal choice to manage these concerns at a WMD incident (Fig. 9-21).

HEAT STRESS

Heat stress or agent exposure can result in severe injuries to response personnel. A responder's monitoring plan will help reduce the chance of injury. EMS responders should work with their local medical control hazardous materials (HAZMAT) team or fire department to establish entry and exclusion criteria. Measures can be taken to prevent or lessen the effects of temperature stress. Measures such as adequate fluid replacement, cooling devices, and proper rehabilitation should all be in place at a WMD incident.

RESPONDER REHABILITATION

Before responders enter the hot zone, EMS personnel should ensure that procedures are in place for responder rest, rehabilitation, and emergency management should a responder be injured. A rest and rehabilitation area and schedule should be established (Fig. 9-22).

The rehabilitation area should be a safe location within the cold zone and should be large enough to accommodate numerous personnel. The area should be easily reached from the decontamination area and should be easily accessible to EMS units for patient loading. It should provide protection from environmental conditions (i.e., a cool, shaded area in warm weather and a warm, dry area in cold weather) if possible. A structure or large vehicle (e.g., bus, truck) located in the cold zone could be used.

Certain supplies and equipment should be available in the rehabilitation area, including fluids for oral replenishment (e.g., cool water, electrolyte solutions) and food. Fruit, stew, soup, or broth will be digested faster than solid food such as sandwiches. Fats and salty foods should be avoided. Medical

equipment will be necessary, including oxygen, blood pressure cuffs and stethoscopes, thermometers, cardiac monitors, IV fluids and administration sets, and advanced cardiac life support (ACLS) medications and antidotes. Support equipment includes tarps and awnings for shade, fans for warm weather and heaters for cold weather, lights for night operations, and extra clothing.

A fixed rehabilitation schedule should be implemented if possible. Many variables must be taken into account when establishing this schedule. The number of technician-trained team members eligible for hot-zone deployment, type of emergency, associated risk factors, level of PPE, and weather conditions must all be considered. A general rule often followed by HAZMAT teams using Level A protective equipment is to take a rest period after each SCBA bottle is used. This will be approximately every 20 to 30 minutes. A rehabilitation schedule also should be established for decontamination team members and support personnel. During the rehabilitation time, team members should move to a safe area and replenish fluids.

PRESERVING EVIDENCE

An incident involving the release of a weapon of mass destruction becomes a hazardous materials response, a mass casualty incident, and a crime scene all in one. The terrorists responsible for the attack may be mixed in with the victims. Victims will be bringing valuable evidence out with them on their clothes and in personal items. Although it is too late to prevent this incident from occurring, law enforcement personnel may be able to prevent the next one by capturing and prosecuting the terrorists.

Paramount to this concern is the collection and preservation of evidence. Medical personnel should have a basic knowledge of this subject. All items removed from patients should be isolated in bags and marked with the information that will link it with the patient. Many triage tags have a tear-off strip that matches the triage tag number. This strip is placed in the bag with the patient's clothing. As much as possible these bags must be isolated and a proper chain of custody followed. Local law enforcement agencies can assist medical responders in developing proper procedures and training programs.

RESOURCES AND PATIENT TREATMENT EQUIPMENT

Certain equipment will be helpful in dealing with mass casualty incidents caused by terrorist attacks or hazardous materials. These include reference sources, patient management equipment, and support equipment.

RESOURCES

Many reference sources are useful for the emergency response to WMD incidents. Many excellent field guides are available, including the companion piece to this book. The Federal Emergency Management Agency's (FEMA) *Emergency Response to Terrorism: Job Aid* is designed in checklist format to guide the initial field response to a WMD incident. Another popular field guide is Jane's *Chem-Bio Handbook.* It is designed to provide quick information on patient management and field procedures. There are numerous military reference sources such as the *Medical Management of Chemical Casualties Handbook* (the "Red Book"), the *Medical Management of Biological Casualties Handbook* (the "Blue Book"), and the *Medical Management of Radiation Casualties.* These are pocket-sized manuals that provide background and treatment information for WMD exposures. Another extremely popular military manual is *The Medical NBC Battlebook.* This manual combines information from many field manuals.

The basic reference source that should be in every ambulance is the *North American Emergency Response Guidebook* (NAERG). Although this manual is designed for response to chemical accidents, it can be used to provide basic response information for WMD agents. The most important individual NAERG guides are:
- Biological agents: Guide 158
- Blister agents: Guide 153
- Blood agents: Guides 117, 125, 131, and 154
- Chemical nerve agents: Guide 153
- Choking agents: Guides 124 and 125
- Irritant agents: Guide 159
- Nuclear and radiological agents: Guides 162, 163, and 164
- Toxic industrial chemicals: Specific guides

The major limitation of the NAERG is that it does not supply detailed information, such as chemical and physical properties, or in-depth patient treatment information. Many other written and computer references supply this information, however. You also have telephone references, such as the Chemical Transportation Emergency Center (CHEMTREC) at 800-424-9300, and your regional poison control center. CHEMTREC provides emergency responders with immediate response information and can contact manufacturers, shippers, and product experts when more detailed information is necessary (Fig. 9-23).

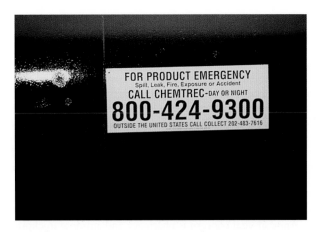

Fig. 9-23
CHEMTREC can contact product experts to obtain detailed information.

Computer references are also available. TOMES Plus is a detailed database available from Thomson Micromedex. It provides detailed response and patient treatment information from numerous databases. The Computer-Aided Management of Emergency Operations (CAMEO) program is a computer database created by the National Oceanographic and Atmospheric Administration (NOAA). It is now available for free download from the EPA. The CAMEO package provides information about more than 3000 chemicals and can predict vapor plume dispersion.

Many other excellent written, telephone, and computer references are available. Responders should find a mix of references that provide assistance in identification, chemical and physical data, emergency response information, and medical management information. No single reference can supply responders with all the information that is necessary. The general rule in using references is to consult a minimum of three and take worst-case data into consideration.

Besides references, EMS responders will find certain support equipment useful. Binoculars or a spotting scope will allow responders to assess the incident from a greater distance and should be part of every ambulance's inventory.

PATIENT TREATMENT EQUIPMENT

Availability of patient treatment supplies for these incidents will be a problem. Mass casualty equipment caches should be located in urban areas where they can be easily acquired and moved. Equipment should include stretchers or backboards, triage and trauma supplies, and decontamination equipment. Large quantities of blankets, towels, and patient gowns should be stockpiled and readily available in case many ambulatory patients must be decontaminated.

Morgan Therapeutic Eye Irrigation Lenses (MorTan, Inc., Missoula, Mont) provide effective ocular irrigation. IV solutions of normal saline and setups also can be used with nasal cannulas to irrigate eyes. The cannula is placed over the bridge of the patient's nose, and the irrigation fluid flows from the cannula across each eye. Disposable medical equipment, such as blood pressure cuffs, stethoscopes, suction units, and laryngoscopes, will save expensive equipment that might not be able to be decontaminated.

Exposure to many biological and chemical agents will result in respiratory compromise requiring ventilatory support. Increased oxygen supplies should be identified for prolonged or multiple-patient situations. Numerous devices are available that allow multiple patients to be treated with oxygen from one regulator. There are also many reasonably priced portable ventilators that can be stockpiled. The military uses a bag-valve-mask unit made by Ambu (Linthicum, Md). It incorporates a chemical–particulate filter on the inlet side and can be used to safely ventilate a patient in a contaminated atmosphere.

Another vital concern is pharmacy and antidote stockpiles. They must be secure and temperature controlled. Some agencies have made agreements with local medical equipment and pharmaceuticals manufacturers to provide equipment and supplies as needed.

Getting fresh supplies to the scene can present problems. Ambulances can drop equipment at the scene before they transport patients to the hospital, and they can replace equipment at the hospital before they return to the scene. Secure, accessible equipment staging areas should be established at the scene.

TRANSPORTATION

These events will likely involve numerous victims. The victims may be ambulatory or nonambulatory. Ambulatory victims will often scatter 360 degrees from the incident. Organized response and decontamination resources will take time to arrive and set up. Many victims may have already exited the area and may be on their way to the hospital before emergency responders have time to arrive and set up at the scene.

Once the news media broadcast the details of the incident, patients who were on the periphery of the incident may think they were exposed and will be calling local hospitals for advice. Early in the incident, hospital emergency departments will be swamped with potentially contaminated patients and requests for information. Obviously, people need information, and they need it as quickly as they can get it.

Patients with known contamination will require decontamination for proper and safe treatment. Unfortunately, it is difficult to determine if the patient is completely decontaminated in the field. Special precautions should be taken to ensure that the patient and crew are protected during transport.

HOSPITAL COMMUNICATION

When responding to a possible terrorist event, early notification and communication with the local hospital's emergency department is essential. Time is needed to carry out research on the weapon (biological, chemical, or radiological) and obtain needed equipment and expertise. Remember that many people may be contacting the local hospital for information and advice. Early communication to the hospital should include the type of agent, any known characteristics of the

agent, and the direction of agent movement, if known. If possible, all hospitals in the area should be contacted. Your base hospital may be able to make the contacts to the other hospitals. The emergency operations center may also be responsible for these contacts.

Receiving hospitals need information on patients being transported by ambulance. They will need to know the number of patients expected. The nature of the agent and expected threats must be communicated. The substance's identity is vital information for proper patient care. Make sure to accurately communicate the name of the agent. The expected route and possible duration of exposure are vital pieces of information for determining population groups at risk of exposure. Some devices use explosives to disseminate the agent. Any associated trauma must be reported. As with any patient, the examination findings and vital signs should be reported.

Because many toxic substances have a delayed onset of symptoms, the symptom trend is important. Both the initial and current signs and symptoms should be noted and reported. The level of decontamination is important. Has the patient been decontaminated? Do you think that the patient will need any further decontamination on arrival? The report should also contain the estimated time of arrival. Remember that it is extremely important to make this contact as soon as possible (Box 9-7).

REDUCING SECONDARY CONTAMINATION

Obviously an exposure potential exists if contaminated patients are transported. Therefore, except in very specific instances, decontamination should always be carried out before transport. In special cases, such as a few patients with severe trauma and low-level particulate radiation exposure or with embedded air- or water-reactive products, proper patient management will

---

Information to Be Communicated to Receiving Hospitals   **Box 9-7**

Number of patients and potential additional patients
Nature of incident
Agent(s) involved
Route(s) of exposure
Duration of exposure
Associated trauma
Victim examination findings and vital signs
Initial signs and symptoms
Treatment administered
Current signs and symptoms
Decontamination carried out?
Need for further decontamination?
Estimated time of arrival

require patients to be isolated and transported before decontamination. Even when patients are decontaminated, a small risk of secondary contamination may still exist. Field decontamination, especially for mass casualties, is carried out in less than ideal conditions. Residual contamination may still exist on the patient.

Postdecontamination patient transportation staging areas should be established. Areas for both ambulatory and nonambulatory patients will be needed. These must be established at a location with easy entry to and egress from the scene. During inclement weather, heated tents or indoor structures will be needed.

There may be an extremely large number of ambulatory patients associated with these incidents. They will have to be transported to hospitals or off-site patient holding or assembly areas. Buses will be useful in transporting ambulatory patients following decontamination. Some patients may have a delayed onset of symptoms, so medical personnel should accompany every transport and be stationed at every holding area. Preplanning activities should include agreements with local transportation and school agencies to provide buses and drivers when necessary. Airport car rental agencies also have access to buses that can be used for this purpose.

Because EMS responders risk secondary contamination when transporting potentially contaminated patients, certain precautions must be taken. The best way to reduce this risk is to decontaminate the patient before transport. Because inhalation is the quickest and most vulnerable route of exposure, adequate ventilation in the transport vehicle is essential. Buses should have all windows open unless weather is extreme.

Nonambulatory patients being transported by ambulance present a greater problem. Their level of contamination was probably greater and the risk of secondary contamination is higher. Ambulances should have both intake and exhaust fans operating to ensure maximum ventilation in the patient care compartment. Some authorities suggest opening all of the windows in the ambulance. Many ambulances do not have windows in the patient compartment, but even with those that do, protection may be inadequate. Windows are bidirectional, allowing some contamination to come back into the ambulance. This may result in inadequate ventilation and an exposure risk. In addition, opening the rear windows may allow exhaust fumes, including carbon monoxide, into the ambulance.

Another suggestion given in many protocols is to completely cover the walls and ceiling of the entire ambulance patient compartment in plastic. Unless time is taken to cut holes for ventilation units and adequately tape down the plastic so there are no flaps, ventilation in the patient compartment will be radically decreased, resulting in an increase of the secondary inhalation hazard to patients and EMS responders. Plastic is useful on the stretcher, floor, and bench to reduce contact exposure from patients who are wet with decontamination water. Precut pieces are useful in reducing excess plastic that may be a tripping hazard. Any water on the plastic also will create a slip hazard.

Another method that sometimes is recommended is reverse isolation (Fig. 9-24). These procedures include postdecontamination isolation of the nonambulatory patient in specially

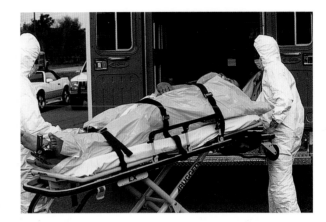

Fig. 9-24
Patient reverse isolation procedures.

designed contaminated-patient transportation bags, plastic, sheets, blankets, or zip-front body bags. Although this process will reduce the risk of secondary contamination of EMS responders, it may increase the risk of further contamination to the patient. When the patient is wrapped up, especially in plastic or a body bag, body temperature will increase, resulting in sweating, open pores, and dilated peripheral blood vessels. If the patient has not been adequately decontaminated, skin absorption may be increased, which 'in turn increases the patient's exposure risk. It has been argued that if adequate patient decontamination has been carried out, there is no need for reverse isolation procedures. Because it is almost impossible to determine if the patient has been adequately decontaminated in the field, a combination of good decontamination and reverse isolation may be useful. Check with your medical control physician and follow his or her recommendations.

EMS personnel may wish to wear respiratory protection and chemical-protective clothing (CPC) when transporting patients who may have been contaminated. Protective equipment should never be used as a reason or excuse not to decontaminate the patient before transport. Lightweight, disposable CPC or body substance isolation equipment can easily be used to reduce the chance of skin exposure and protect the responder's uniform and shoes. Two pairs of gloves (examination and chemical) can provide hand protection.

Respiratory protection is not nearly so easy. Many EMS responders have not been trained and fit-tested to wear air-purifying respirators (APRs) other than disposable high efficiency particulate air (HEPA) respirators commonly used for protection against tuberculosis. HEPA respirators will provide protection against particulates but not chemical vapors or gases. APR filters and cartridges must be specific for the chemical threat. It is difficult and expensive to try to stock a complete selection of respirator cartridges on the ambulance. Remember that some chemicals cannot be filtered or rendered harmless by APRs. Respiratory protection with APRs cannot be ensured unless the responder has been fit-tested into that specific brand, model, and size of respirator. Air-supplied units

(SCBA or air lines) are almost impossible to use during transport unless your ambulance has been specially designed with an air-line system, which is expensive.

In addition to the logistical concerns, the use of chemical-protective equipment, such as respirators and heavy chemical gloves, will complicate patient care procedures. If protective equipment is to be used, responders should practice with the equipment before actual use. In all cases, responders should never attempt to wear respirators or protective clothing unless they have received specific training and fit testing, as necessary, on that piece of equipment. Consider coordinating with the HAZMAT team for training and provision of the proper types of protective equipment.

AIR TRANSPORT

Transporting patients from these incidents by air involves risk. The helicopter may travel through an unsafe area, or the rotor wash from the helicopter may affect vapors or fumes at the scene. If decontamination is not complete, the flight crew could be exposed. Because of this, air transportation of patients from a HAZMAT emergency or WMD incident involving chemicals usually is contraindicated unless rapid transport is absolutely necessary and the patient is *completely* decontaminated or was exposed to a chemical with no risk of secondary contamination.

POSTINCIDENT CONCERNS

After the incident, numerous issues must still be addressed. Procedures must be in place to prevent secondary contamination after the incident is concluded. Residual contamination may still exist on the ambulance and patient care equipment and may present a significant hazard. An incident debriefing and postincident analysis and review should follow every terrorism or HAZMAT response. Response procedures should be assessed. Procedures also should be in place to deal with any emotional stress created by the incident.

CONTAMINATION CONTROL

All articles that might be contaminated must be isolated for further testing and for proper decontamination or disposal according to federal, state, and local regulations. These items may include patient clothes and personal possessions, any contaminated patient care equipment, and the responder's contaminated uniforms or PPE. Patient clothes and personal possessions isolated during the response will most likely be turned over to law enforcement as evidence. If they are not, they must be completely decontaminated before being returned to the owner or disposed of properly.

Contaminated uniforms or PPE must be handled properly. Contaminated clothing should never be taken home and laundered or disposed of. It should be disposed of as hazardous waste or isolated for cleaning at a designated facility.

Patient care equipment is another concern. If equipment is to be reused, decontamination must be complete. The local or state health department, CHEMTREC, or the Agency for Toxic Substances and Disease Registry (ATSDR) may be able to provide advice on complete decontamination procedures. Wipe samples from decontaminated surfaces can be sent for laboratory analysis to ensure that decontamination is complete. Most laboratories will provide sample wipes, containers, and instructions on how to obtain and preserve the sample.

Any contaminated items that cannot be decontaminated must be disposed of as hazardous waste. Contaminated items should be isolated and left at the scene for proper cleanup and disposal. Items that must be removed from the scene, such as responder uniforms and patient care equipment used during transport, should be isolated and a responsible party contacted for pickup and disposal. The hazardous waste division of your state health department can offer valuable assistance and advice on handling hazardous waste properly.

The ambulance also may be contaminated. Returning the unit to service prematurely will expose EMS personnel and create a hazard for other patients. The unit should be isolated until it can be decontaminated, including a thorough decontamination of the patient compartment, as well as mechanical and exterior decontamination if needed. Tests, such as wipe sampling, can be carried out to ensure proper decontamination. In most cases a bleach solution or soap and water are adequate for vehicle decontamination. CHEMTREC, ATSDR, and the local health department can assist with decision making. This is another reason to ensure safe scene practices and adequate decontamination before transport. If patients are clean and ambulances remained a safe distance from the release, then ambulances and equipment also will be clean.

EMS responders also must undergo decontamination as necessary. Responders should take all steps to avoid contact with the agent. If the responders were contaminated or their protection from contamination was uncertain, they should follow a procedure that will ensure proper decontamination. Detailed decontamination procedures can be found in Chapter 13. Contaminated articles (clothing, personal possessions, equipment) should be isolated in polyethylene bags or hazardous materials drums until they can be properly decontaminated or disposed of as necessary. All scene responders should shower and change into clean clothes as soon as possible after the incident response is terminated.

MEDICAL FOLLOW-UP

Medical follow-up for EMS personnel should be carried out as needed. The Occupational Safety and Health Administration (OSHA) Hazardous Waste Operations and Emergency Response (HAZWOPER) regulation requires exposure-specific examinations for any personnel who were exposed and injured during a hazardous materials response; a WMD incident is considered a hazardous materials response. Every EMS responder should complete a personnel exposure record. This record should include the type of agent involved in the incident. Any possibility of exposure and the type of PPE used should be recorded. Any signs and symptoms that are experienced and the type of immediate medical care received also should be recorded.

POSTINCIDENT DEBRIEFING

Fortunately, we have not experienced many WMD incidents. However, this lack of experience does present problems. We have not had the opportunity to adequately test procedures and maintain proficiency of special skills. Therefore every exercise and certainly every incident should be followed up with specific termination procedures. All responders should be debriefed immediately following the incident so that they know what agents they have been exposed to and so that any necessary precautions can be taken. Any equipment that was damaged or needs specialized decontamination also should be taken care of. Responsibilities can be assigned for gathering information for a postincident analysis and review. The need for a critical incident stress management meeting should be assessed.

POSTINCIDENT ANALYSIS

The second step is to conduct a postincident analysis (PIA). The PIA is an in-depth look at the response from start to finish. One purpose of the PIA is to ensure that the incident has been properly documented and reported. It also establishes a clear picture of the response practices and procedures for further study. It provides a foundation for developing formal investigations and establishes information that can be used to guide the incident review.

INCIDENT REVIEW

The final step is to hold an incident review. Because multiple agencies are involved at these incidents, there may be multiple agency reviews, with key personnel participating in an agency-wide review. Communications during the incident should be examined. A major problem at many large incidents is a lack of essential personnel, equipment, and supplies. Reviews can give administrators a realistic list of equipment and other resources that were actually needed at the incident.

An incident review can identify what areas of an emergency response plan need changing. Emergency response plans should constantly be rehearsed or examined after an incident, changed as necessary, and rehearsed again. One very important note: The review must be well managed, and it should never be used to assign blame. The review should promote teamwork and be a valuable learning experience.

CRITICAL INCIDENT STRESS MANAGEMENT

Another factor to consider is the effect of stress on EMS personnel. Stress factors will be extraordinarily high because of the nature of the incident and its many complicating factors. The inability to intervene at the scene because of inadequate equipment or training is a major factor. Medical training has always emphasized the need for quick intervention and transport. In WMD incidents, EMS personnel may find themselves waiting for an extended period for patients to be rescued

and decontaminated. Multiple victims will necessitate making triage decisions, leading to increased stress. Concerns for response team member safety may have been a factor at the scene. There may also be questions and concerns regarding possible exposure and delayed health effects. The services of a qualified critical incident stress management team should be obtained. In long-duration incidents, on-scene critical incident stress management procedures should be considered. Detailed information on critical incident stress management can be found in Chapter 14.

BIBLIOGRAPHY

Agency for Toxic Substances and Disease Registry: *Managing hazardous materials incidents, emergency medical services: a planning guide for the management of contaminated patients,* Atlanta, 2001, U.S. Department of Health and Human Services.

Andrews LP, editor: *Emergency responder training manual for the hazardous materials technician,* New York, 1992, Van Nostrand Reinhold.

Bowen JE: *Emergency management of hazardous materials incidents,* Quincy, Mass, 1995, National Fire Protection Association.

Bronstein AC, Currance PL: *Emergency care for hazardous materials exposure,* ed 2, St Louis, 1994, Mosby.

Bronstein AC, Currance PL: Module 4: emergency medical operations. In Ayers S, Christopher J, editors: *Medical response to chemical emergencies,* Washington, DC, 1994, Chemical Manufacturers Association.

Buck G: *Preparing for biological terrorism,* Albany, NY, 2002, Delmar.

Currance PL: *Hazmat for EMS,* St Louis, 1995, Mosby (videotape and guidebook).

Currance PL, Bronstein AC: *Hazardous materials for EMS,* St Louis, 1999, Mosby.

Department of Transportation: *2000 North American emergency response guidebook,* Office of Hazardous Materials Transportation, Research and Special Programs Administration, Washington, DC, 2000, U.S. Department of Transportation, http://www.tc.gc.ca/canutec/erg_gmu/erg2000_menu.htm, retrieved September 20, 2004.

EMS sector standard operating procedures. In Tokle G, editor: *Hazardous materials response handbook,* ed 2, Quincy, Mass, 1993, National Fire Protection Association.

Environmental Protection Agency: *Computer-aided management of emergency operations,* http://www.epa.gov/ceppo/cameo/, retrieved September 20, 2004.

Federal Emergency Management Agency: *Emergency response to terrorism: job aid,* Washington, DC, 2000, Federal Emergency Management Agency, http://www.usfa.fema.gov/fire-service/c-terror/download-jobaid.shtm, retrieved September 20, 2004.

Guidelines for public sector hazardous materials training, HMEP Curriculum Guidelines, Emmitsburg, Md, 1998, National Emergency Training Center.

Hawley C: *Hazardous materials incidents,* Albany, NY, 2002, Delmar.

Laughlin J, Trebisacci DG, editors: *Hazardous materials response handbook,* ed 2, Quincy, Mass, 2002, National Fire Protection Association.

National Fire Protection Association: *NFPA 471, Recommended practice for responding to hazardous materials incidents,* Quincy, Mass, 2002, National Fire Protection Association.

National Fire Protection Association: *NFPA 473, Standard for professional competence of EMS responders to hazardous materials incidents,* Quincy, Mass, 2002, National Fire Protection Association.

Noll GG, Hildebrand MS, Yvorra JG: *Hazardous materials: managing the incident,* ed 2, Stillwater, Okla, 1995, Fire Protection Publications.

Occupational Safety and Health Administration: *29 CFR 1910.120, Hazardous waste operations and emergency response;* Final rule, March 6, 1989; Washington, DC, 1989, U.S. Government Printing Office.

Strong CB, Irvin TR: *Emergency response and hazardous chemical management: principles and practices,* Delray Beach, Fla, 1996, St Lucie Press.

Varela J, editor: *Hazardous materials handbook for emergency responders,* New York, 1996, Van Nostrand Reinhold.

Chapter **10**

Hospital Management of a Mass Casualty Incident

LANA BLACKWELL AND WENDY HOUT

CHAPTER OBJECTIVES

At the conclusion of this chapter the student will be able to:

- Discuss the need for emergency operations planning for the mass casualty incident related to WMD.
- Explain the Hospital Emergency Incident Command System (HEICS) and the versatility of using HEICS in the emergency management plan (EMP).
- Discuss Joint Commission on Accreditation of Healthcare Organizations (JCAHO), National Institute for Occupational Safety and Health (NIOSH), and Occupational Safety and Health Administration (OSHA) regulations related to emergency management planning for MCIs in acute care facilities.
- Explain the importance of preplanning and hazard vulnerability assessment in developing the EMP.
- Describe the essential components of an EMP.
- Discuss the decontamination process for ambulatory and nonambulatory victims and for special populations.
- Discuss specific health care facility planning and special considerations for casualties of biological, chemical, and nuclear incidents.

CASE STUDY

It was a Saturday afternoon, and approximately 10,000 people had gathered downtown at the capital for a political protest. Media, onlookers, security, police, and Emergency Medical System (EMS) personnel were everywhere. Suddenly a loud explosion was heard coming from the middle of the crowd; someone had just set off an explosive device. Immediately people began running and screaming in a panic. Many casualties were seen around the immediate area of the explosion. The thousands of other protesters began running in all directions. Police officers activated their emergency operation procedures, including notification of all local emergency medical providers and local hospitals. EMS providers began to triage the casualties and begin transport. Local fire departments arrived to set up an incident command post in conjunction with officials at the scene. Information was spilling into the local hospitals in bits and pieces.

The local hospitals were already operating at full capacity in their urban communities. When notified of the incident, the hospitals activated their emergency management plans including their Hospital Emergency Incident Command System. Calls started to come into the local emergency departments. First reports coming in pointed toward the use of a dirty bomb. Victims at the scene had multiple injuries from the blast and they were exhibiting signs and symptoms of an exposure to an unknown agent.

What type of agent might this be?

What type of decontamination is necessary for this agent?

What type of symptoms and injuries will these victims have?

What level of personal protective equipment (PPE) must hospital personnel use if they are to decontaminate victims of this agent?

What positions are necessary in the first few hours of the mass casualty using the hospital incident command system?

Is your facility prepared to answer the questions in this case study? How would your facility respond to this mass casualty incident? A *mass casualty incident* is "any large number of casualties produced in a relatively short period of time, usually as the result of a single incident such as an aircraft accident, hurricane, flood, earthquake, or armed attack that exceeds local logistical support capabilities."[11]

Health care facility response to a mass casualty incident has been a source of discussion and planning, and these plans are slowly being refined into a workable format. Health care facilities, including hospitals and clinics, have realized the need for more extensive planning. It has become more evident that all workplaces and all communities risk the threat of domestic terrorism as well as natural disasters. Potential targets include amusement and entertainment venues, government facilities and buildings, hospitals, hotels, industrial plants, private office buildings, shopping malls, sporting events, transportation systems, and utilities.

Those involved in making emergency management plans are preparing for an event that *will*, not *might*, happen in their community (Fig.10-1).

EMERGENCY MANAGEMENT PLAN

JCAHO, NIOSH, and OSHA are requiring health care facilities to adopt an emergency management plan (EMP) that can work for *any* number of victims for *any* incident. In addition, the JCAHO and the American Hospital Association have specifically recommended policies and procedures for mass casualty and biological weapons planning and response. Included in this emergency management plan, health care facilities must prepare to accept many patients at any one time *and* be able to decontaminate these patients in the event of a hazardous materials or WMD event.

Before health care facilities prepare to decontaminate victims, the staff must be aware of and recognize signs and symptoms of biological, chemical, and radiological exposures. Only then can proper decontamination and appropriate care take place. This requires extensive training of all health care personnel involved, from the emergency department staff to the environmental staff. The training should all be outlined in the emergency management plan. The following material identifies key areas necessary for a functional emergency management plan.

PHASES

Disaster preparation is often overwhelming. An emergency management plan is essential, and preparation can be simplified by dividing the plan into phases. The emergency management plan is often divided into four phases: mitigation or risk-vulnerability assessment, preparedness, response, and recovery. Incident command is a major component of the EMP that guides a system through the challenges of these phases. Under

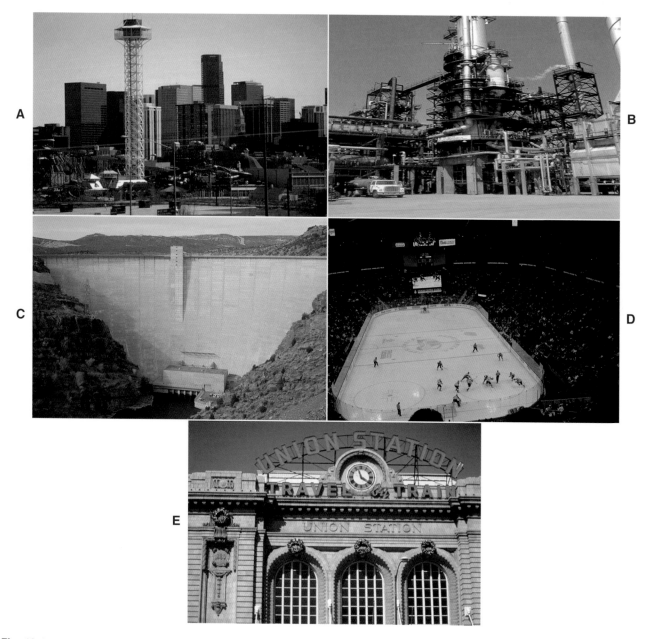

Fig. 10-1
Many different locations are considered terrorist targets.

these sections, details will develop into a functional emergency management plan. Although each facility has its own customs, the basics are the same. This chapter first addresses the primary sections of the EMP and then gives details that can assist your facility in making or revising your plan for dealing with weapons of mass destruction.

Phase one of an emergency management plan is *mitigation*. In this phase, the facility tries to determine what it might be dealing with, identifying the facility's risks and vulnerabilities,

and thereby reducing the severity and impact of a potential emergency. Appendix C gives a list of questions that can help your facility determine its risks and then develop the plan from there. Many commercial tools are also available to assist facilities with this step. Now that terrorism is in the front of our minds, rethink this part of your EMP and look for any necessary revisions. Use all available resources to make a comprehensive risk analysis. Talk with your local police, fire, public health service, and FBI officials. Do not try to reinvent the wheel; they may have information that is valuable in planning for terrorism. This step will also open up lines of communication and begin the process of community involvement.

Phase two is the *preparedness and improvement* phase. It is the time to replace processes that do not work and to build on other processes that do work. It is also a time to identify available resources. This is when involvement and input from all areas of the facility become crucial. Listen to those who deal with these issues on a routine basis. Review regulatory standards, measure progress, and consider what changes or adaptations must be made to the EMP. Changes are often identified through actual incidents, drills, or table-top exercises.

Phase three is the *response or implementation* phase of the EMP. Make this phase as simple as possible. Make role and responsibility cards and checklists for all team members to follow. Disaster management kits are available for purchase that can help in this organizational phase. In some cases it is just as easy to make your own role cards to fit your needs. If personnel have checklists to follow during an MCI, chaos and missed steps can be avoided.

Recovery is the fourth and final phase of the overall EMP. Recovery needs just as much planning as the other phases do. If your facility has been contaminated or suffered physical damage, for example, does your plan provide for back-up facilities? The plan must consider maintaining the overall operations of the facility and managing an MCI at the same time.

HOSPITAL EMERGENCY INCIDENT COMMAND SYSTEM

Efficient use of the incident command system can steer the facility through all phases of the EMP. The Hospital Emergency Incident Command System (HEICS), a system developed in the 1990s in California, is an "emergency management system which employs a logical management structure, defined responsibilities, clear reporting channels, and a common nomenclature to help unify hospitals with other emergency responders."[14] In 1999, JCAHO revised its Standard EC, Environment of Care, to include the following regarding a facility's emergency management plan: "A plan addresses emergency management . . . [and] should address four phases of emergency management activities: mitigation, preparedness, response, and recovery."[7] HEICS was developed to address such issues as managing an emergency and directing facilities in their MCI response through the incident command system (Fig. 10-2).

HEICS is similar to the prehospital emergency management system that has existed for years in the fire service, the Incident Command System (ICS). The ICS is discussed in Chapter 8. HEICS or some form of it is being adopted by facilities across the nation because of its compatibility with the ICS system. The compatibility of these two systems improves communication among health care facilities, EMS, police departments, and fire agencies. During revisions of your current emergency operation plans, make the ICS your standard operating procedure when any plan is activated.

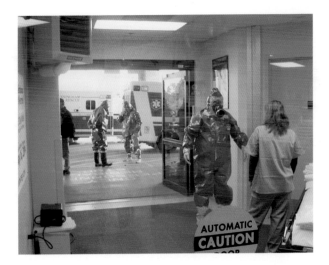

Fig. 10-2
Hospitals need an identified incident command system just as much as prehospital responders do.

HEICS provides a predictable chain of management, a flexible organizational chart, prioritized response checklists, accountability of position function, reliable documentation, common language to promote communication and facilitate outside assistance and a cost effective emergency plan.[14]

HEICS is not meant to be the entire emergency management plan of a facility, but it can provide organized structure to an otherwise chaotic MCI.

At first glance, the HEICS organizational chart is overwhelming with its 49 operational positions. Each position has a checklist of responsibilities that are divided into immediate, intermediate, and extended functions. The advantage of the HEICS plan is its flexibility: It uses only the positions that are required in each individual emergency. For example, the HEICS plan may be fully activated for a catastrophic, extended MCI, such as an earthquake, that could take hours or even days, but the majority of MCIs require the activation of far fewer positions. Therefore, during the initial activation of the HEICS plan in an MCI, one person may be filling multiple positions, and other positions might not be used. As the MCI continues and more personnel arrive, positions can be redistributed and more positions can be used. As the crisis dissipates, the positions can slowly be eliminated until finally the HEICS plan is discontinued.

HEICS is but one area of a complete emergency management plan that requires preplanning. Many other areas also require preplanning. See Appendix D for an outline of medical facility preparedness and preplanning guidelines that will be covered under essentials of the EMP.

During the preplanning and revision phases of the EMP, clearly define all areas in policies and procedures. Preplanning is not just an important part of the emergency management plan; it is a requirement by JCAHO and OSHA. In addition, safety officers and personnel who perform decontamination must be trained to the level required by OSHA's Hazardous Waste Operations and Emergency Response regulations.[4] OSHA's regulations address employee safety, personal protection, decontamination, and training. JCAHO also requires the facility to perform two drills to test the facility's EMP every year. Other components of the preplanning process include fit-testing and maintenance of PPE, maintenance of decontamination equipment, and ease of procurement of equipment that will be needed during an MCI.

The other standard requirement that is critical to the EMP is community involvement. The plan must define the organization's role within the community-wide emergency response plan. This includes integration with other emergency response systems and crucial coordination of media and security issues that can arise during an MCI. Jurisdictional issues and regional issues must be discussed and resolved before a terrorist event or WMD incident to make for smooth transitions and communication during an MCI.

ESSENTIAL COMPONENTS OF AN EMERGENCY MANAGEMENT PLAN

Essential components of an emergency management plan all require preplanning. These same components make a successful plan for an MCI involving terrorism or weapons of mass destruction. Planning should be more important than the actual written document. Planning brings people into the process and allows for personal contacts that can affect how the final product looks. Research shows that predisaster contacts result in a smoother emergency operation when an incident occurs. Initiation of the actual EMP must be practiced over and over to establish trust and an understanding of others' roles and responsibilities and to provide success for the process.

MITIGATION, VULNERABILITY, AND RISK ASSESSMENT

Disasters are not just large emergencies. Research shows that disasters present unique problems that require different strategies, especially for MCIs involving terrorism or WMD.

Every plan must start by knowing what risks to prepare for. Mitigation is the part of the plan that helps the facility avoid becoming a part of the disaster. This plan is valuable to the facility only if it can anticipate the problems that are likely to be faced and then plan for cost-effective and realistic countermeasures. For example, preplan for special events that could result in an MCI in your community and be aware of the National Terrorist Alert System. Remember that the goal of terrorism is not necessarily mass casualties but inciting fear. Mass casualties may just be the outcome.

Be alert to promotions of political, economic, military, ethnic, or religious agendas identified in your community. Keep in mind these predictions from the Chemical and Biological Arms Control Institute: Use of chemical agents is more likely than use of biological agents; use of industrial chemicals is more likely than use of military chemicals; dispersal is most likely in enclosed areas. Then consider vulnerability and look at population demographics, geographic location, and shelter-

ing areas. The Government Accounting Office in 1998 suggested looking at these same areas for threat and risk assessment. Presidential Decision Directive 62 recommends that a threat and risk assessment also be performed on such targets as telecommunications and financial infrastructures.

One of the lessons learned from disaster literature is that most complications arise from a lack of interjurisdictional and interorganizational coordination and communication. We are at greatest risk of failure if health care facilities and organizations plan in isolation. Contact your local emergency management office and become a part of the community disaster planning. If possible, through your local officer of emergency management or community contacts, gain access to as much nonclassified intelligence as you can from local and federal law enforcement sources.

This is just the beginning of the plan for MCI related to terrorism and WMD. How do you then actually manage the incident?

ACTIVATION AND DEACTIVATION

Some form of hospital incident command system answers the question of management. HEICS is designed for any hospital emergency. This includes MCIs involving WMD, but how and when is the system activated? Activation and deactivation responses of the EMP must be clearly defined. The health care facility must define who initiates the response and where, how, and when the response is initiated. Deactivation of the response is just as important as activation and requires the same criteria. Who decides when and how deactivation takes place must also be clearly defined.

Residual effects of a mass casualty are not clearly defined, but research tells us that they can last for weeks or months. The many operational positions in the HEICS will provide valuable input for the decision to deactivate. All of these decisions must be practiced and valued by all of those who could be involved in these decisions at some time or other.

COMMUNICATION MODEL

One of the most important internal functions that is often put off until an MCI occurs is communication. Communication is also the frequent subject of research issues in an MCI. One recurring lesson in disaster response is the lack of mutual aid radio frequencies for two-way communication. How are departments going to communicate with one another *and* incident command during the MCI? What if the phone lines are tied up by people calling in or out of the hospital? Health care facilities can arrange to have priority with a telephone company when lines are jammed, but what if the phone lines are down because of a terrorist attack?

A number of backup systems can be used. Keep in mind that ground and cell phones are the first form of communication lost or overloaded during an MCI. Often there is only one telephone operator on the night shift, and if the MCI occurs at night the operator will immediately be overwhelmed with call volume and require immediate backup. The engineering and telecommunications departments must plan redundancy into communication systems so they are ready for any disaster.

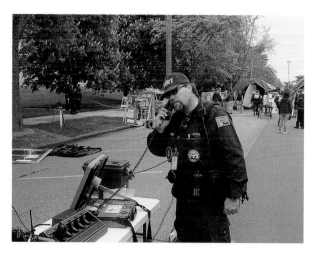

Fig. 10-3
Several forms of communication should be identified. A responder uses a satellite phone to establish contact with the hospital.

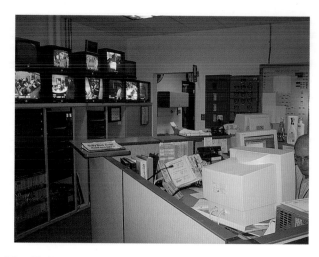

Fig. 10-4
The hospital incident command post can be located separate from the emergency department. The security office might be a good choice.

Handheld radios are a good form of communication, but only a limited number of channels are available. Handheld radios are also a great backup to the internal wireless phones because they do not depend on any infrastructure. The disadvantage of the handheld is that it can handle only one transmission on a channel at a time. Handhelds are often not programmed to interface with outside responding agencies.

Another choice is the all-in-one digital phone. Internal wireless phones are a very good resource and can be used on a day-to-day basis. Because personnel are familiar with how to use them, they are a good system for an MCI. They can provide many services, such as text and numerical pages, two-way radio communication, and Internet. This phone lets you talk to one person or transmit to a group. It has become a very popular mode of communication in busy or large units and can easily be adapted for an MCI.

Do not forget internal resources for communication from outside the facility such as battery-operated radios, televisions, and hand-held radios that provide severe weather alerts. Satellite phones can be another option. Satellite telephone systems can be effective because they are portable, can operate anywhere, and are no longer too expensive to own (Fig. 10-3).

Another resource that is often forgotten is the amateur radio network. A disaster seldom destroys the amateur radio network.

When all else fails, return to the basics. Devise a manual communication system using runners and communication forms, and assign someone to log all messages.

Whatever system the facility chooses, redundancy and the capability for two-way communication internally and externally is essential. Remember that this communication system may be the link to the outside world. It is now common for the facility's command center to be located separate from the main building (Fig. 10-4).

Does your system accommodate all these facets? Backup hardware is essential to the communications plan. Study your community to make the most of your plan. Most facilities will have to research all options and consult an expert in communications to provide the system or systems needed to survive a true terrorist MCI. This is money well spent.

Equipment is essential for communication, but so are the people using the system and what they are communicating. There must be someone responsible for collecting critical information and getting that information to all the key organizational structures in a timely manner. For example, during an MCI involving terrorism and WMD, the facility needs to know what the agent is, how many casualties it can expect, and when to expect them. Who in the field is responsible for getting this information to the facilities? The prehospital ICS must be prepared to pass this information along. This is another example of community-wide training that can have a great impact on the outcome of MCIs. Community involvement and interacting with outside agencies is a key to successful communication in an MCI.

COORDINATED PATIENT CARE

When the news of the MCI reaches the health care facility, policies and procedures regarding coordinated patient care must automatically take effect. A response should be planned for patient care in and out of the facility. This includes transfers out of the facility following the appropriate regulations of the Emergency Medical Treatment and Active Labor Act (EMTALA). Developing a policy that waives regulatory requirements under conditions of an MCI may be worth the time. Clarify the applications of EMTALA, HIPAA (Health Insurance Portability and Accountability Act), and EPA (Environmental Protection Agency) regulations during the time of crisis. Remember that the site of the disaster can

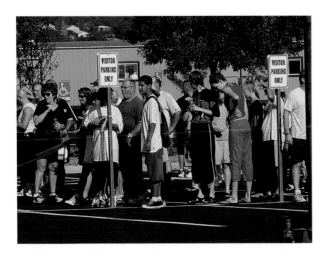

Fig. 10-5
Many patients will self-refer to the closest hospital
when an incident occurs.

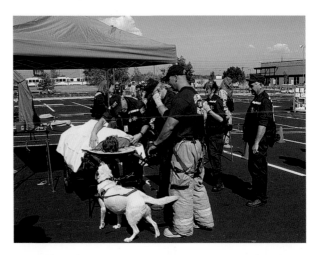

Fig. 10-6
The needs of special populations must be addressed,
including decontamination of service dogs, if necessary.

determine where the greater number of patients will self-refer. If the incident is nearest your facility, you will have to initiate the procedures for rapid discharge and transfer of patients because the majority of victims are coming your way (Fig. 10-5).

Policies for rapid discharge of inpatients on the floor or in the emergency department have to be predetermined so that staff can act without immediate medical direction or with minimal direction by phone if available. Standing orders for patient management and care must go into effect when communication systems are down.

Scrutinize the EMP for the following concerns: Are patients able to leave by a route that is not affected by the influx of victims from the disaster? Do you need a discharge center to manage this process? An evacuation plan that is comprehensive, well thought out, and practiced must be in place in case the facility itself is affected, such as by contaminated patients. Do the stairwells have lighting on backup generator? Can you find enough flashlights to get staff around the unit at night? Do you have agreements with agencies that can provide transport during an incident? Do you have gurneys or backboards that can carry patients down from the top floor of your facility without using the elevators?

JCAHO asks facilities to define their surge capacity in the EMP. Can your facility expand care during a sudden MCI? Contact local emergency planning agencies to become aware of any geographical surge capacity planning. This involves looking at space for potential patient care that is not normally used on a daily basis for such purposes. Identify in the EMP latent space and human resources that can be used during an MCI. Standardization of equipment, supplies, and medications can be of great importance during an MCI when staff are put into unfamiliar situations. Answering these questions can make for a coordinated plan of patient care when evacuation is required.

Although the capacity to handle victims with multiple traumas is important, most research indicates that many injuries

in an MCI are minor and could be managed in medical facilities other than hospitals. According to the Disaster Research Center, only 20% of casualties have to be admitted, on average.[6] If your facility has attached physician medical offices or clinics, consider making them a part of your EMP for coordinated patient care of minor injuries or illnesses.

Victims who seek care for conditions other than trauma must also be covered by your EMP. Victims may have lost their usual source of care, for example, custodial home care or prescription medications. Facilities must maintain the ability to provide routine care even while an MCI is occurring. Exacerbations of chronic medical conditions such as asthma or diabetes will also bring patients into the facility. Preplanning for routine services during an MCI reduces the burden of MCI victims on the hospital and allows MCI victims and routine patients to be treated in tandem.

Special populations must also be considered in coordinated patient care. The young, the elderly, the homebound, and the disabled will require special consideration in your EMP. Think about their needs and how to accommodate them without consuming your time and space. Work out plans for decontamination procedures for these patients (Fig. 10-6). Consider the disabled, wheelchair-bound victim who is exposed and requires decontamination. The very expensive wheelchair now must be decontaminated or secluded as waste. Does your EMP provide for systems that can accommodate the deaf and blind during an MCI? Multilingual personnel and personnel fluent in sign language are invaluable and must be included in preplanning. Establish support systems for this population. This again requires knowing and interacting with the community so that the facility is not overwhelmed during an MCI.

RESOURCE MANAGEMENT

Immediate and long-term planning for an MCI must be considered in the EMP. The general EMP should provide for enough medication, food, water, and shelter to cover the

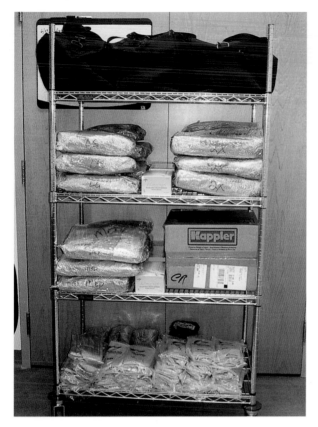

Fig. 10-7
Mass casualty supplies should be readily available.

facility's needs during emergency operations for at least 48 to 72 hours. Exclusive prearranged contracts or memoranda of agreement must be made with agencies to provide service after 72 hours to sustain the facility during an MCI. It is often assumed that resources during an MCI are lacking; to the contrary, however, unsolicited donations of supplies of all kinds are common. Define in the risk analysis what human, equipment, and supply resources are truly available during an MCI (Fig. 10-7).

Sometimes donations require staff resources to track and manage them, especially if they are perishable. Pharmaceutical donations become a problem for several reasons. Often the medications are in quantities not needed, they might be outdated, and they are usually not sorted or organized. During an incident involving weapons of mass destruction, specific antidotes and other medications will be required. Offers of blood donations can overwhelm the system; blood banks are often unprepared for so many volunteers.

Be sure to include in your plan the ability to store, move, and transport these incoming resources. The security of this site and of the loading dock should also be covered in this plan when an incident involves terrorism.

Research shows facilities report having more regular staff and volunteers than they could effectively use. We don't know

if that will prove true during an incident involving nuclear, biological, or chemical incidents. (See also Volunteers.)

MANAGING HUMAN RESOURCES

A good EMP includes preplanning for managing human resources. It is very important to repeatedly practice your emergency management plan. One reason is to be able to efficiently manage personnel when they show up at the facility during an MCI. This includes medical staff, visitors, volunteers, and the media.

Medical Staff. Most facilities have a disaster call down list for each unit of the hospital. This call down list will be activated for response to the MCI. Most call lists are kept at the facility; duplicate lists should be kept elsewhere. Administrators in Houston found during the floods of 2001 that they were unable to get to their facilities to activate the call down lists. They now keep their call lists with them at all times in a personal digital assistant (PDA). The list can also be centrally located in the facility and accessible 24 hours a day to someone responsible for initiating the call down. Depending on the situation, communication may be limited to radio or television. Remember that the media can be a help and a hindrance at the same time.

It is also important to instruct staff not to report directly to their unit but to the designated holding area. Arrange a designated holding area where all the regular staff members will report. If phone lines are working, the facility can have a hotline for staff to call to get information about when and where to report. This hotline can direct them to safe travel routes, specify staff parking lots, and tell them how to respond to the call down list.

Some facilities have set up Internet disaster response communications to use if the Internet is operating during a crisis and to allow for two-way communication. Before an incident, inform the staff that they could be at the facility for 48 to 72 hours at a time for work, for facility lockdown, or because it is unsafe to leave. Remind them to bring a survival bag of food, water, medications, change of clothes, and a pillow.

There will probably be a significant response to the call for help during a crisis involving weapons of mass destruction. In using HEICS for this personnel response, the operations chief and the planning chief will delegate placement of staff. As the operations chief or the planning chief gets a request for more staff, staff can be pulled from the holding area. This is a very efficient, controlled, and coordinated way to use the available staff because staff are needed in many different areas. The operations and planning chiefs will try to use them in the places they are most familiar and comfortable with, but staff must know that they will be expected to go where the needs are. This type of plan also provides for ease of tracking staff entering and exiting the facility.

The operations chief and planning chief must keep the hospital in 24-hour operation. Worker fatigue is often not recognized until workers crash from lack of rest. If a lot of staff show up at the beginning of the MCI, will there be adequate staff for relief in 8 or 12 hours? Unfortunately, this point is generally not recognized until many hours into the MCI, when the relief staff have responded to the disaster call down and are currently at the facility helping, leaving no relief shift available.

When the medical staff arrive, good security will be needed at the designated staff entrance. Here all staff IDs must be checked before allowing entry. During a crisis many well-intentioned people want to help. With a good disaster plan, the staff know that they must have ID or they will not be allowed in the hospital. This must be practiced and reinforced every time the facility practices the EMP, and it must become second nature, *even for physicians*. Administration support can help in implementing this rule.

Volunteers. In major MCIs, including the bombing in Oklahoma City and the attacks on the New York World Trade Center and the Pentagon, one of the recurring issues was the number of people who showed up to help. People often show up at the incident or a facility and say they are medical professionals but do not have their credentials. This can cause problems and has in many cases.

Make a plan to have these people help elsewhere. You can even establish a policy with different ID systems for medical versus nonmedical volunteers. Health care facilities should develop common policy and procedures for checking in, checking credentials, and providing worker's compensation and liability for all volunteers who enter the facility. Predeveloped waivers may be in order for this population. Community planning and immediate assessment of needs and communication of these needs to the public using the media is critical to maintain a manageable volunteer pool.

Family. Management of the family and friends of victims, as well as family of staff members, will also be needed when they arrive at your facility. This is a more sensitive area. Where do you place the family? Where does the information for keeping them updated come from? Are media and the families separated?

The EMP should identify a separate holding area for family and friends of arriving victims. The holding area must meet certain basic requirements, such as access to a working phone, television for updates, and food, water, and bathroom facilities. This holding area must be separate from the media to allow for privacy. If at all possible, a smaller separate area would be nice for family to receive updates on the status of their family members. Confidentiality does not disappear with an MCI.

If family are allowed anywhere else in the facility, such as critical care or the emergency department, then they must be given an obvious family or visitor identification badge when they arrive at the facility. A specified holding area allows physicians and nurses to know where to find families, give status updates, and keep the emergency waiting area clear. When the patient is admitted, the family may be allowed to go to the patient's room.

All of this management requires another staff member to monitor and track the visitors and family and function as a liaison among all departments. The liaison must have knowledge of the facility that will allow him or her to give proper directions to certain areas and knowledge of how the EMP operates to maintain a calm environment. This could be an appropriate area for volunteers to assist in.

The other part of family management involves the staff itself. Some plans allow for an immediate break for on-duty staff to contact their family before an incident overwhelms the facility. Off-duty staff might not be able to respond to the call down unless they can bring their children or pets with them. Some MCIs will require staff to remain at the facility for 48 to 72 hours.

A separate area must be designated for children and pets, and another survival bag will be required. This area must also meet the basic requirements of food, water, bathroom, and sleep areas, with phone, TV, and other entertainment if possible. A specific supply cart or delivery must be made available to this area. A reliable person, possibly a volunteer, must be delegated to this area. Staff must be able to trust that their family is under the watchful eye of someone they know, otherwise how can they concentrate on the task ahead?

Media. Dealing with the media can be a difficult balancing act during an MCI. They can be very helpful in alerting the public to the disaster. Along with this alert, they can provide the public with medical information that can differentiate between real and somatic symptoms of the incident, and they can provide information about what to do and the best place to go at the time of the announcement. The media can also reach non–English-speaking populations; know the languages of your community. All of this can help distribute the population to different facilities and prevent complete chaos. "Trusted media representatives may fulfill a vital function by delivering simple, salient, and repeated messages regarding matters of concern to the public."[1]

Therefore plan *with* the media, because they will be there. Plan for a media holding area that will be staffed by a public information officer (PIO). In your plan, assign more than one person to fill this role; a true MCI will last longer than 24 hours and the PIO will require qualified backup. The PIO immediately establishes a rapport and explains to the media how the situation will be handled. The persons assigned to be PIO must be familiar with current departmental policy, government laws, and any directives that relate to providing information to the media. Confidentiality does not go away during an MCI.

The PIO will also be in charge of verifying official media credentials and establishing an ID system for the media. The holding area can actually be in a separate section of the facility. It must meet the basic requirements of food, water, and bathroom access to keep reporters from wandering all over the facility. In addition, the media and the PIO will require fax machines, electrical outlets, and phone access if this is available during the incident.

The PIO reports directly to and communicates frequently with the hospital's incident commander. The incident command staff preapproves all press briefings. The PIO needs to release accurate updates on a scheduled basis. If the PIO gains the media's trust, the media can help your facility. If the PIO does not keep the promise for scheduled updates, the media will find their own information and it may not be what the PIO wants released. This part of the EMP must also be practiced. General statements of the EMP process within the facility can be prepared prior to an actual incident.

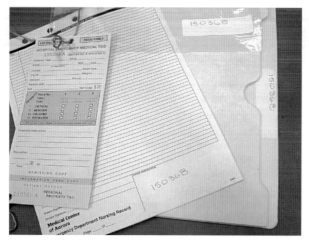

Fig. 10-8
Hospitals should develop patient tracking packets as a preplanning task.

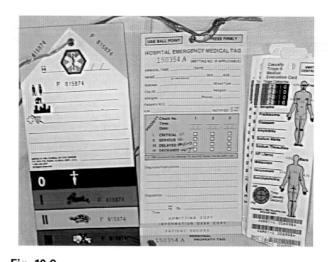

Fig. 10-9
Triage tags are the first step in patient tracking. The tag on the right is designed for use during decontamination.

During table-top exercises, always include the PIO. Have the PIO practice releasing information so that it will be second nature when the actual incident occurs.

DATA MANAGEMENT

Data management includes victim and personnel tracking as well as sharing the data between staging areas. Victim tracking begins when the patient arrives and ends with the patient's discharge from the facility, which is really no different from everyday functions. The difference occurs when normal tracking systems are no longer functioning (Fig. 10-8).

Identification and tracking often becomes a manual process unless multiple laptop computers or other wireless systems with long battery life are available and can communicate with multiple network areas. For victims who are in critical condition and not able to talk, the only form of data management may be the triage tag (Fig. 10-9). The triage tag number *must* remain with the patient, the chart, and all other forms of the medical record at all times. All employees must be familiar with the triage tag system.

Victim tracking can be done on manual forms as victims enter the facility. Individual Polaroid snapshots or videos can also be useful for documentation. Bar-code patient-tracking systems are being developed and tested to manage data from field to hospital during an MCI. This documentation may become part of a forensic or legal document if the incident involves weapons of mass destruction rather than a natural disaster.

Personnel tracking systems are crucial for knowing who entered the facility, when they entered, and where they are currently located in case of a secondary incident. Personnel tracking and contacts with specific victims may be used by the Centers for Disease Control and Prevention (CDC) during a biological event. Therefore, long-term tracking mechanisms

could be essential for worker's compensation claims and medical reimbursement. Tracking for payroll will be important to the employees later and may prevent unnecessary time lags at the end of an event.

All this information must then be communicated among areas in a timely manner. You don't want to lose a staff member in your own facility. It is crucial to plan for these tracking mechanisms if you are to prevent chaos and confusion.

SECURITY MEASURES

Security measures are both internal and external. During a WMD incident the protection of the employees and the facility depends on well-planned security. Facilities must follow the national terror alert levels and respond with appropriate awareness and security measures. When employees practice security awareness on a daily basis, it will be second nature during an MCI. Most facilities have instituted lock-down procedures that restrict access to a single secure entrance. Working with internal security resources to secure the inner perimeter in a timely manner can prevent contamination of the entire facility.

The concept of scene safety is not common in health care facilities. They are no longer regarded as havens; they can also be considered targets. In an MCI involving WMD, remember the following:
- All terrorist attacks are crimes, and evidence preservation is crucial.
- Terrorist targets are mainly civilian, and health care facilities are not off limits.
- Secondary devices are present about half the time.
- Terrorist acts are not accidents, they are intentional actions designed to inflict civilian casualties.

Security staff could be on the frontlines of greeting victims of WMD and will need to be included in the training sessions for PPE and decontamination processes. Security will play a

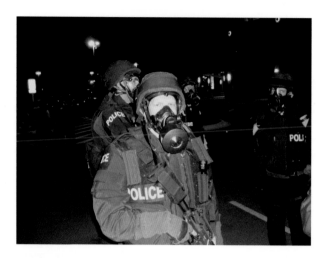

Fig. 10-10
Cooperation with law enforcement is mandatory.

big role in this area of safety and should be trained to perform sweeps and to recognize secondary devices.

Triage of the many arriving victims in a terrorist MCI should take place outside the facility to prevent contamination and damage from a possible secondary device. Law enforcement officers may also be victims, and they may be carrying weapons. Staff should be taught how to safely remove a weapon and how to secure the weapon.

Many facilities are taking further measures to protect themselves against assaults. Recent protective measures include fenced-off access as well as entrances and exits that can be secured or controlled. Other measures include securing loading docks and other means of entry. Some facilities have disguised air intakes that provide fresh air to the heat and air conditioning systems.

External security measures may involve outside law enforcement or security agencies. Community planning with these agencies can also be critical to the safety of the facility. Practicing these plans during a drill can work out many problems and bring in many ideas. If resources are available and a plan is in place, the outer perimeter of the facility can be secured to prevent excessive access and traffic to the health care facility itself. The outer perimeter can be the first ID checkpoint for employees, family, or media. Ambulances, family, and staff can be directed down the road and traffic jams can be avoided.

It can be useful to have a contract with local police agencies to have them posted at main entrances or even the loading dock area (Fig. 10-10). They can assist or relieve internal security, conduct body searches, and control access. Think about your needs and individualize your plan.

FACILITY AND PROPERTY MANAGEMENT

Facility and property management continues even during an MCI. Issues discussed under security and resource management are also key to property management. Proper policy and procedures for decontamination, controlled ventilation, and runoff collection are essential for keeping the facility clean and functioning. Clearly delineated lines of clean and dirty zones for nuclear or chemical incidents and functioning isolation rooms and procedures should also be included in property management. A large part of property management may take place in the recovery phase when things begin to slow down. This might include assistance from the EPA, CDC, FBI, and other government agencies to clean, transport waste and wastewater, and gather evidence. Continue with proper policy and procedures until the end.

IDENTIFYING LOCAL, STATE, AND FEDERAL RESOURCES

Your local, state, and federal resources should be included in your EMP. This can be the difference between success and failure during a WMD incident. Weapons of mass destruction can overwhelm the capabilities of state and local resources. Contact your local and state emergency operations management planning offices and learn how to gain access to all the services available to your facility. Establish interagency, interjurisdictional, and interorganizational disaster plans for major disasters.

Include directions for using the Federal Response Plan (FRP). Decisions to mobilize federal resources are usually made by the president under the Stafford Disaster Relief Act. The process begins when the governor asks for federal assistance during a major disaster. The Federal Emergency Management Agency (FEMA) evaluates the request and makes a recommendation to the president, who then decides whether to declare an emergency or not. Upon the president's approval the federal assets move to meet the needs of the states.

FEMA has primary responsibility for coordinating federal emergency preparedness, planning, and management functions. The CDC assists with assessing health and medical effects, collecting and analyzing samples, and providing protective actions during a nuclear, biological, or chemical exposure. Other specialty teams (see Chapter 1) are available to provide mental health services, disaster mortuary services, and veterinary medical assistance.

Local and state resources may be the same agencies already listed, such as the local CDC, and include the Red Cross agencies and local poison control centers. Metropolitan Medical Response Systems (MMRSs) are local teams that are located in terrorist-targeted cities and are funded to respond to WMD incidents. Most cities and states have an Office of Emergency Management (OEM). Get to know your resources and make contact before you need them.

EDUCATION AND TRAINING

Failure to provide the necessary resources is one reason things don't go according to plan. For example, time and money are often not budgeted for development of training programs or the overtime needed to complete the training or drills. According to the American Hospital Association, only one quarter of the hospitals in the United States are at "some state of readiness for a chemical or biological incident."[13] Training grants are available from many sources, including the federal government.

So many organizations and individuals are trying to develop training programs to meet the needs of the responders that it becomes confusing to know where to turn. While waiting for external programs to be developed, the facility must shoulder the burden of training its personnel. Where does the hospital start? JCAHO Standard EC 1.4 notes that the EMP must provide an orientation and education program for all personnel. (See Appendix E.) How do you find qualified programs and personnel to teach your employees?

The hospital must define its role in community emergency response by preplanning and coordinating with other local emergency response organizations, providing guidelines and ideas for training. It must be familiar with the ICS used by other local organizations during emergencies and should participate in training and practice sessions using HEICS or some form of ICS. All personnel who are expected to respond in emergencies involving hazardous substances must be trained to handle contaminated victims, objects, and body fluids. Training must be based on the duties and expected responsibilities of each employee. Facilities should have access to a database to provide immediate information to staff about the hazards associated with exposure to toxic materials, and all staff must be trained to use this database.

The medical personnel who set up the decontamination system must be trained to the Operations Level, and they must be trained to use PPE and to perform decontamination.[9] Responders who are trained to the Operations Level must first be trained to the Awareness Level. Then they must have 8 hours of additional training, which includes basic hazard and risk assessment, PPE selection, containment and control procedures, decontamination, and standard operating procedures. Facilities may train medical personnel with their own course after these personnel have taken the standard Operations Level course[9] (Fig.10-11).

Medical personnel who are not trained to the Operations Level still should receive training if they might be exposed to hazardous materials during an emergency. These personnel must know the hospital's plan for such an emergency, must be trained to use PPE, and must participate in scheduled drills.[9] JCAHO requires facilities to implement their response plan, either by drill or an actual emergency, twice a year.[8]

Practice Drills and Table-Top Exercises. Invest generous amounts of time in the training drills and table-top exercises. This is where the EMP will be challenged and improved. Make your drills as realistic as possible, using live victims and possible scenarios developed from the risk assessment. Remember to practice on every shift, on different days of the week, and using all areas of the facility and covering all sections of the EMP. JCAHO requirements are found in Standard EC section. At a minimum, at least one drill must include simulated victims and one must include the community relevant to the priority emergencies based on the hazard vulnerability risk assessment. Community emergency preparedness agency participation is crucial to this phase of operation.

Personal Protective Equipment. PPE is the part of a hospital's response to decontamination that takes the greatest amount of preparation and training. There are many factors to consider in the training in and maintenance of PPE (Fig. 10-12).

Employee turnover is a huge hindrance in the maintenance program and training. If the staff is not stable, how can the training be monitored and documented? The proper use of PPE requires considerable training by a competent person and is required under OSHA standard 29 CFR 1910.132. According to OSHA 3152, wearing PPE without proper training can be extremely dangerous and potentially fatal.[9] The person designated to complete fit-testing must also meet certain training requirements to monitor, test, and document this process for the facility. Be sure to review OSHA and NIOSH requirements for completing the proper training.

Communications. Another crucial area that is often overlooked in a training program is education on appropriate use of available communication tools and appropriate

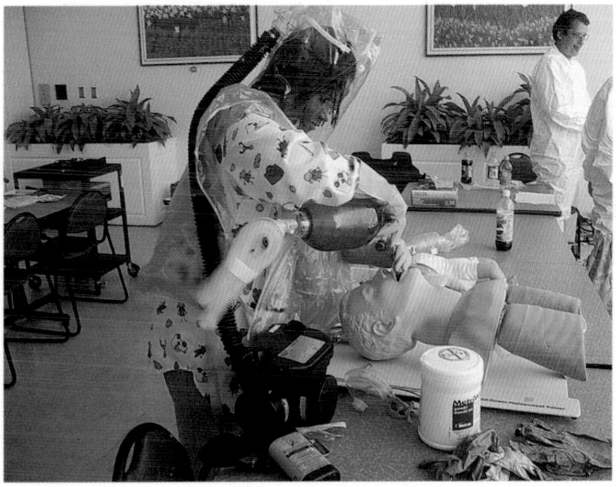

Fig. 10-11
Hospital personnel should attend a training course that meets their needs.

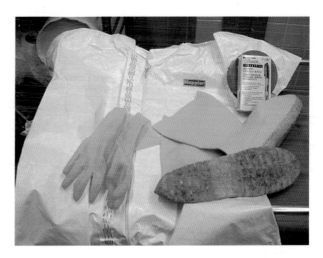

Fig. 10-12
Proper protective equipment must be selected.

terminology. During the disaster is not the time for staff to test and learn to use their communication tools. Use of common terminology and avoidance of jargon should be stressed. Discipline in information sharing will keep channels free for emergency traffic. The training plan must include the call (identification) signs for each team leader. A preprinted list of the call signs can be included for each area so staff will know whom they are conversing with. Develop a communication model, teach staff how the model works, and train staff to use the communication tools.

Preserving Evidence. Preservation of forensic evidence is very important in a terrorist incident. The subject of terrorism must be in the front of our minds during mass casualty incidents. In the current environment an MCI involving WMD should be treated as a criminal act until proven otherwise. When victims begin to arrive at health care facilities, processes for preserving evidence must begin and then follow the proper chain of evidence throughout the facility until discharge. Forensic evidence can be crucial in identifying the terrorists and in charging and convicting them.[15] Although medical personnel are not expected to act as law enforcement, they are expected to have a basic knowledge of this subject.

Some items, such as bullets and shrapnel, are obvious evidence, but other items are not. It therefore becomes necessary to keep everything and let professional law enforcement officers sort it out at the end. Education in this area becomes crucial. Basic chain of evidence and preservation are required along with an understanding of the triage-tag system and the patient-belongings bagging system during the decontamination process. Staff should also have a clear understanding of the data management processes. When staff understand the basics of evidence preservation and collection they can merge their procedures for decontamination and patient care into this process.

Triage. *Triage* is the French word meaning "to sort or select." Accurate triage allows the medical staff to provide the best care for the largest number of patients. There is no universal triage system.

There are four types of triage: field triage, emergency department triage, interhospital triage to specialized care facilities, and mass casualty triage. Emergency department triage and mass casualty triage are discussed here.

In the emergency department, triage is a rapid way to classify patients on the basis of priority and treatment needed. This classification is based on the nature and severity of the illness or complaint, history, signs and symptoms, general appearance, vital signs, and a brief physical assessment. The emergency department triage nurse relies on three areas:

- The assessment, taking into account the history given by the patient or those with the patient; vital signs; and a brief exam
- Knowledge of pathophysiology, staff, department capabilities, and resources
- Experience, sensitivity, and observation

With these things in mind, the triage nurse quickly classifies patients *one at a time.*

Who should be the triage officer and who makes up the primary triage team? The controversy is between the highest

---

Helpful Hint	Box 10-1

Have this information printed on laminated cards for the members of the triage team.

Helpful Hint	Box 10-2

If you run out of triage tags, you can use colored surveyor's tape (Fig. 10-13). Always plan on redundancy!

---

skilled or the lowest skilled staff. Members of the triage team must remember the goals: rapid and effective triage, triage tagging and routing of patients, and morgue operations. This is a physically and emotionally demanding job to perform, especially while in PPE. Backup must be ready to support this team at any time. This team must determine and communicate about the resources available (or not available) to make good triage decisions. For example, how many ventilators are in the facility and how many patients are being triaged into the red treatment area who need assisted ventilation? Frequent communication is the key to success.

Of course, all patients can't be treated at once, so they must be triaged and routed to different staging areas. START triage is one system that can be used in the MCI. This system is described in Chapter 9. START triage was developed specifically for MCIs where rapid triage of many victims is needed. Ambulatory victims should immediately be moved into one location, and then START triage should be performed on the nonambulatory victims (Box 10-1).

In a mass casualty incident, especially when decontamination is needed, the normal triage system may have to be altered and another system implemented. The health care facility must have a plan to shepherd victims through the established triage system. The Disaster Research Center has shown that more than half of the casualties arriving within 60 to 90 minutes after the incident are transported by means other than ambulance. This is obviously the key time for planning in the triage area. An area must be rapidly identified with scene tape or cones. Triage tags must be prepackaged and easily accessible for the staff in PPE to administer promptly (Box 10-2, Fig. 10-13).

There are other special triage considerations for victims of WMD. Triage tags must be used, and if decontamination is necessary, triage tags must be waterproof. Triage tags used during decontamination must be applied to the patient and go through decontamination without being destroyed or taken off the patient (Fig. 10-14).

Another triage consideration is that victims may be suffering additive effects and increased mortality because they are contaminated by radiation, just as in the case study at the beginning of the chapter. Additionally, some victims might not be stable enough to go through decontamination. If there is a question whether the patient will survive decontamination without medical intervention, triage personnel have to decide whether to treat or to send the victim to an area designated for

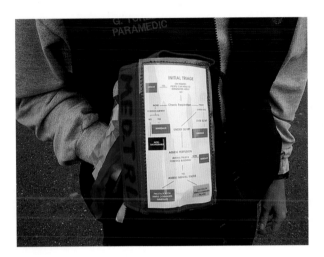

Fig. 10-13
Colored surveyor's tape can be used if you run out of triage tags.

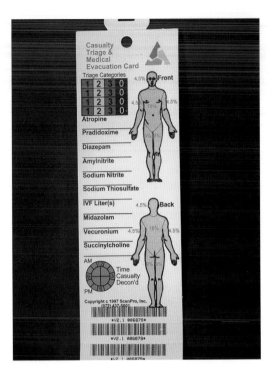

Fig. 10-14
Special triage tags are needed if the patient will be going through decontamination.

black-tagged patients (patients who are not expected to live). It is here that the triage officer must have experience and knowledge of chemicals, remembering that some have delayed effects. The triage team must ask themselves what type of medical intervention is necessary and if they have the resources to supply that medical intervention without jeopardizing other victims. If they do not, the patient should be black tagged until all other victims are treated.

Once the patient has gone through decontamination, there should be a nurse to triage the decontaminated patients and direct them to an appropriate location in the facility. Victims should be triaged at each stage of the process. It may be necessary to retag patients because of status changes. When making the emergency management plan, it will be necessary to designate different staging areas of the facility for the different types of patients.

The patients who only need decontamination and who have no medical complaints or whose complaints are very minor (tagged green) can go to a holding area where they can be seen after the more seriously injured patients have been cared for. Physicians who respond to the MCI can be sent from the pool to run an urgent care clinic with these victims. The setting for these patients can be as simple as the outpatient or ambulatory care clinic or physician's office, where they can be treated and released with standard discharge instructions.

Although green-tagged patients will be the last ones to arrive at the hospital from the field triage, the greatest number of victims of an MCI fit into this category. Generally the hospital emergency department will be overrun with yellow-

tagged and red-tagged patients by the time the green-tagged patients arrive. If the hospital has an active disaster plan that has been well practiced, the yellow-tagged patients will also go to a designated area and leave the emergency department open for the most critical red-tagged patients. The postanesthesia care unit, for example, could handle most yellow-tagged patients, unless many patients require surgery. Whatever system used, it must remain flexible and manageable.

CRITICAL INCIDENT STRESS MANAGEMENT

Critical incidents, such as MCIs, have an emotional impact on the victims and the responders, and this effect can overwhelm the usual coping mechanisms and cause significant distress in otherwise healthy people. Add to this the uncertainty of terrorism and potential for nuclear, biological, and chemical events, and usual coping mechanisms are quickly overwhelmed. If this stress is not addressed in a timely manner, its cumulative effect could render the victim and the responder helpless, which will add to the chaos of the immediate situation. The two groups with mental health issues to consider during a mass casualty incident are those victims who have a psychological response to the MCI and the responders who take care of these victims. Valuable information can be found in Chapter 14.

Critical incident stress management is necessary for the mental health of the responders. Stress-management teams are designed and implemented to specifically address the needs of emergency personnel, allowing for ventilation of emotions and other reactions to a critical event. They also provide educational information and constructive pathways to minimize the impact of stress-producing situations and their effects on emergency service personnel.

Critical incident stress management is a comprehensive program involving the entire organization and possibly the community that has experienced an MCI. The goal is to return responders and victims to their preincident state of mental health by mitigating the effects of this extreme type of stress, thereby accelerating the recovery period. As with all other aspects of the facility's emergency management plan, the stress-management program must be planned.

The organized training of specific persons within the organization and community must take place before an actual event. During the acute crisis phase, the goal of stress management is to capture the bigger picture of immediacy during a critical incident. Acute crisis planning must focus on the immediate mental health needs of the victims and responders. A good EMP can take care of many of these mental health needs just by providing organization and structure. It does not take the place of crisis intervention or of family, responder, or community recovery.

Postcrisis planning should take place on a larger scale. Information must be made available in the planning phases for MCIs. If information is not available before the MCI, the cumulative human and financial loss following the MCI can be staggering. History has taught us that facilities must plan to see and treat this form of stress following an MCI; after a WMD incident, the mental health issues can be even worse.

Fear can cause a variety of somatic syptoms.[1] Following a bioterrorist attack, people may experience an increased heart rate and shortness of breath and then attribute these symptoms to an exposure instead of recognizing them as a stress response to the event. Experienced triage personnel must distinguish between somatic symptoms and actual symptoms of exposure. A very good history of the proximity to the WMD attack will help the triage personnel to know if this is a true exposure or a response to stress. If the symptoms are diagnosed as a traumatic stress response, patients should to be sent to an area where experienced personnel can keep an eye on them in case their symptoms worsen.

A mass casualty incident creates a disparity between demand for and availability of resources. A bioterrorist attack can easily cause an overwhelming demand for medical care.[1] Medical responders to a WMD attack must be prepared to deal with many people who seek care even though they have not been exposed. They must treat these persons with respect and know what resources are available for them. When the president declares a national disaster, many federal resources for coping and recovery can be set into motion. Red Cross disaster assistance, community mental health centers, social workers, home health nurses, and hospice care providers can provide long-term help.

These groups should be part of the EMP. They can be included as actual participants, or their activation processes can be noted and tested. Practice this response in your drills, and search for community resources for the worried well. Spending time on this in the planning stage will be worth its

weight in gold during the recovery phase because in the end it decreases the burden on the health care facility.

SPECIAL SITUATIONS: WEAPONS OF MASS DESTRUCTION

BIOLOGICAL CASUALTIES

Bioterrorism is the deliberate release of pathogenic micro-organisms (bacteria, viruses, fungi, or toxins) into a population with the intent of creating illness and incapacitating or killing humans, animals, or plants. A biological attack may be a covert act of terrorism; we may not even be aware that an attack has occurred. The 2001 anthrax attacks, along with other recent terrorist events, have forced the medical community to be more aware of the threat of bioterrorism. The most likely diseases associated with bioterrorism are anthrax, smallpox, botulism, plague, and tularemia. These agents are discussed in detail in Chapter 5.

FACILITY PLANNING

Biological agents pose a great threat to the population because they are easy to produce and deliver, and they can kill or injure many people.[3,6,10] In 2001 most facilities were required to develop or revise their emergency management plans to include plans for biological agents. Review your current plan to see that it protects personnel, patients, and the community. The plan should alleviate the spread of infectious disease related to the incident. The structure of these plans should include easily accessible and specific treatment pathways for personnel to follow during a declared bioterrorism event.

Standard precautions plus a respirator with a HEPA (high-efficiency particulate air) filter constitute adequate PPE. If the HEPA filter is properly fitted, it should protect the wearer against biological agents. Reverse isolation rooms may or may not be used depending on your facility's policy and individual patient requirements.

Health care facilities must coordinate their emergency management plan with federal, state, and local directives to ensure the highest possible level of safety for patients and personnel. It is also essential that facilities maintain a list of their own laboratory capabilities and access to other laboratory resources for specialty testing that may be required in these instances.

Another list that health care facilities must maintain is the list of pharmacy cache; they must determine whether this meets the needs of their internal and external community. Research the availability of the National Pharmaceutical Stockpile. (See Appendix F for details of the National Pharmaceutical Stockpile.)

Reducing the incidence of transmission of infectious agents to medical personnel, patients, and the community depends on many factors that must be considered in the EMP. For example, incidence reduction depends on how quickly victims of a biological exposure can be triaged, isolated, and given appropriate medical treatment. Therefore educational information, specific guidelines, and all tools related to triage, diagnosis, treatment, and isolation procedures must be in place and practiced during drills and table-top exercises.

SPECIAL CONSIDERATIONS

The key to rapid intervention is for emergency responders to maintain a high level of vigilance not only in our health care facilities but also in community clinics, where many exposures may first become evident. Signs and symptoms of biological agents are usually vague. The initial symptoms are flulike and mild and nonspecific, such as malaise, cough, and fever. Because of this, an extensive patient history must be taken to identify the agent involved. This history includes an occupational, work, and environmental assessment in addition to the regular admission history.

Because the symptoms can be vague, medical personnel can easily fail to recognize the signs of a bioterrorist attack.[3,10,12] A bioterrorism event may be suspected when increasing numbers of otherwise healthy persons with similar symptoms seek treatment over a period of several hours, days, or weeks. An exposure history now becomes important. At a minimum the exposure history contains information about current and past exposures to possible hazards and an assessment of the patient's typical day and any deviations in routines. The work history, at a minimum, contains a description of previous jobs, including short-term, seasonal, and part-time employment and military service. An environmental history includes assessment of present and previous home locations, personal hobbies, and water supply. Include in your patient history any recent travel or contact with others who have been ill or have died recently of a fatal illness. Box 10-3 lists further potential signs of a bioterrorist attack.

The early clinical symptoms of infection for most bioterrorism agents may be similar to those of common diseases seen by health care professionals every day. The hospital infection control practitioner plays a significant role in rapidly identifying an outbreak and notifying local health departments. Daily surveillance of admissions to the hospital and to the intensive care units is vital to the early recognition of a bioterrorism event. All hospital units, including the emergency department, should communicate any unusual infectious disease patterns to the infection control practitioner as soon as they are noticed.

Advanced trauma life support has developed an expanded secondary ABCD survey that will help identify a biological agent:

Anticipate: There may be clues to a bioterrorism attack; see Box 10-3.

Be careful: Emergency personnel must protect themselves. Although some may prefer Level C PPE or greater, standard precautions and a HEPA filter mask provide sufficient protection from most biological agents.

Continue: Continue the primary survey; continual reassessment is necessary.

Decontaminate: Decontamination is rarely needed with a biological attack. An exception may be an announced release of a biological agent, with gross surface contamination of victims by a confirmed agent or material. In cases where decontamination may be warranted, showering with soap and water is sufficient.

A sick patient who reports to the emergency department and is suspected of being symptomatic from a bioterrorism agent should be placed in isolation with infection control precautions (preferably an isolation room) to reduce the risk of transmitting infection. Infection control and public health departments must then be notified.

Most victims will not be symptomatic for days after exposure, and in the interval they will have bathed and otherwise removed the agent, so decontamination will not be necessary. In rare cases of victims who are heavily contaminated, removing the clothing and then showering with soap and water will effectively remove almost all agents.

Once the path of a possible biological attack is started, the diagnosis, treatment, and public health interventions will center on the victims. Because the epidemic caused by a bioterrorist attack is not natural, public health officials are essential to containing it. Therefore it is necessary for the facility to prepare to assist in an epidemiological investigation.[5]

Demographic and epidemiological information must be obtained for each patient and documented on an epidemiology tracking form. This tracking information can then be recorded into a computer tracking program and made available to those making daily decisions and evaluations. This tracking program can also contain other documents required for the incident; reporting requirements; contact information for local, state, and federal agencies; laboratory criteria; and other useful information. As part of the Federal Response Plan, the CDC's Emergency Preparedness and Response Branch has a 24-hour help line at 770-488-7100. All of this information can help facilities reduce their vulnerabilities to the threat of bioterrorism, and it prepares the same facility for other threats related to weapons of mass destruction.

CHEMICAL CASUALTIES

The aim of the medical management in chemical disasters is to provide the greatest benefit for the greatest number of

---

Potential Signs of a Bioterrorist Attack   **Box 10-3**

Rapid increase in disease incidence in a normally healthy population

Epidemic curve that rises and falls during a short time

Unusual increase in the number of people seeking care for symptoms such as fever and gastrointestinal complaints

Endemic disease that emerges rapidly at unusual times or in an unusual pattern

Clusters of patients arriving from a single locale

Large numbers of rapidly fatal cases

Increased incidence of illnesses among outdoor populations versus indoor populations victims to achieve a critical reduction in mortality and morbidity. This is only possible if the facility or community uses a good emergency management plan and the plan is practiced routinely. Medical treatment for chemical exposure is limited and largely supportive; antidotes are available for only a few substances. (See Chapter 6.)

FACILITY PLANNING

Every health care facility should be able to assess, decontaminate, and treat victims of chemical incidents. This procedure is most often performed in the emergency department. How many contaminated patients can you accommodate at one time efficiently and safely? Can you accommodate ambulatory and nonambulatory patients simultaneously? Most systems can accommodate only 3 to 5 patients at one time.

In a WMD incident the operation is monitored by the safety officer, who advises the incident commander of procedures that can reduce the risk to the facility and employees. Medical personnel are trained to get in there and care for victims, but WMD events require a different approach. Before staff can enter the hot zone, they must be cleared by the safety officer. The safety officer must also monitor staff and see that they are given relief when needed. The safety officer must know hospital policy and procedures related to WMD; OSHA safety standards 29 CFR, part 1910; infectious disease control procedures (OSHA 29 CFR, part 1920.1030); the hospital incident command system; and the identified PPE and decontamination units. The safety officer also must understand the processes completely. The safety officer has the authority to stop any operation that becomes life threatening to personnel.

Personal Protective Equipment. Appropriate selection of PPE also relates to safety. Choosing PPE is not an easy task for a facility. Selection should be based on research by your facility in conjunction with the vulnerability analysis and fit-testing. Health care personnel should use Level B or Level C PPE when caring for chemically contaminated patients. Level B PPE includes a supplied-air respirator or a self-contained breathing apparatus (SCBA). Level C PPE (which provides less protection than Level B) includes a full-face mask with a powered or nonpowered canister filter (Fig. 10-15).

The type of canister or cartridge must be specific for the agent. There is no one cartridge that can filter every type of agent. If the agent cannot be identified, use a HEPA or an organic vapor filter.[2] The facility must make an educated and informed decision before purchasing PPE. New WMD or domestic preparedness filters are designed to provide protection against a wide range of nuclear, biological, and chemical threats.

Communication is difficult while wearing PPE. Plan for this with small communication boards and other communication systems placed in the hot zone. Some respirators have internal communication systems.

Many factors must be taken into consideration when the facility is selecting and purchasing PPE. Chapter 12 has detailed information. Once PPE is chosen and initial training and fit-testing is complete, then work can begin on the decontamination plan.

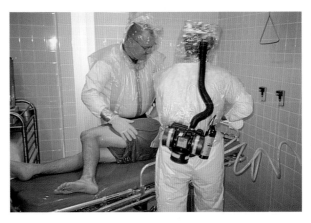

Fig. 10-15
Responders use Level C protection with a powered air-purifying respirator (PAPR) while decontaminating a patient.

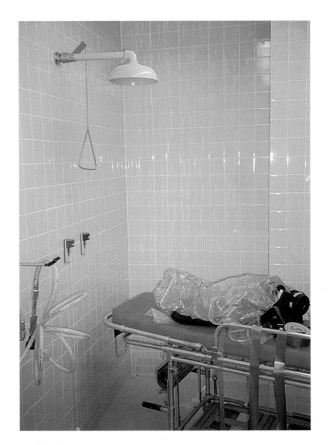

Fig. 10-16
Many hospitals have decontamination rooms.

Decontamination. Location and choice of decontamination units has become as complicated as choosing the correct PPE. All facilities that have the potential to receive contaminated patients must provide an area for decontamination (Fig. 10-16).

A proper decontamination room has many architectural requirements, which are discussed in detail in other texts. Some of these include location of the intake and exhaust vents in the hospital and separate entries and exits. The overall goal is to prevent spreading contamination outside of the decontamination room.

Runoff must be contained separately from the regular facility drainage system unless the EPA has declared a catastrophic emergency or during a true MCI. This self-contained tank must be accessible for drainage and must handle the large number of victims from a MCI. Many facilities are looking at portable units that can take the decontamination process away from the building or complement the internal unit.

The most attractive decontamination units are portable ones that can easily be set up in the hospital parking lot by assigned personnel (Fig. 10-17). These portable units provide shelter from the elements and protection of the victims from the public eye.

Whatever the unit, internal or external, the decontamination process must be accessible to a warm water tap or have a portable water heater. Even in warm weather, contaminated patients who are frightened and in shock will require and appreciate the warm water.

SPECIAL CONSIDERATIONS

Decontamination is the process of removing accumulated contaminants and is critical to the health and safety of health care providers by preventing secondary contamination. All staff who might use the decontamination unit must be trained to perform decontamination and to use the equipment. Staff must practice the decontamination procedure while wearing their PPE. The decontamination plan should establish procedures and educate employees about decontamination procedures, identify the equipment needed and methods to be used, and establish methods for disposing of contaminated materials.

The extent to which decontamination is performed depends on the exposure situation. Removing and bagging the victims' clothing can eliminate much of the contamination and minimizes the risk of spreading the contaminant. To be effective, decontamination must include a minimum of two steps: (1) removing the clothing and jewelry and then rinsing the patient with water. (2) It is generally accepted that a mild soap and clean water rinse will complete the decontamination procedure for most patients. There are actually two types of decontamination: that for the ambulatory victims and that for the nonambulatory victims.

Ambulatory Decontamination. The preplanning phase must determine where the hot, cold, and warm zones will be established. (For more detail in decontamination processes and procedures, refer to Chapter 13.) In general, the hot (dirty) zone is contaminated and requires the highest PPE level, the warm zone is where the victims are decontaminated, and the cold or clean zone is where victims are treated.

The first step of the process is to clearly delineate the hot zone and not allow crossing back and forth between the cold zone and the hot zone. The hot zone is where the ambulatory victims get undressed and put their belongings into individual bags. It is important to remember that most of the contaminants will be removed with the clothes because contaminants cling to the clothing.

Control of the hot zone and direction of the victims is crucial in the hot zone. This is where internal and external security and others assigned to this zone become an integral part of the process. The first responders into the hot zone will be there to control the crowd and direct the victims and incoming EMS to the triage area. Everyone will demand direction and require information upon entering the hot zone. If the facility is not yet prepared to administer decontamination for the waiting victims, then victims should be distracted with tasks.

Begin with a general triage system and identification instructions. There are many ways to distract people; one is a

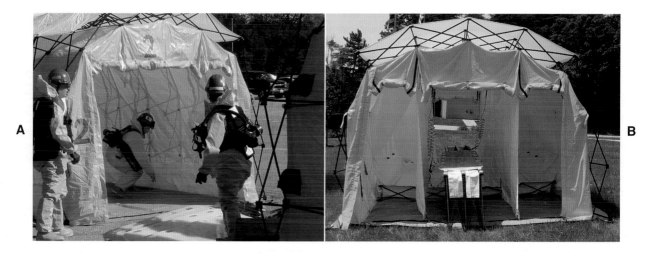

Fig. 10-17
There are many commercial decontamination units that can be easily and quickly set up. **A,** Responders setting up a tent. **B,** A tent with both ambulatory and nonambulatory corridors.

predecontamination kit that can be handed out to the victims. This kit will give the victim a temporary outfit, usually a large paper poncho, and a bag in which to put all of his or her clothes and valuables. These kits can be purchased or prepacked by the facility. At this point, health care personnel can determine who might have the potential for primary contamination or secondary contamination. Victim ID bands and triage tags can be distributed at this time if the bands and tags can tolerate going through decontamination. There are generally four steps to the ambulatory decontamination unit: disrobing, washing, rinsing, and redressing.

The first step in decontamination is the removal of clothing. These belongings should be identified for each victim and left at the entrance of the hot zone as directed by staff. Provide a separate zippered bag for belongings such as jewelry and identification (e.g., driver's license) if these items are not grossly contaminated. This allows for controlling and identifying the victims. Victims can be given directions for bagging and labeling their clothes and other belongings in many ways; for example, a prerecorded message in different languages can be set up on a simple public address system to provide direction (Box 10-4).

While the victims are getting out of their clothes, the decontamination unit and staff can be readied. Once the decontamination unit is ready, the crowd will be instructed to move toward the decontamination unit. If they have already used a predecontamination kit, they can step into the decontamination unit and take the temporary outfit off and throw it in a trash bag.

The second step of the decontamination process is the soap or decontamination solution stage. Once the victims have moved through the soap stage of the decontamination, they proceed to the third step, which is the clean water rinse. The fourth step is to dry off and redress when they come out the other end of the decontamination unit (Fig. 10-18). They will need some type of clothing to put on so that they can proceed into the facility for a second triage and possible treatment. Many facilities are stocking boxes of disposable paper jump suits that have feet and hood attachments all in one, in large sizes to fit all.

No medical treatment has been initiated at this point. At this time the victims are considered clean and can enter the facility. Once they are dressed, the victims must be directed into the facility and guided to where they should go next. This is the cold zone of the decontamination area, and some type of spot checking should take place. Chemical agent monitors (CAMs) or other monitoring devices can be used to check patients to see if they are clean or free from the agent or chemical. Although most facilities have not yet purchased air-monitoring equipment, it is highly recommended in identified high-risk areas. (Refer to Chapter 11 for detailed information on available systems.)

Nonambulatory Decontamination. While the ambulatory victims are moving to another area waiting for the decontamination unit, medical personnel must get into place in the hot zone to triage patients for decontamination. The triage team will assist the victims to the nonambulatory side of the decontamination unit.

Decontamination personnel from the facility should be set to receive the victim and cut off the clothes, remove jewelry, and use the same decontamination process as described for the ambulatory patients. There should be soap or decontamination solution and a clean water rinse area, and then the victim should be put on a clean gurney and transported into the facility. During this process basic medical care can be provided based on the number of victims, the available supplies, and the capabilities of the decontamination staff (Fig. 10-19). Have blankets available to prevent hypothermia.

The entire decontamination procedure must be practiced with staff wearing PPE. The process must be reviewed extensively on a regular basis to protect the staff and the clean area of the facility.

RADIOLOGICAL CASUALTIES

Among the terrorist threats are radiological exposures. The case study at the beginning of this chapter is an example of the current threats. These threats can range from the dirty bomb to a nuclear weapon. The dispersal method will affect delivery of care. Refer to Chapter 4 for detailed information.

FACILITY PLANNING

Principles of radiation exposure remain the same: Exposure depends on time, distance, and shielding. Therefore the EMP must include training on working quickly to minimize radiation exposure. Staff rotation and planning for this

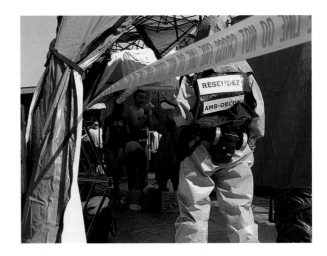

Fig. 10-18
A responder waits to check patients for residual contamination after they complete decontamination.

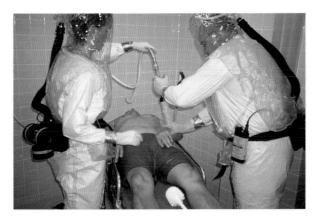

Fig. 10-19
Medical responders should be available to provide essential treatment during the decontamination process.

concern must also be a part of the plan. PPE for radiation is no different from PPE for other agents; those doing the primary decontamination need the most protection, and PPE can be downgraded after this process. Respiratory protection is required during the decontamination process to prevent inhalation exposure. Radioactive particles adhere to dust and other materials and become airborne, so it is crucial that the ventilation system be controlled and separate from the rest of the facility.

Spot checks by qualified personnel should be a part of this process to ensure that decontamination is complete before patients enter the cold zone. Once decontamination of all victims is complete, decontamination of staff and proper disposal of PPE is crucial to prevent the spread of contamination. Policies must be in place for decontamination water runoff and waste disposal.

SPECIAL CONSIDERATIONS

When a terrorist incident involves a dirty bomb, the patients may have trauma in addition to radiation injuries. Trauma in conjunction with radiological contamination is an emergency and requires decontamination to minimize internal contamination. The other issue for immediate consideration is the possibility of a secondary device.

Gross dry decontamination should take place outside the health care facility to prevent facility contamination. Take care to avoid contaminating wounds during decontamination. Remembering the principles of wound care, cover wounds once they are clean, and finish the decontamination process.

Actual radiological syndromes may not appear for hours or even years depending on many factors, such as radiation dose exposure. Therefore trauma victims with radiation exposure should be triaged the same as other MCI victims. Because the extent of the radiation injury may not be apparent, triage should be based on the other injuries. For patients known to be experiencing a high-dose radiation exposure, the treatment is emergent. Victims may have fever, delirium, bloody diarrhea, and profuse diarrhea and vomiting within the first 2 hours.

(See Chapter 4 for complete details.) Health care facilities must be prepared for the multitude of "worried well" who may present themselves for treatment.

A detailed exposure history is important; remember that triage decisions should always reflect the available resources at that time. Victims with obvious symptoms of radiation syndrome soon after exposure are not likely to recover, and resources must be conserved.

Reference sources for health care facilities are the state health departments, the Radiation Emergency Assistance Center/Training Site (REAC/TS), and the CDC.

CHAPTER SUMMARY

Health care facility response to a mass casualty incident has been a source of discussion and planning over the past few years. With the help of OSHA, JCAHO, NIOSH, and other regulatory agencies, these plans are slowly being refined into a workable format. Health care facilities, including hospitals and clinics, have recognized the need for more extensive planning for MCIs involving WMD. It has become more evident that all workplaces and all communities are at risk for domestic terrorism. A good offense is always the best defense; your defense is your emergency management plan, which includes specifications for biological, chemical, and nuclear terrorist attacks.

A facility's response to a mass casuality incident must be a well-executed plan. A detailed emergency management plan using the hospital emergency incident command system is one path to success. If the facility does its research and repetitively practices and revises the EMP, when the MCI happens, processes will fall into place with little effort. Chaos will be the exception and not the rule. Every employee from the CEO to the new hire must be involved in order for the plan to be effective and well executed. This preparation requires an extensive education plan for all employees.

REFERENCES

1. Benedek DM, Holloway HC, Becker SM: Emergency mental health management in bioterrorism events, *Emerg Med Clin North Am* 20:393-407, 2002.

2. Geller RJ et al: Nosocomial poisoning associated with emergency department treatment of organophosphate toxicity—Georgia, 2000, *J Toxicol Clin Toxicol* 39:190-111, 2001, http://www.cdc.gov/mmwr/preview/mmwrhtml/mm4951a2.htm, retrieved September 23, 2004.

3. Gwerder LJ, Beaton R, Daniell W: Bioterrorism: implications for the occupational and environmental health nurse, *AAOHN J* 49:512-518, 2001.

4. Gum R, Hoyle J, Selanikio J: *CBRNE—chemical warfare mass casualty management*, 2002, http://www.emedicine.com/emerg/topic895.htm, retrieved September 23, 2004.

5. Henretig FM et al: Medical management of the suspected victim of bioterrorism: an algorithmic approach to the undifferentiated patient, *Emerg Med Clin North Am* 20:351-364, 2002.

6. Hogan DE, Burstein JL: *Disaster medicine*, Philadelphia, 2002, Lippincott Williams & Wilkins.

7. McGlown J, Moore A: *New JCAHO emergency management standards for health care facilities*, edited version of November

22, 2000 transcript, http://www.emforum.org/vforum/lc001122. htm, retrieved August 25, 2002.

8. O'Brien K: *Disasters: the role of the nurse in responding*, 1998, http://ironbark.bendigo.latrobe.edu.au/~obrien/LN-DN.htm, retrieved September 23, 2004.

9. Occupational Safety and Health Administration: *Hospitals and community emergency response—what you need to know*, 1997, http://www.osha-slc.gov/Publications/OSHA3152/osha3152. html, retrieved September 23, 2004.

10. Persell DJ et al: Preparing for bioterrorism, *Nursing* 32:36-43, 2002.

11. Powers R: *Mass casualty (definition)*, http://usmilitary.about. com/library/glossary/m/bldef03847.htm, retrieved September 23, 2004.

12. Salazar MK, Kelman B: Planning for biological disasters— occupational health nurses as "first responders," *AAOHN J* 50:174-181, 2002.

13. Salvatore S, Zewe C: *Most U.S. hospitals found unprepared to handle chemical, biological attack*, CNN.com, January 11, 2000, http://www.cnn.com/2000/HEALTH/01/11/bioterrorism.02/, retrieved September 23, 2004.

14. San Mateo County Emergency Medical Services Agency: *Hospital emergency incident command system*, ed 3, vol 1, 1998, San Mateo County (funded by the California Emergency Medical Authority).

15. Technical Working Group for Bombing Scene Investigation: *A guide for explosion and bombing scene investigation*, Washington, DC, 2002, National Institute of Justice.

BIBLIOGRAPHY

Are we ready to respond? Assessing nursing's bioterrorism preparedness, *Am Nurse*, November/December 2001 (editorial), http://nursingworld.org/tan/01novdec/respond.htm, retrieved September 23, 2004.

Broward County EMS: *Critical incident stress management*, http://www.browardems.com/tmi02712.htm, retrieved September 23, 2004.

Broward County EMS: *Mass casualty incidents and START triage*, http://www.browardems.com/tmi02719.htm, retrieved September 23, 2004.

Caine RM, Ter-Bagdasarian L: Early identification and management of critical incident stress, *Crit Care Nurse* 23:59-65, 2003.

Carlson-Fell D: Terrorist Danger—Part One and Two, *Nurseweek* Feb 3 and 17, 2003.

Collins J: *Training America's emergency responders: a report on the Department of Justice's Center for Domestic Preparedness and the U.S. Public Health Service's Noble Training Center*, Washington, DC, 2000, Center for Strategic and International Studies, http://www.csis.org/burke/hd/reports/FirstResponders. html, retrieved September 23, 2004.

Currance P, Bronstein A: *Hazardous materials for EMS: practices and procedures*, St Louis, 1999, Mosby.

Joint Commission on Accreditation of Healthcare Organizations: *Health care at the crossroads—strategies for creating and sustaining community-wide emergency preparedness systems*, Oakbrook Terrace, Ill, 2003, JCAHO.

Kim DH, Proctor PW, Amos LK: Disaster management and the emergency department, a framework for planning, *Nurs Clin North Am* 37:171-187, 2002.

Latrobe University (2001). *Lecture notes: triage*, http:// ironbark.bendigo.latrobe.edu.au/`obrien/LN-TRIAGE.htm, retrieved July 27, 2002.

Maniscalco PM, Christen HT: *Mass casualty and high impact incidents: an operations guide*, Upper Saddle River, NJ, 2002, Prentice Hall–Brady.

Nextel. *Digital phone systems*, http://www.Nextel.com, retrieved March 2003.

O'Connell KP, Menuey BC, Foster D: Issues in preparedness for biological terrorism: a perspective for critical care nursing, *AACN Clin Issues* 13:453-469, 2002.

Saksen L: Bioterror response requires targeted disaster plan, *Hosp Case Manag* 10:39-42, 2002.

Williams S: Be prepared: unpredictability of Mother Nature—and human nature—prompts more hospital to examine and upgrade their emergency response systems, *Nurseweek* January 30, 2003, http://www.nurseweek.com/news/features/03-01/disaster print.html, retrieved September 23, 2004.

Weapons of Mass Destruction Detection Devices

PHIL CURRANCE

CHAPTER OBJECTIVES

At the conclusion of this chapter the student will be able to:

- Discuss the need for air monitoring and detection equipment at a WMD incident.
- Discuss the limitations of field instruments.
- Describe the function, use, and limitations of explosive detection devices and radiological, chemical, and biological detection equipment.

CASE STUDY

An unknown chemical agent has been released inside an upscale shopping mall. Numerous employees and shoppers were exposed while trying to escape the building. Emergency Medical System (EMS) responders are on the scene. Patients are being treated after decontamination. The hazardous materials (HAZMAT) team has deployed responders with air monitoring equipment to assess the extent and severity of the release. The incident commander is consulting with EMS responders and public health personnel regarding the extent of patient exposure and need for further evacuation. In addition, the number of patients who were possibly exposed is overwhelming the capability of EMS and hospital resources.

Can data from air-monitoring equipment be used to assist with evacuation decisions?

Can this air-monitoring data assist with triage decisions (who was exposed and level of exposure)?

Which air-monitoring devices will be useful?

What limitations must be considered when assessing data supplied by air-monitoring devices?

At an incident involving weapons of mass destruction, responders must determine the identity and the amount of the released material and the extent of spread of the material so decisions can be made about the types of personal protective equipment (PPE) that responders will need. Responders must identify the chemical and the extent of exposure so specific medical treatment can be provided.

Both patient and equipment decontamination effectiveness must be evaluated. Responders must not rely on a visual assessment alone. Many threats are invisible to the eye, and threats that are visible are usually in very high concentrations. Detection and air-monitoring equipment can aid in these decisions by supplying data. This data can be used to:
- Determine the extent of the release
- Establish the boundaries of the hot zone
- Assist in identifying unknown products
- Define the source of a release
- Assist in selecting PPE
- Help to assess changes in conditions and ensure safety of responders
- Assist in triage decisions by identifying by location which patients have a greater exposure risk

- Guide specific medical treatment modalities
- Determine decontamination effectiveness

This chapter looks at common portable equipment used by hazardous materials response teams and special operations teams to detect, identify, and monitor environments containing chemical, biological, and radiological hazards.

EQUIPMENT SELECTION AND LIMITATIONS

Direct-reading instruments are often complex electronic devices. Before using such instruments, training is essential for understanding their limitations, selecting the proper instrument, ensuring proper use and calibration, and interpreting the data.

To get maximum benefit from these instruments, responders must be aware of their capabilities and limitations. Some equipment is used for air monitoring and other equipment is used for air sampling. There is a difference between air monitoring and air sampling.

AIR SAMPLING

Air sampling is done to ascertain the identity and quantity of agent in the sample, and the sample is analyzed in a laboratory. Because emergency responders need immediate information, sampling has very limited application. The larger response teams use complex instruments that allow field analysis of samples. These devices are complex and expensive and not usually available to first responders. Even when support teams arrive with this type of equipment, time is still required to collect and analyze samples.

AIR MONITORING

Direct-reading air-monitoring instruments and detection devices are designed to supply immediate information by way of a readout or gauge. The information may not be totally accurate, and in some cases exact identity of the product cannot be established.

As monitoring devices have become more sophisticated, we have often incorrectly assumed that they are telling us exactly what agent and how much of the agent is present. In reality, direct air-monitoring devices are extremely limited. Some monitors only assess flammability; others monitor oxygen concentration or toxicity levels. Some devices work only with organic compounds. Responders must understand these limitations and use appropriate caution when assessing the data supplied by direct-reading air-monitoring and detection equipment. The use of more than one type of instrument will improve the quality of data used for hazard assessment (Fig. 11-1).

Air-monitoring equipment used for emergency response situations must meet certain criteria (Box 11-1). A major concern is if the instrument presents an ignition source if used in the presence of flammable gases or vapors. Instruments operated in these areas should be certified as intrinsically safe or explosion proof. Minimum standards for inherent safety in hazardous atmospheres have been defined by the National Fire

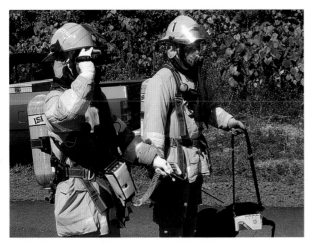

Fig. 11-1
Multiple instruments should be used to detect all possible hazards.

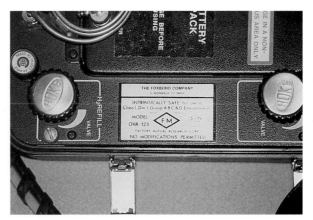

Fig. 11-2
Detection equipment should be rated as intrinsically safe.

Criteria for Air-Monitoring Equipment	**Box 11-1**
Air-monitoring equipment should be:	
Easy to use	
Accurate	
Reliable	
Able to generate a fast response	
Easy to interpret	
Portable	
Able to withstand weather conditions	
Approved for HAZMAT use	
Easy to decontaminate	

Protection Association (NFPA) in the National Electric Code (NEC). Instruments are certified as intrinsically safe for specific classes and groups of flammable atmospheres by Factory Mutual Research Corp. (FM) or Underwriter's Laboratory (UL) (Fig. 11-2).

DETECTION PRIORITIES

An important consideration is the suspected or known contaminant. Does the agent present a radioactive or explosive threat? Is the agent chemical or biological? Detection priorities should be established. Because protective equipment does not provide reliable protection from radiation or explosive devices, these devices are usually considered the first and second priority. Detection of chemical agents should be considered next and then detection of biological agents as necessary. The responders carrying out monitoring and detection activities should use proper PPE and limit their exposure.

DETECTING RADIATION

Whenever radioactive materials might be encountered, radiation detection devices should be employed. Radiation monitors include personal dosimeters and radiation survey instruments.

PERSONAL DOSIMETERS

Personal dosimeters monitor the radiation dose responders are exposed to and should be carried by all personnel who could be exposed to radiation. Numerous dosimeters are available for emergency response work. One is the pen type, which must be used with a battery-operated charger base (Fig. 11-3). The base charges the pen and sets the scale to zero. The accumulated dose can be determined by looking through the pen much like a telescope. Other dosimeters resemble pagers and are equipped with digital readouts and alarms. Some dosimeters are equipped with two alarm settings. The first alarm sounds when low levels of radiation are detected, and the second alarm indicates a potentially dangerous level of exposure.

RADIATION SURVEY INSTRUMENTS

Radiation survey instruments are used to detect surface contamination (Fig. 11-4). Normal background radiation should be measured to determine areas of higher concentration and contamination. Using this information, patient and equipment decontamination efficiency, safe work practices, and protective equipment needs can be determined.

Radiation survey instruments measure ionizing radiation. Detectors containing an ionizable detection medium are commonly used. The ions produced in the medium are counted electronically, and a relationship is established between the number of ions and the quantity of radiation present. Different probe types may be used to determine the type of radiation present (Fig. 11-5).

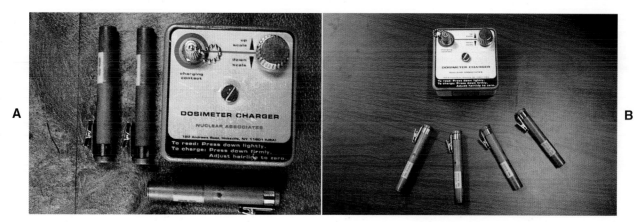

Fig. 11-3
Charger base and pen dosimeter.

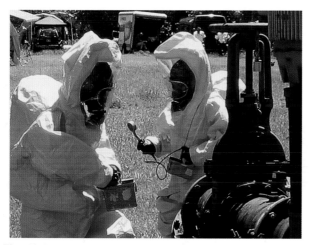

Fig. 11-4
Responders using radiation survey instruments.

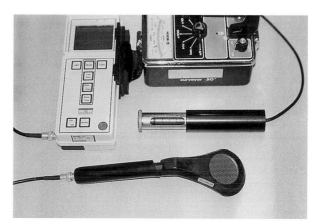

Fig. 11-5
The correct radiation instruments and probe must be selected.

TYPES OF PROBES

Pancake or end-window probes with a mica window are used for alpha radiation. For beta and gamma radiation the most common type of probe is the Geiger-Mueller detector. A side window allows beta radiation to pass through, and a movable metal shield is used to cover the window and allow for gamma radiation monitoring. There are also special probes designed for detecting neutron radiation.

Radiation survey instruments are factory calibrated and usually returned to the factory or manufacturer for recalibration. One can use a cesium-137 source that can be obtained from the manufacturer to perform calibration checks.

INTERPRETATION OF DATA

Radiation instruments measure radiation in various units. Roentgen equivalent in man (rem) or radiation absorbed dose

(rad) are dose-related exposures. Gamma radiation is typically measured in milliroentgens per hour. Some instruments measure millisieverts per hour. These units express an exposure rate, or the amount of radiation that a person would be exposed to at the point of measurement. Alpha and beta detectors typically measure in counts per minute. Both counts per minute and milliroentgens are functionally related.

As a general rule, when the radiation level increases to three to five times the background level, responders should withdraw and assess the need for special procedures. OSHA regulations state that when radiation exceeds 0.2 milliroentgens per hour, protective measures must be taken (Box 11-2).

When interpreting the data, keep in mind that radiation detectors may be sensitive to radio waves, microwaves, magnetic fields, and electrostatic fields. The radiation level is dependent on distance from the source. What is considered a safe level at one location may be unsafe as the responder moves closer to the source. Thus when radioactive materials are suspected, a systematic and thorough search of the area must be made.

DETECTING EXPLOSIVES

The two most common types of explosive detection devices available to emergency responders are ion mobility spectrometry (IMS) and mass spectrometry. In IMS a device with a radioactive source is used to ionize a test sample. This results in ion clusters traveling at different speeds. The device measures the time of flight (TOF) of the ions and compares it to element signatures stored in the instrument's memory (Fig. 11-6). With mass spectrometry a wipe sample is taken with a specially designed wipe, and the instrument measures the weight of the materials on the wipe and compares it to a sample library in the instrument. Both of these technologies are expensive.

Many new explosive detection technologies are currently under development. Most devices of this class will detect the presence of explosive agent or residue. They do not identify the exact explosive compound or the amount of explosive agent present.

DETECTING CHEMICAL AGENTS

Many chemical agent technologies are available. They include:
- Detection papers and kits
- Colorimetric indicator tubes
- Combustible gas indicators
- Oxygen meters
- Gas-specific sensors
- Photoionization detectors (PIDs)
- Flame ionization detectors (FIDs)
- Ion mobility spectrometry (IMS)
- Non–hand-held devices

DETECTION PAPERS AND KITS

M-8 PAPER AND M-9 TAPE

M-8 paper and M-9 tape are military-designed detectors especially for chemical warfare agents. They provide a rapid (less than 1 minute) and inexpensive test for the presence of liquid mustard and/or nerve agents.

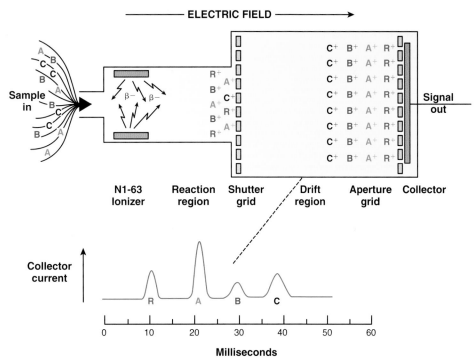

Fig. 11-6
Ion mobility spectrometry instrument.

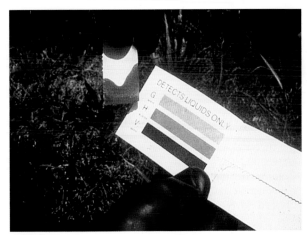

Fig. 11-7
M-8 paper can be used to detect the presence of blister and nerve agents.

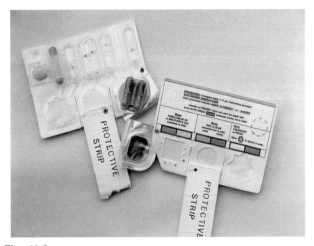

Fig. 11-8
The M256A1 kit can be used to detect vapor exposure to cyanide, vesicants, and nerve agents.

M-8 paper is tan and is usually found in a tear-out book format (Fig. 11-7). It is a preliminary detection test for the presence of liquid agents on nonporous surfaces. The paper strip is blotted on a suspected agent and observed for a color change. G-type nerve agents (sarin, soman, tabun) turn the paper yellow, VX turns it dark green, and blister agents (mustard) turn it red.

M-9 tape is an adhesive-backed tape placed on the outside of protective suits and other equipment. The color changes from green to red or pink when contacted by a liquid chemical warfare agent. Unlike M-8 paper, M-9 tape doesn't identify the type of agent.

Both the M-8 paper and M-9 tape should be considered screening tests only. Both frequently show false positives when in contact with substances such as petroleum products and antifreeze. Results must be verified with more accurate methods of detection.

M256A1 KIT

Another military detector kit is the M256A1. This kit includes enzyme-based detector cards (tickets) with multiple tests (Fig. 11-8). This detector has specific tests for vapor exposure to cyanide, vesicants, and nerve agents. Use of the kit requires the operator to be in the vapor exposure area. The tests take approximately 15 to 20 minutes. Sensitivity for lower concentrations is low. False negatives may result even at up to levels of 500 times the acceptable exposure level.

OTHER DEVICES

Besides the military papers and kits, there are many commercially available devices. Paper test strips are available for measuring pH and other features of an agent. The accuracy of paper test strips depends on the ability of the user to determine the color change compared to standard color charts. Hand-held meters are available for testing pH, temperature, and oxidation-reduction potential. Field test kits are available for determining the concentration of specific liquids. Hazard

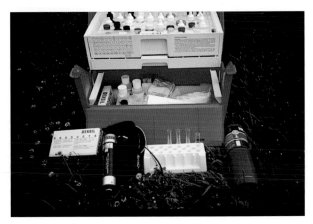

Fig. 11-9
The HAZCAT kit can be used to identify certain unknown products.

categorization kits, designed for identification of unknown products, are useful for identifying liquids and some solid agents (Fig. 11-9). In order to use any of these devices the responder must come into direct contact with the chemical. Because the product has not been identified, protective equipment may not be adequate. Extreme caution must be used.

COLORIMETRIC INDICATOR TUBES

Colorimetric indicator or detector tubes are a type of gas-specific monitor. The tubes are specific for a certain compound or family of chemicals. There are approximately 400 different tubes that can be used to identify almost 1000 chemicals. Some tubes are specific for detection of chemical warfare agents such as nerve agents, pulmonary agents, and vesicants (Fig. 11-10). The tubes contain chemically treated granules that react with the contaminant to produce a stain or color change.

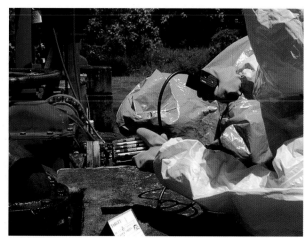

Fig. 11-10
Colorimetric tubes can be used to detect most chemical weapons of mass destruction and many industrial chemicals.

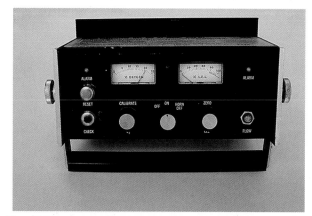

Fig. 11-11
The CGI/O_2 monitor can be used to determine flammability risk.

Most tubes are marked with a scale to indicate the approximate concentration of vapor that is drawn through the tube.

This air-monitoring system consists of a hand-operated piston or bellows pump and detector tubes. Battery-powered pumps are also available. Responders using colorimetric tubes must be properly trained. Each type of tube requires a certain number of pump strokes and a minimum amount of time between each stroke. Manufacturers' instructions must be carefully followed to ensure that the proper volume of air is drawn through the tube. If responders do not use these tubes properly, the data will not be accurate. Different manufacturers' tubes are not interchangeable.

Many manufacturers market a special selection of tubes in kit form that may be helpful in assessing unknown chemicals. A selection of tubes is used and results are compared to a decision tree. The test may be able to identify the family of chemicals involved and allow for more effective patient assessment and treatment and a better selection of responder PPE.

Calibration of colorimetric tubes is not necessary, but the pump must be periodically checked for leaking valves. Additionally, the pump should be volumetrically calibrated on a regular basis.

Colorimetric tubes have a shelf life that is marked on the box containing the tubes. Storage under hot conditions may reduce shelf life. Temperature and humidity may affect the tubes' accuracy.

There is a military version of colorimetric tubes known as the M-18 detection kit. It has specific sensor tubes for cyanide, phosgene, lewisite, sulfur mustard, and nerve agents. Tests for each chemical take 2 to 3 minutes but must be conducted serially.

INTERPRETATION OF DATA

The length of the color change within the tube corresponds to the gas concentration. This color change should be examined immediately. The length of the color stain may change after just a few minutes, which can cause responders to misread the results and can severely affect the quality of the data.

Tubes are marked in either percent or ppm (parts per million). Unfortunately, the color change is commonly not a straight line but a jagged or faded edge. Estimates should always indicate the worst-case scenario.

If detector tubes are used when more than one gas is present, cross-sensitivity may occur. This means that a gas other than the one of interest can cause a color change within the tube. Possible cross-sensitivity problems are identified on the instruction sheet that accompanies the tubes.

These limitations substantially affect the accuracy of the colorimetric tubes. As a general rule, the error factor can range from 25% to 50%. Because of this, many response teams use the tubes as a qualitative rather than a quantitative detection device. In other words, the tubes are used to detect and identify the type of agent, not the amount of agent present. As with specific gas monitors, the action level may be set at the specific chemical's PEL/TLV (permissible exposure limit–threshold limit value), IDLH (immediately dangerous to life or health) value, or LOC (level of concern) value.

COMBUSTIBLE GAS INDICATORS

Combustible gas indicators (CGIs) are some of the most widely used field instruments found in emergency response operations (Fig. 11-11). CGIs are also known as explosion meters or lower explosive limit (LEL) monitors. These instruments use a circuit called a Wheatstone bridge that burns the gas sample on two filaments. One filament is coated with a catalyst that enhances combustion and creates an imbalance. The degree of imbalance in resistance is translated to a percentage of the lower explosive limit (Fig. 11-12).

The majority of CGIs read in percentage of LEL. Therefore they cannot be used to determine if an atmosphere is too rich to burn. When the meter reads 100%, you are at the agent's LEL.

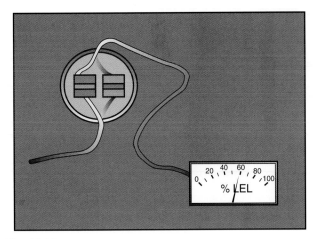

Fig. 11-12
Wheatstone bridge.

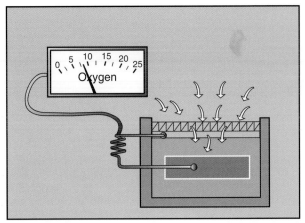

Fig. 11-13
Oxygen sensor.

INTERPRETATION OF READINGS

CGI readings are relative to the calibration gas. Pentane, methane, propane, and hexane are common calibration gases. The device will be accurate only when it is sensing the gas that it was calibrated for. When measuring a different gas, the instrument works the same but the LEL reading will not be accurate. Most manufacturers provide a graph or table showing the response of their instruments to various gases and vapors. This response curve can be used to more accurately interpret the monitoring data. Calibration should be checked on a daily basis. With some units, calibration is checked every day and a full recalibration is done every month (follow manufacturer's instructions).

Because the CGI operates by burning gases, appropriate levels of oxygen are required for accurate results. CGIs are not useful for determining toxicity because they are not chemical specific or sensitive at low concentrations.

Because of the inherent inaccuracy of CGIs and the presence of possible mixtures of gases or vapors, action levels should be established. At the action level, personnel must evacuate the area or take special precautions. The action level usually referred to for CGIs in outdoor operations is 20% to 25% LEL. OSHA has established 10% LEL as the action limit in confined spaces.

OXYGEN METERS

In many conditions oxygen concentrations are abnormal. High concentrations of other gases may displace oxygen, or combustion or chemical reaction may deplete the oxygen supply. Chemical reactions, chemicals that act as oxidizers, and a release from an oxygen supply may increase the level of oxygen. Oxygen levels must be determined in order to select protective equipment, to ensure proper operation of CGIs, to assess flammability hazard, and to determine the possible mechanism of injury. Oxygen meters determine the percentage of oxygen in the air and are usually calibrated to detect concentrations

between 0% and 25% oxygen; some may detect up to 50% oxygen. In many cases the CGI and oxygen meter are combined in a single meter. (See Fig. 11-11.)

Oxygen meters work on an electrochemical principle. Air is drawn into a detector cell, and oxygen molecules diffuse though a membrane into electrolyte solution. A chemical reaction between the oxygen and the electrolyte within the cell produces a small current that is proportional to the sensor's oxygen content. The current passes through an electronic circuit, and the resulting signal is displayed on a readout (Fig. 11-13). When oxidizers are in the atmosphere being monitored, they react with the sensor in addition to oxygen, resulting in an above-normal oxygen response.

The electrolyte in the oxygen meter begins to wear out from the time the unit is first used. The sensor should be replaced according to the manufacturer's recommendations.

INTERPRETATION OF DATA

OSHA has established 19.5% as the minimum amount of oxygen necessary for workers. Below 19.5%, air supplied respirators (SCBA or air line with escape bottle) must be used. Because of increased flammability in atmospheres with high oxygen concentrations, 25% is considered the upper safe limit. Oxygen-enriched environments must be vented before workers can enter. In confined spaces, OSHA has established 19.5% as the minimum and 23.5% as the maximum allowable concentrations of oxygen.

GAS-SPECIFIC SENSORS

Many gas-specific monitors are available. These are commonly found combined in the same instrument with a CGI and oxygen monitor. Monitors are available that include CGI-oxygen and one, two, three, or four specific-gas sensors (Fig. 11-14).

Specialized instruments can detect vapors such as chlorine, ammonia, hydrogen sulfide, and carbon monoxide. These instruments function in an electrochemical manner similar to

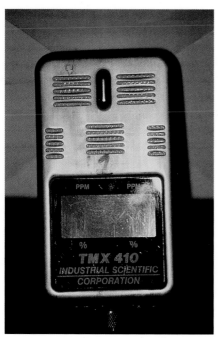

Fig. 11-14
Gas-specific monitor.

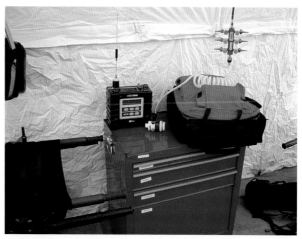

Fig. 11-15
The photoionization detector is used to determine the concentration of ionizable vapors in the air. This device also radios the information to a receiver in the cold zone.

the oxygen meter. Chemically reactive sensors produce electrical signals that are converted to vapor concentration on the monitor.

Use caution when interpreting data supplied by these monitors. Other gases or vapors may interfere with the device and cause an inaccurate reading. Other chemicals may not be detected. For example, most four-gas meters are set up to read combustible gas, oxygen levels, carbon monoxide, and hydrogen sulfide. If other toxic gases are present, this device probably will not provide adequate warning or information.

Some gas monitors are specific for chemical warfare agents. The Surface Acoustic Wave (SAW) MiniCAD, a commercially available pocket-sized instrument, and the new Joint Chemical Agent Detector (JCAD) can monitor for trace levels of sulfur mustard and G nerve agents. The SAW MiniCAD can also detect some toxic industrial chemicals. These instruments use a pump and thermal concentrator to provide enriched vapor sample concentrations to a pair of high-sensitivity coated SAW microsensors. These sensors detect changes in the properties of acoustic waves as they travel at ultrasonic frequencies in piezoelectric materials. Multiple sensor arrays with multiple coatings and pattern recognition algorithms provide the means to identify agent classes.

INTERPRETATION OF READINGS

Gas-specific sensors measure products in ppm. They are not useful for interpreting flammability. Because these devices are designed to measure a specific gas, they are not very useful for identifying unknown chemicals. The identity of the released chemical should be ascertained so that the proper device can

be selected. As with oxygen sensors, these devices should be calibrated under local conditions.

The action level for gas-specific sensors may be set at the specific chemical's PEL/TLV, IDLH limit, or LOC. These values are explained in Chapter 2.

PHOTOIONIZATION DETECTORS

Photoionization detectors (PIDs) are probably the most commonly used field instruments for detecting chemical WMD agents by hazardous materials teams and first responders.

A PID is used to determine the concentration of ionizable vapors in the air. PIDs detect most organic and a few inorganic vapors. They are used for general monitoring, characterizing plumes, determining agent travel, and detecting situations where protective equipment is needed. Many manufacturers are producing four-gas monitors (O_2, LEL, two toxic gases) and a PID in the same unit. One manufacturer produces a four-gas monitor (O_2, LEL, two toxic gases) and a PID that can send the data to a remote computer receiver by radio (Fig. 11-15). The receiver can monitor up to 16 units as far away as 2 miles. This allows one person to monitor multiple locations. It also allows for fence-line monitoring: Monitors can be placed in front of the decontamination line or in front of a sensitive area to detect agents moving in that direction.

Air is pumped into an ionization chamber that is flooded with ultraviolet (UV) light. The light provides the energy to split uncharged molecules into charged ions. The ions are attracted to a metal grid within the ionization chamber. The grid conducts a small amount of current, and the ions attracted to the grid produce a change in current. This change is displayed as a ppm equivalent (Fig. 11-16).

Anything that interferes with light transmission can affect PID readings. Any water vapor in the ionization chamber acts

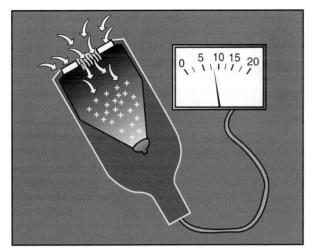

Fig. 11-16
Photoionization detector chamber, ultraviolet light, and grid.

Table 11-1
Interpreting Photoionization Detector Data

Chemical	eV Lamp Required	Correction Factor
Arsine	10.6	1.9
Hydrogen cyanide	Not detectable by PID	
Cyanogen	Not detectable by PID	
Lewisite	10.6	1
Mustard (HD)	10.6	0.6
Nitrogen mustard (HN-1)	10.6	1
Phosgene	11.7	2
Sarin (GB)	10.6	3
Soman (GD)	10.6	3
Tabun (GA)	10.6	0.8
VX	10.6	0.5
GF	10.6	3
DMMP	10.6	4.3
Triethylphosphate	10.6	3.1
Methylsalicylate	10.6	0.9

like a fog and scatters and reflects the UV light back toward the source. Because of this, PIDs may not function adequately in close proximity to decontamination setups. Also, gases that cannot be ionized act in a similar manner.

INTERPRETATION OF DATA

The PID measures all ionizable vapors within the range of the energy supplied by the UV light source. Therefore the instrument can ionize only those vapors that have an ionization potential (IP, measured in electron volts [eV]) equal to or less than the electron volts emitted by the UV lamp. For example, a PID having a UV lamp of 10.6 eV will not detect any vapors that have an ionization potential greater than 10.6 eV. The interchangeable UV lamps in PIDs generally range from 9.6 to 11.7 eV. The 11.7 eV bulb has an extremely short shelf life and is expensive. The most common lamp is the 10.6 eV. This lamp will detect almost all chemical warfare agents and many toxic industrial chemicals.

A PID is usually calibrated to isobutylene. Some instruments can electronically change the calibration to be accurate with other agents. Correction factors are also available to obtain a more accurate reading when detecting other chemicals with a PID calibrated to isobutylene. The readout is multiplied by the correction factor to obtain a more accurate reading. Table 11-1 demonstrates the PID bulb strength needed to detect common chemical threat agents and the correction factor when using a 10.6 eV–bulb PID calibrated to isobutylene.

Some simple compounds, such as methane, cannot be detected by a PID. Zero ppm on the monitor should never be interpreted as no chemicals present. There may be toxic chemicals present that the monitor cannot ionize.

The PID detects all vapors within its ionization range; it cannot identify individual vapors or tell the operator which vapor is present. Therefore the PID is of greatest use when the specific chemical has been identified. Some PIDs are equipped with a gas chromatograph feature. The gas chromatograph, in

the hands of an experienced operator, may be able to identify specific chemicals. Once the chemical has been identified and the instrument properly calibrated, the action level for the PID may be set at the specific chemical's PEL/TLV, IDLH, or LOC.

FLAME IONIZATION DETECTORS

Flame ionization detectors (FID), sometimes called organic vapor analyzers (OVA), are similar to the PID in that they detect ionizable vapors. The operational theory of an FID is similar to the PID's, with one important difference. The energy source for the FID is a hydrogen flame that generates 15.3 eV, enough energy to ionize any compound containing carbon.

Gases are pumped into a detection chamber containing a hydrogen flame. The ions that are produced are attracted to a grid within the detector. An electrical current is generated proportional to the ionic concentration. The change is then displayed as a ppm equivalent.

The FID detects only organic compounds. Additionally, there must be sufficient oxygen in the air to support combustion. The instrument must also be intrinsically safe. As with PIDs, zero ppm on the monitor should never be interpreted as no chemicals present. A popular instrument with many WMD response teams is a device that combines a 10.6 eV PID and an FID in the same unit. The FID detects organic vapors and the PID detects some inorganic compounds (Fig. 11-17).

The FID is typically calibrated to methane. Like the PID, this instrument has a span setting that can electronically recalibrate the instrument for a specific gas.

INTERPRETATION OF DATA

The FID measures total ionizable vapors that the hydrogen flame can ionize. Most instruments are unable to distinguish the type of vapor detected. Similar to PIDs, some FIDs are

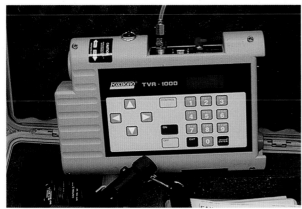

Fig. 11-17
This instrument combines a photoionization detector and a flame ionization detector into one instrument.

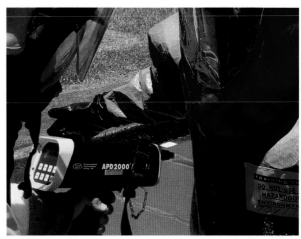

Fig. 11-18
The advanced portable detector detects the presence of nerve agents, blister agents, riot control agents, and gamma radiation.

equipped with a gas chromatograph feature that will identify specific compounds. FID action levels are set at the specific chemical's TLV/PEL, IDLH, or LOC.

ION MOBILITY SPECTROMETRY

Ion mobility spectrometry (IMS) technology can also be used to detect chemical agents. The chemical agent monitor (CAM) or newer advanced portable detector (APD), the automatic chemical agent detection alarm (ACADA-M22), and others are devices that detect chemical warfare agents (Fig. 11-18).

These devices can be used to detect chemical nerve agents and blister agents. The APD can also detect riot control agents and gamma radiation. They are point monitors used to determine if patients or equipment are contaminated with these agents. Air is pulled from an area approximately 10 cm from the tip. The APD 2000 can function as an area detector, but most of the others cannot determine the amount of agent in the air.

IMS devices operate like the PID and FID by producing ions. These devices use a radioactive source (usually nickel-63) as the ionization energy. The agent ions travel through a charged tube where they collide with a detector plate and a charge is registered. A plot of the current generated over time provides an ion mobility spectrum with a series of peaks. The intensity of the peaks indicates the class of agent and relative concentration. Their readout is in units that represent an increasing level of hazard. Response times can take up to 60 seconds. Due to their function, they can show false-positive readings with a number of organic compounds. Because of the extreme toxicity of chemical warfare agents, any reading should be considered a sign of possible contamination if the use of chemical warfare agents is suspected.

NON–HAND-HELD DEVICES

All of the instruments discussed so far have been hand-held, direct-reading devices. Although they are portable and fairly easy to operate, most have low sensitivity and cannot identify

the specific agent in question. There are larger, much more accurate devices. These devices are usually laboratory-based instruments, but vehicle-mounted and even portable versions are available for field use.

INFRARED SPECTROSCOPY

Infrared (IR) spectroscopy measures the absorption of infrared light by a substance. Portable spectrometers can provide infrared analysis in the field. They are relatively simple to operate. A sample of the suspected agent is obtained in the hot zone, isolated in a sample container that is decontaminated, and transferred to a laboratory or to a portable unit in the cold zone. The sample is measured and compared against reference libraries of known compounds for identification. Infrared technology can also identify nerve and blister agents, some toxic industrial chemicals, and explosives in solid or liquid form.

FOURIER TRANSFORM INFRARED

Fourier transform infrared (FTIR) spectrometry devices, such as the Joint Services Lightweight Standoff Chemical Agent Detector (JSLSCAD), identify compounds that are separated by gas chromatography. After the separation of compounds, the sample is exposed to an infrared beam. The adsorption of the infrared light is measured. The JSLSCAD can detect nerve and blister agent vapor clouds at a distance of up to 5 km.

GAS CHROMATOGRAPHY

Gas chromatography (GC) coupled with a mass spectrometer is a laboratory technology that is used to positively identify suspected agents and compounds. The gas chromatograph–mass spectrometer combination is commonly used to identify unknown agents.

The compound is separated by chemical and physical properties and compared to a standardized library of compounds. While this procedure is commonly carried out in offsite

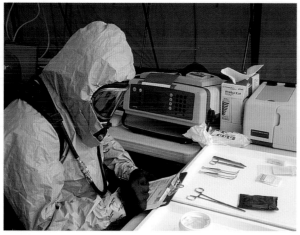

Fig. 11-19
A gas chromatograph–mass spectroscopy device can be used to identify unknown chemicals in the field.

laboratories, specialized units such as the National Guard Civil Support Teams use these units in the field (Fig. 11-19). The equipment is expensive and requires specialized training.

BIOLOGICAL DETECTION

In a covert attack using a biological agent, the first indications may be an unusual distribution or number of cases of a disease. This will usually be long after the agent has been dispersed or degraded. Because there will be no immediate emergency response to these covert attacks, the need for rapid detection devices is not as important as it is in a chemical attack. Testing can be helpful in identifying an agent when a release is ongoing or immediately discovered. Testing also is important in cleanup activities after an attack with spore-forming agents such as anthrax. Real-time detection in the environment is a difficult task due to the vast number of potential agents, the nature of the agents, and the similar microorganisms that are normally present in the environment.

The same wet chemistry test kits that are used to identify unknown chemical substances can be used to rule out common materials such as drywall dust, talcum powder, and powered sugar that are often used in biological agent release hoaxes.

One test kit manufacturer has developed a wet chemistry kit specifically for WMD agents, including biological and radiological agents. The testing procedure is fairly complicated and requires extensive training.

IMMUNOASSAY TEST STRIPS

Immunoassays are test strips that can bind specific antigens with corresponding antibodies. Many immunoassay tests are in the form of a strip that changes color, similar to home pregnancy tests. Other systems using immunoassays may use readers, which tend to be more accurate. A sample is obtained, mixed in a liquid medium, and exposed on the test surface. A color

change provides a positive or negative indication within 15 minutes. Tests are available for *Yersinia pestis, Francisella tularensis, Bacillis anthracis, Vibrio cholerae,* staphylococcal enterotoxin B (SEB), ricin, botulinum toxins, and *Brucella* spp. There can be a high frequency of false positives and some false negatives with these tests. The CDC suggests that assays should be used only for preliminary field screening and should not be used to make determinations about patient care. Confirmatory laboratory testing should be carried out.

POLYMERASE CHAIN REACTION

Another biological testing technology is polymerase chain reaction (PCR). PCR uses a gene-based system to detect the presence of the DNA of bacterial or viral agents. This technology is very sensitive and very specific.

LABORATORY ANALYSIS

Obtaining samples in the field and transferring them for laboratory analysis is the most accurate way to identify biological agents. Because samples may be critical evidence in a criminal case, chain of custody procedures should be followed. Mass spectrometry is a common laboratory analysis method.

BIOLOGICAL INTEGRATED DETECTION SYSTEM

Some military units have more sophisticated biological testing units such as the biological integrated detection system (BIDS). This system continuously samples ambient air and determines the background distribution of aerosol particles. Particles are concentrated and analyzed for biological activity. At present this system includes tests for *Y. pestis, B. anthracis,* SEB, and botulinum toxin A. Research and development is under way to develop reliable and accurate real-time detection for biological agents in the environment.

STAND-OFF DETECTION SYSTEMS

Stand-off detection systems designed to detect agents from a distance are also available. These devices detect the plume before it reaches the detector. Typically, these instruments use laser remote sensing, so the instrument must be in the line of sight of the plume.

CHAPTER SUMMARY

Detection and monitoring equipment allow responders to make decisions regarding the identity and amount of the released material, the extent of spread of the material, the types of protective equipment needed, and decontamination efficiency. EMS responders can use the data supplied by direct-reading air-monitoring equipment to assist in triage and patient management decisions. To accomplish this, the appropriate device must be chosen, the instrument must be used properly, and the results must be properly and accurately assessed.

Typically, responders use combustible gas monitors, oxygen meters, and radiation survey instruments in an initial survey. If chemical warfare agents are suspected, PIDs, FIDs, colorimetric indicator tubes, or specific gas indicators may also be used. Ion mobility devices such as the CAM or APD can be used to determine the efficiency of decontamination if nerve or blister agents were used. Remember that all devices have major limitations and might not detect the presence of certain gases or vapors. If solid or liquid contaminants are present, detector strips or field test kits may be helpful. Field screening tests and laboratory analysis are available for biological contaminants.

Responders must be able to identify the limitations associated with these devices in order to accurately use the data to make decisions and guide treatment. Air monitoring should be an ongoing process throughout the response. Conditions may change without warning and present extreme hazards.

Remember that each instrument has limitations. Never interpret a device or test's failure to detect anything as evidence that no agent is present. Different types of detectors may need to be used to detect certain agents. Multiple detectors should always be used to verify results. All instruments must be properly calibrated and maintained to ensure their efficacy. Detection instruments can provide invaluable information to emergency response personnel, but only if they are used properly and in conjunction with adequate risk-assessment procedures.

BIBLIOGRAPHY

Andrews LP, editor: *Emergency responder training manual for the hazardous materials technician,* New York, 1992, Van Nostrand Reinhold.

Committee on Research and Development: *Chemical and biological terrorism,* Washington, DC, 1999, National Academy Press, http://books.nap.edu/books/0309061954/html/index.html, retrieved October 4, 2004.

Emergency Film Group: *Detecting weapons of mass destruction,* Edgartown, Mass, 2003, Detrick Lawrence.

Hawley C: *Air monitoring and detection devices,* Albany, NY, 2002, Delmar.

Hawley C: *Hazardous materials incidents,* Albany, NY, 2002, Delmar.

Laughlin J, Trebisacci DG, editors: *Hazardous materials response handbook,* Quincy, Mass, 2002, National Fire Protection Association.

Maslansky CJ, Maslansky SP: *Air monitoring instrumentation,* New York, 1993, Van Nostrand Reinhold.

National Fire Protection Association: *NFPA 471, recommended practice for responding to hazardous materials incidents,* Quincy, Mass, 2002, National Fire Protection Association.

Noll GG, Hildebrand MS, Yvorra JG: *Hazardous materials—managing the incident,* ed 2, Stillwater, Okla, 1995, Fire Protection Publications.

Occupational Safety and Health Administration: *29 CFR 1910.120, hazardous waste operations and emergency response, final rule, March 6, 1989,* Washington, DC, 1989, U.S. Government Printing Office.

Strong CB, Irvin TR: *Emergency response and hazardous chemical management—principles and practices,* Delray Beach, Fla, 1996, St Lucie Press.

United States Fire Administration: *Guidelines for public sector hazardous materials training,* Emmitsburg, Md, 1998, Federal Emergency Management Administration.

Varela J, editor: *Hazardous materials handbook for emergency responders,* New York, 1996, Van Nostrand Reinhold.

Chapter **12**

Personal Protective Equipment

PHIL CURRANCE AND CHRIS MAILLIARD

CHAPTER OBJECTIVES

At the conclusion of this chapter the student will be able to:

- Explain the use and limitations of standard and specialized emergency medical services (EMS) protective equipment in weapons of mass destruction (WMD) incidents.
- Identify three types of respiratory-protective equipment and discuss their limitations.
- Describe respiratory-protective equipment fit-testing procedures.
- Discuss the difference between vapor-protective and splash-protective clothing.
- List the four Environmental Protection Agency (EPA)-designated levels of protection, and discuss the use and limitations of each.
- Identify the limitations of structural firefighter's protective equipment in WMD incidents.
- Discuss military WMD protective equipment.
- Describe donning and doffing procedures for personal protective equipment.

CASE STUDY

An explosive device has been detonated in a six-story office building; the building has collapsed. The building was constructed in the 1960s, and asbestos may have been present in the building. The bomb may have contained a chemical or radiological agent. Firefighters are performing rescue operations in the demolished shell of the building, and EMS responders are providing treatment to both ambulatory and nonambulatory patients. Some patients have been transported to hospitals by private vehicles.

What type of protective equipment is needed for this incident?

Do responders performing decontamination and providing treatment to nondecontaminated patients need the same protective equipment as those inside the building?

Will air-purifying respirators provide adequate protection?

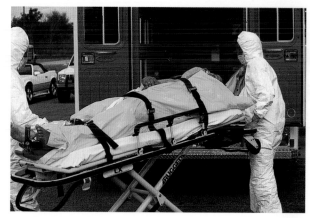

Fig. 12-1
EMS responders in body-substance isolation personal protective equipment.

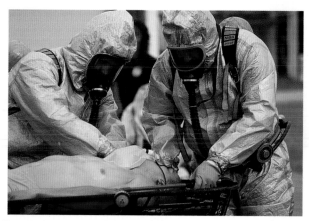

Fig. 12-2
EMS responders in chemical-protective personal protective equipment.

Responders at WMD incidents must be adequately protected from potential exposure and injury. The purpose of personal protective equipment (PPE) is to shield or isolate persons from chemical, physical, radiological, and biological hazards.

Protective equipment concerns must be addressed before any response activity. Protective equipment decisions must be based on responder involvement. Activities in clean, safe areas, such as management of decontaminated patients, can be safely carried out in PPE commonly used for body substance isolation. This will include gloves, mask, eye protection, and a suit to keep liquids from contacting the responder's uniform.

This type of PPE is not adequate for use in the contaminated area or for use during primary decontamination activities. In these areas, specialized protective equipment is needed. Chemical-protective equipment includes chemical-resistant clothing and gloves that are specifically compatible with the chemical plus an air-purifying respirator (APR), a self-contained breathing apparatus (SCBA), or a supplied-air respirator (SAR). The use of this equipment requires specific training and selection by a knowledgeable, experienced person (Figs. 12-1 and 12-2).

Responders should not attempt to use PPE without proper preplanning, training, medical examinations, and fit-testing as required. Selection of equipment by an informed and knowledgeable person using appropriate reference sources is essential. Having equipment is not enough. The equipment must be compatible with the hazard. Chemical-protective equipment usually does not provide protection against fire or heat. Initial hands-on training and repeated practice with all the protective equipment is essential for safe and effective use.

In addition to EMS responders' protection, knowledge of protective equipment concerns is vital for the support of the other responders at the incident. The use of PPE can itself create significant worker hazards such as heat stress; physical and psychological stress; and impaired vision, mobility, and communication. In general, greater levels of PPE protection can cause the associated risks to increase. For any given situation, equipment and clothing should be selected that provides an adequate level of protection. Gross overprotection, as well as underprotection, can be hazardous and should be avoided.

No single combination of PPE and clothing is capable of protecting against all hazards. Thus PPE should be used in conjunction with other protective methods. All potential hazards should be identified. Once identified, as many hazards as possible should be mitigated. Examples of hazard mitigation include:

- Ventilation of structures or confined spaces
- Use of foam to suppress vapors
- Control of ignition sources
- Avoidance of contact with hazardous substances as much as possible
- Adequate decontamination before removal of PPE

RESPIRATORY PROTECTIVE EQUIPMENT

The most vulnerable route of exposure is inhalation. Responders must have adequate respiratory protection. Respiratory protection can be provided by air-purifying respirators (APRs), positive-pressure SCBA, or positive-pressure SAR or air lines.

Occupational Safety and Health Administration (OSHA) standard 29 CFR 1910.134 cites specific requirements for respirator use. These include a written program, proper selection of respirators, medical monitoring, fit-tests, user training, and storage and inspection. Proper-use procedures, such as restrictions on facial hair, also are included in the standards. The selection of the proper respirator is based on several factors:

- Oxygen concentration in the area
- Identity of the substance
- Concentration of the substance
- Chemical and physical properties of the substance
- Warning properties of the substance
- Area in which responders must operate
- Specific tasks to be completed

The level of protection that can be provided by a respirator is indicated by the respirator's protection factor (PF). This number, which is determined experimentally by measuring face piece seal and exhalation valve leakage, indicates the relative difference in concentrations of substances outside and inside the face piece that can be maintained by the respirator. The PF is multiplied by the chemical's exposure limit to determine the maximum use concentration (MUC) of the respirator. The chemical's exposure limit is the permissible exposure limit time-weighted average (PEL-TWA) or the threshold limit value time-weighted average (TLV-TWA). APRs should never be used at concentrations above either the chemical's IDLH (immediately dangerous to life and health) value or MUC (PF × PEL-TWA = MUC). Above these levels, SCBA or SAR is required.

Several factors can affect the proper fit of a respirator and reduce the PF. These factors are:

- Facial hair that contacts the sealing surface
- Facial deformities
- Extreme heat or cold
- Eyeglasses with temple bars or straps

AIR-PURIFYING RESPIRATORS

APRs use filters or sorbent materials to remove harmful substances from the air (Fig. 12-3). APRs consist of a face piece and an air-purifying device, which is either a removable component on the face piece or an air-purifying apparatus worn on a body

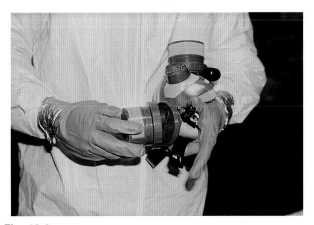
Fig. 12-3
Air-purifying respirator and combination cartridge (HEPA and organic vapor).

harness and attached to the face piece by a corrugated breathing tube. APRs selectively remove airborne contaminants by filtration, absorption, adsorption, or chemical reactions. They are approved for use in atmospheres containing specific chemicals up to designated concentrations. The use of APRs in the contaminated area is limited, especially for emergency response operations, and is only appropriate when:

- Atmospheric oxygen is greater than 19.5%
- The chemical substance is known
- The chemical substance can be filtered, absorbed, adsorbed, or neutralized
- The chemical substance has an adequate warning property (odor, irritation, or taste detectable below the PEL and consistent to above the IDLH)
- The airborne concentration of the chemical substance is known
- The airborne concentration of a chemical substance does not exceed 1000 ppm, the calculated MUC, or the established IDLH
- There is a NIOSH-approved cartridge
- No firefighting activities are involved
- Users have been properly trained and fit-tested and have undergone medical monitoring

Warning: Some contaminants cannot be removed by APRs. These respirators are *not* used in oxygen-deficient or IDLH situations or when the contaminants are unknown. During emergency response operations, initial entry into the contaminated area or hot zone must be considered an IDLH situation, and atmosphere-supplying respirators must be used. Once the substance has been identified and quantified and all criteria are met, APRs may be used. In these circumstances they may be used during decontamination or in low-risk cleanup activities.

Escape-only air purifying respirators are also available for victims escaping from contaminated areas. These are usually hooded respirators that provide a limited time of protection (usually 15 minutes). They do not require fit testing. Certain high-risk terrorist target areas are providing these for staff in case of attack. They should only be used to escape the contaminated area. They do not provide adequate protection for rescue or patient-care activities.

Air-purifying cartridges and canisters are designed for specific materials at specific concentrations. The respirators that EMS personnel use to protect against tuberculosis are particulate cartridges. They are available in different filtering efficiencies. N95 filters are the type most often used by medical personnel. The most efficient particulate filters are the high-efficiency particulate air (HEPA) filters. The new designation for the HEPA filters is *P100*. These respirators may provide protection against asbestos and other particulates, but they will allow gases and vapors to pass through.

To aid the user, manufacturers have color-coded the cartridges and canisters to indicate the chemical or class of chemicals against which the device is effective.
- Purple: Particulates (HEPA) or P100
- Black: Organic vapor
- White: Acid gas
- Yellow: Combination of organic vapor and acid gas
- Green: Ammonia
- Blue: Chlorine
- Silver: Mercury

Cartridges can be stacked. A common combination is a HEPA (particulate) and acid gas–organic vapor stack. Recent improvements have resulted in what many companies refer to as their domestic preparedness or WMD cartridges. These cartridges are effective against particulates, chemical warfare agents (nerve, blister, and choking agents), ammonia, chlorine, pesticides, acid gases, organic vapors, and a few other chemicals depending on the manufacturer. The color coding on these cartridges is usually black or gray depending on the manufacturer. Check the compatibility of the exact cartridges you have with the manufacturer's printed data.

Cartridges and filters will eventually plug up with particulates or saturate with chemical vapors. The National Institute for Occupational Safety and Health (NIOSH) recommends that the use of a cartridge not exceed one work shift. However, if breakthrough of the contaminant or breathing difficulty occurs first, then the cartridge or canister must be replaced immediately. Breakthrough occurs when the adsorbent bed becomes saturated. Vapors and gases then pass through the cartridge. The user will detect the warning property (odor, taste, or irritation) of the chemical. Particulate filters (N95 and P100) eventually plug up with the contaminant, and breathing resistance increases.

POWERED AIR-PURIFYING RESPIRATORS

Powered air-purifying respirators (PAPRs) are very similar to APRs. The only difference is that the PAPR uses a fan to push the air into the face piece (Fig. 12-4). A PAPR uses a face piece similar to an APR's or a hood that can be worn by responders who cannot wear a face piece because of facial hair or framed eyeglasses (Fig. 12-5).

Tight-fit masks offer more protection than the hooded type. Also, the tight-fit type will continue to protect the user

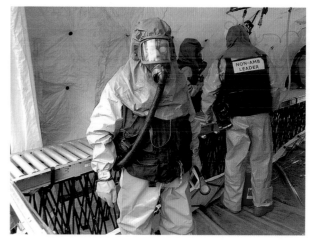

Fig. 12-4
Responder wearing powered air-purifying respirator with tight-fit mask.

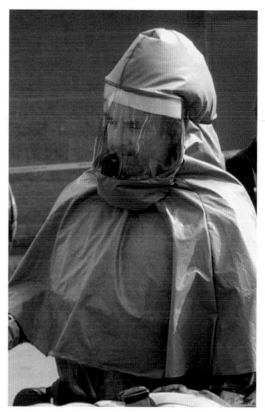

Fig. 12-5
Hood-type air-purifying respirator.

in cases of battery or unit malfunction. Both of these attach with a hose that is connected to the power-and-filter unit. The power unit is worn on a belt or vest and contains a battery and two or three cartridges used to filter the air. The PAPR uses the same cartridges as an APR, and all the same precautions must be taken when using a PAPR.

One advantage of a PAPR is much less breathing resistance due to the powered airflow. The second advantage a PAPR has over an APR is that the cool air inside the face piece provides an added degree of comfort as well as keeping the lens clear of fog. The disadvantages of a PAPR when compared to an APR are increased weight and a more complex unit.

Even though standard PAPRs use a fan to push air into the mask, they cannot guarantee a positive pressure inside the mask at all times, as a positive-pressure SCBA does. With the SCBA, the regulator maintains a slight positive pressure inside the mask at all times. If a face fit leak develops, the positive pressure air inside the mask will push contaminants out. With the PAPR, a deep breath may overcome the positive airflow to the mask, resulting in a momentary negative pressure. This is why OSHA gives the same protection factor to PAPRs with a tight-fit mask and to a standard full-face APR.

At present one manufacturer has designed a positive-pressure PAPR. The SE400 designed by S.E.A. Group (Australia) uses a computer chip to measure the user's demand on the system and a variable speed fan motor. As the user demands more air, the fan speed increases to provide more airflow to the mask. This unit will maintain a positive pressure in the mask under all but the most extreme conditions. An indicator light informs the user if the mask goes into a negative pressure state. Even in the negative pressure state the unit provides the same protection as a standard APR.

HOSPITAL/DECONTAMINATION PERSONNEL USE

There has been a great deal of discussion on the use of APRs and PAPRs for protection of decontamination personnel, especially in the hospital setting (Fig. 12-6). At the heart of this discussion is the OSHA requirement of identifying the chemical and concentration present before an APR or PAPR can be used. Recent communications from OSHA have helped to answer some of these questions.

OSHA's current position is that the requirement to wear SCBA, until the exact identity and concentration of the chemical can be identified, "applies to employees under an Incident Command System who are engaged in emergency response with the intent of handling or controlling the release."[1] OSHA further states,

> In contrast, hospital staff members who decontaminate a patient at the hospital are removed from the site of the emergency and the point of release. Normally, these personnel do not need to be trained or equipped for the same level of control, containment, or confinement operations as required for the hazardous materials (HAZMAT) team. Potential exposures to hospital staff usually result from proximity to, or contact with a patient whose skin

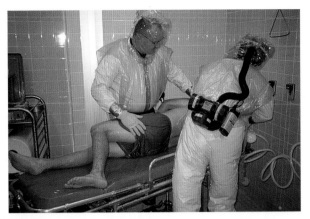

Fig. 12-6
Hospital personnel using powered air-purifying respirators.

and/or clothing may be contaminated. The hospital staff's personal protective equipment must be sufficient for the type and exposure levels an employee can reasonably anticipate from such incidents.[2]

These opinions can be found in answers to interpretation questions asked by Roth and Hayden. These letters are on the OSHA website (www.osha.gov). Because of these interpretations, many hospitals protect their patient-decontamination personnel with hooded PAPRs equipped with domestic preparedness or HEPA–organic vapor–acid gas cartridges. The Soldier Biological and Chemical Command (SBCCOM) carried out extensive testing on PAPR units and found that they offered high levels of protection against various chemical warfare agents. More detailed information can be found by visiting the SBCCOM website at www.ecbc.army.mil/hld/ip/pf_papr_download.htm.

ATMOSPHERE-SUPPLYING RESPIRATORS

Atmosphere-supplying respirators supply certified breathable air to the face piece from a clean air source other than the surrounding contaminated atmosphere (Fig. 12-7). Atmosphere-supplying respirators come in three types: SCBA, SARs or air lines, and escape-only respirators. These respirators must be operated in a positive-pressure or pressure-demand mode.

Pressure-demand respirators maintain a positive pressure in the face piece during both inhalation and exhalation. In these respirators, a pressure regulator and an exhalation valve on the mask maintain the mask's positive pressure. If a leak develops in a pressure-demand respirator, the regulator sends a continuous flow of clean air into the face piece, preventing penetration by contaminated ambient air. This is in contrast to negative-pressure respirators such as APRs.

In a negative-pressure system the user inhales, creating a negative pressure inside the mask and allowing air to move through the filter medium to the inside of the mask. If there are any facial-fit leaks, contaminated air will be drawn into the mask.

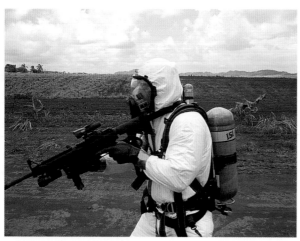

Fig. 12-7
Law enforcement responder using self-contained breathing apparatus.

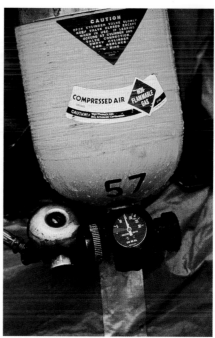

Fig. 12-9
Open-circuit self-contained breathing apparatus.

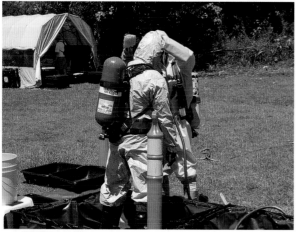

Fig. 12-8
Open-circuit self-contained breathing apparatus.

SELF-CONTAINED BREATHING APPARATUS

Self-contained breathing apparatus (SCBA) respirators are the most common respiratory protection devices used by emergency responders. SCBA respirators can be purchased with open-circuit or closed-circuit design. An open-circuit SCBA exhausts exhaled air directly into the environment (Fig. 12-8).

Air is supplied by either a single-stage (conventional) or a two-stage National Aeronautics and Space Administration (NASA) regulator. Single-stage regulators reduce the air pressure from the air cylinder only once before reaching the wearer. This type of SCBA usually is characterized by a corrugated low-pressure tube connecting the face piece to the regulator. Two-stage regulators are characterized by an initial reduction of cylinder air pressure immediately exiting the air cylinder. A second regulator then is placed at the face piece.

Open-Circuit Apparatus. Open-circuit SCBAs provide respiratory protection from most types and levels of airborne contaminants. However, the air supply is a limiting factor. The duration of the air supply is limited by the amount carried in the tank (tank pressure pounds per square inch [psi]), the rate of consumption, and the type of work being done. The size, physical condition, breathing rate, and lung volume (tidal volume) of the responder using the equipment determines the rate of consumption.

Open-circuit SCBAs typically are described as high-pressure or low-pressure systems. Low-pressure systems with standard-size bottles, commonly referred to as *30-minute units,* have service pressures of 2216 psi; high-pressure systems with standard-size bottles, commonly referred to as *1-hour units,* have service pressures of 4500 psi. High-pressure units also are available with smaller bottles that are rated at 30 or 45 minutes. Most users will not get the 30-, 45-, or 60-minute use time. A good general rule is 1 minute for each 100 pounds of pressure in a standard-size cylinder.

An alarm (e.g., bell, whistle, or vibrator) is set to signal when 25% of the service pressure (approximately 500 psi for low-pressure bottles) is reached (Fig. 12-9). While working in a contaminated area, the responder should not depend on the alarm as a signal to withdraw from the contaminated area.

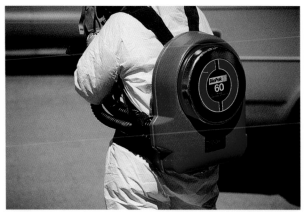

Fig. 12-10
Responder using closed-circuit self-contained breathing apparatus.

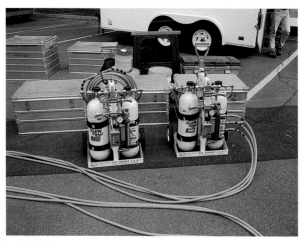

Fig. 12-11
Air-line system.

Personnel will have to be decontaminated before removing the respirator face piece. Time must be allocated for exit from the contaminated area and decontamination.

Other negative aspects of open-circuit SCBAs are bulk and weight. Responders wearing SCBAs may be unable to operate in tight spaces. These units provide EMS personnel with the highest level of protection during patient decontamination, but the weight and bulk limit the responders' ability to carry out some patient-care activities. The weight of the SCBA will contribute to the physical and heat stress of the wearer. An increased risk of back injuries exists and is a result of a change in the wearer's center of gravity when wearing SCBA. Also, because of the time limitations, SCBAs will be difficult to use when attempting to decontaminate the multitude of patients expected at WMD incidents. Trying to keep enough bottles for all responders operating at a WMD incident for an extended period of time presents numerous logistical problems.

Closed-Circuit Apparatus. A closed-circuit breathing apparatus recycles the wearer's exhaled air (Fig. 12-10). Closed-circuit units consist of a carbon dioxide (CO_2) scrubber unit and a bottle of compressed oxygen. These units have one tube that carries air to the mask and a second tube that carries exhaled air back to the unit. The CO_2 is chemically removed, and fresh oxygen is introduced. This type of breathing apparatus is commonly referred to as a *rebreather.*

Advantages of a closed-circuit unit are lighter weight and longer service duration (up to 6 hours in some units). Disadvantages include higher prices, higher operating costs, and heat build-up caused by the exothermic reaction in the CO_2 removal process, which can add to heat stress in the responder. Some response agencies are adding closed-circuit units to their inventory for special operations such as confined-space rescues and search and rescue operations in large buildings.

SUPPLIED-AIR RESPIRATORS

Supplied-air respirators (SARs), or air lines, provide clean air to a face mask through a connecting hose from a tank of certified breathing air or a certified breathing air compressor located in a safe, clean area (Fig. 12-11). A safety escape bottle must be part of the equipment in IDLH conditions. OSHA regulations state that the air line cannot exceed 300 feet.

Advantages of air-line systems include an increased work time and reduced weight and bulk. Disadvantages include the close proximity of the air source to the contaminated area and the vulnerability of the air line. The air line can be damaged by chemicals or cut by sharp edges or debris, or it can kink, cutting off the air supply. In addition, responders have limited mobility. They must retrace their steps to exit the area. This limits the responders' escape routes. Additional responders must be assigned to manage the air source and air lines.

Air lines may be useful for responders carrying out decontamination activities or rescue in confined spaces. Air lines also can be combined with open-circuit SCBAs. This combination can provide for mobility and increased work time in isolated areas or increased time for decontamination.

ESCAPE-ONLY RESPIRATORS

Escape-only respirators provide continuous airflow from a small bottle to a plastic hood that goes over the head. Escape bottles typically have 5-minute or 10-minute duration. They supply direct, continuous-flow air but are not pressure-demand units. They are used by otherwise nonprotected personnel to escape from hostile areas.

They are also used to rescue patients from contaminated areas or confined spaces (Fig. 12-12). The escape-bottle hood is placed over the head of the spontaneously breathing patient, giving the patient 5 or 10 minutes of clean air during the rescue. Most of these units have hoods that are tightened by a drawstring around the neck. Spinal immobilization can be maintained by a responder stabilizing the head and neck from the front while another responder applies the hood. The second responder slides the hood over the patient's head and the first responder's hands.

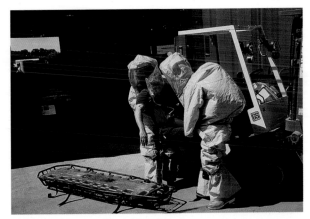

Fig. 12-12
Responders performing a rescue using an escape-only respirator.

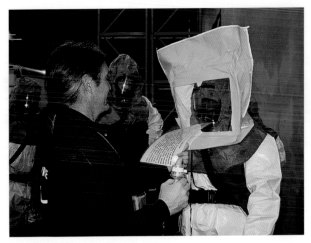

Fig. 12-13
Qualitative fit-testing.

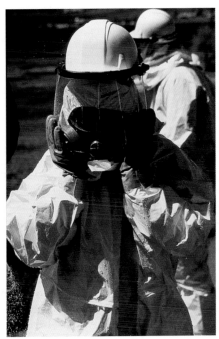

Fig. 12-14
In a negative fit-check, inward rushing of air indicates a poor fit.

Once the hood is in place the second responder takes over immobilization, and the first responder removes the hands and tightens the drawstring.

RESPIRATOR FIT-TESTING

All users of tight-fitting respirators must be fit-tested to ensure proper face piece–to-face seal of the respirator. The fit-test should be accomplished using standard OSHA methods. Fit-testing can be conducted by qualitative or quantitative testing, depending on the respirator type.

In qualitative testing the wearer is exposed to isoamyl acetate vapors (banana oil), irritant smoke, or saccharin. During the test the wearer reads aloud and conducts simple exercises (Fig. 12-13). A failure occurs if the wearer can detect the test agent. In quantitative testing a computerized device attached to the mask is used to detect face-piece leaks. Quantitative testing is more accurate.

Personnel should be tested into a specific brand, model, and size of respirator. Fit-testing must be conducted annually. Fit-testing also is required if the user gains or loses 20 pounds or more, has facial or dental surgery that would interfere with the facial fit, or changes to a different brand or model of respirator.

In addition to the annual fit-test, a fit check should be performed every time a respirator is donned. The purpose of this check is to ensure that a proper fit is possible and to check the patency of the mask's exhalation valve. This is accomplished by means of a positive-negative fit check. To conduct a positive fit check, gently exhale while covering the exhalation valve to ensure that a positive pressure can build up. Failure to build a positive pressure indicates a poor fit. To conduct a negative-pressure check, close the inlet part with the palm or squeeze the breathing tube so it does not pass air, and gently inhale for about 10 seconds (Fig. 12-14). Any inward rushing of air indicates a poor fit or failure of the exhalation valve.

RESPIRATOR MAINTENANCE

Respirators should be inspected before and after each use. OSHA regulations state that respirators that are not used routinely must be inspected at least monthly. Emergency responders routinely inspect their respirators on a daily basis. Inspections should include a check of the tightness of the connections; a check of the face piece, valves, connecting tube, and filters (in APRs); and a check of the regulator, warning devices, and air pressure on SCBAs for proper functioning.

Respirators should be cleaned and disinfected after each use. Maintenance should be performed by factory-trained personnel, or the respirator should be returned to the factory for service. APRs can be stored in sealed plastic bags. Filters or cartridges should not be stored with the respirator but should be unsealed and installed just before use. SCBAs can be stored in quick-don racks or in their factory cases.

PROTECTIVE CLOTHING

When activities are conducted at sites in which chemical, biological, or particulate radiological contamination is known or suspected to exist, chemical-protective clothing (CPC) must be worn. Street clothing or uniforms offer little or no protection from these exposures. The predominant physical and chemical or toxic properties of the agent will dictate the type and degree of protection that is required. The maximum level of protection can only be determined when complete identification of a hazard has been made.

VAPOR-PROTECTIVE CLOTHING

Vapor-protective clothing is designed to provide the highest level of protection against skin-destructive and skin-absorbable substances. It consists of a fully encapsulating, vapor-tight suit and the highest degree of respiratory protection (pressure-demand SCBA or SAR with escape bottle).

CHEMICAL-SPLASH PROTECTIVE CLOTHING

Chemical-splash protective clothing is designed to provide protection against liquid splash or particulates. It provides very limited protection against vapors. Tape often is used with splash-protective clothing to seal openings, gloves, and boots. Sealing splash-protective suits with tape will not make them vapor tight. A key component with splash-protective clothing is the type of respiratory protection used. Splash-protective clothing can be used with either an APR or SCBA.

EPA PROTECTION LEVELS

The Environmental Protection Agency (EPA) has divided protective clothing and respiratory protection into four categories according to the degree of protection afforded.

LEVEL A PROTECTION

Level A protection should be worn when the highest level of respiratory, skin, eye, and mucous membrane protection is needed (Fig. 12-15). This level usually is used for protection against skin-toxic or corrosive vapors. It also is needed when gross liquid contact is possible, such as when working on leaking overhead pipes, and for extremely hazardous materials. PPE for level A includes the following:

- Positive-pressure (pressure-demand) SCBA (approved by the Mine Safety and Health Administration [MSHA] and NIOSH)

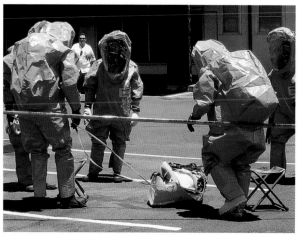

Fig. 12-15
Responders using Level A vapor-protective suits.

- Fully encapsulating, vapor-tight, chemical-resistant suit, inner gloves, chemical-resistant outer gloves, and chemical-resistant boots with steel toe and shank
- Underwear (cotton, long-john type) (optional, as needed)
- Hard hat (under suit) (optional, as needed)
- Cooling vest (optional, as needed)
- Coveralls (under suit) (optional, as needed)
- Two-way radio communicators (that are intrinsically safe) (optional, as needed)

Even if Level A protection is used, responders should try to keep any contact with the substance to an absolute minimum.

LEVEL B PROTECTION

Level B protection should be selected when the situation requires the highest level of respiratory protection but a lower level of skin and eye protection (Fig. 12-16). This level usually is used for protection against inadvertent liquid splash or particulates. A relatively new style of splash-protective suits is a fully encapsulating, non–vapor-tight suit that offers a higher degree of skin protection and protects the SCBA. PPE for this level includes the following:

- Positive-pressure (pressure-demand) SCBA (approved by the MSHA and NIOSH)
- Chemical-resistant clothing (overalls and long-sleeved jacket; coveralls; hooded, two-piece, chemical-splash suit; disposable, chemical-resistant coveralls; or fully encapsulated, non–vapor-tight suit)
- Coveralls (under splash suit) (optional, as needed)
- Inner gloves
- Chemical-resistant outer gloves, taped to suit
- Chemical-resistant boots with steel toe and shank
- Cooling vest (optional, as needed)
- Two-way radio communicators (that are intrinsically safe) (optional, as needed)
- Hard hat (optional, as needed)

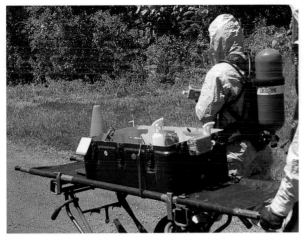

Fig. 12-16
Responders using Level B splash-protective personal protective equipment.

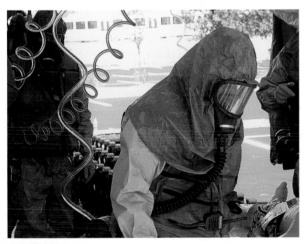

Fig. 12-17
Responders using Level C personal protective equipment: splash suit and powered air-purifying respirator.

LEVEL C PROTECTION

Level C protection should be selected when the type of airborne substance is known, its concentration has been measured, the criteria for using APRs have been met, and skin exposure is unlikely (Fig. 12-17). Periodic monitoring of the air should be performed when this level of protection is used. PPE for this level includes the following:
- Full-face APR or PAPR (MSHA/NIOSH approved)
- Chemical-resistant clothing (one-piece coverall; hooded, two-piece chemical-splash suit; disposable, chemical-resistant overalls)

Personal Protective Equipment	**Box 12-1**
for Emergency Medical	
Activities	

Standard Protective Equipment

Body substance isolation equipment for cold zone operations:
- Eye protection
- Mask
- Gloves (latex undergloves and chemical-resistant outer gloves)
- Fluid-resistant gowns or suits
- Fluid-resistant shoe covers

Specialized Protective Equipment

For warm or hot zone operations:
- Self-contained breathing apparatus or
- Air purifying (APR) or powered air-purifying respirators (PAPR)
- Chemical-resistant gloves (with latex under gloves)
- Chemical-resistant suits
- Boots or shoe covers

Source: Pavlin JA: *Emerg Infec Dis* 5:528-530, 1999.

- Inner gloves
- Chemical-resistant outer gloves, taped to suit
- Chemical-resistant boots, with steel toe and shank
- Coveralls (under splash suit) (optional, as needed)
- Two-way radio communicators (that are intrinsically safe) (optional, as needed)
- Cooling vest (optional, as needed)
- Hard hat (optional, as needed)
- Escape mask (optional, as needed)

LEVEL D PROTECTION

Level D protection is primarily a work uniform. It should not be worn in any location where respiratory or skin hazards exist (Fig. 12-18).

In many cases the initial survey of a contaminated area is done in a minimum of Level B protection. If skin-toxic chemicals are present or suspected, Level A protection should be used. The level of protection is then upgraded or downgraded accordingly as information becomes available. The type of equipment used and the overall level of protection should be constantly reevaluated as additional information about the incident is obtained and as responders are required to perform different tasks (Box 12-2).

NATIONAL FIRE PROTECTION ASSOCIATION STANDARDS

A weakness of the EPA levels of protection is that they provide only a design specification instead of a performance specification. A suit might meet EPA-designated Level A standards, but users have little idea if it meets their protection need.

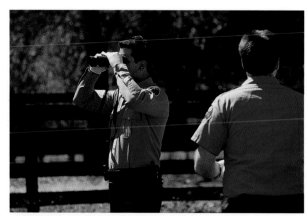

Fig. 12-18
Responders wearing Level D personal protective
equipment: street uniforms (no protection).

Choosing Protection Level   **Box 12-2**

Reasons to upgrade protection levels include:
- Known or suspected presence of chemicals that can cause skin damage
- Occurrence or likely occurrence of gas or vapor emission
- Change in work task that will increase contact or potential contact with hazardous materials

Reasons to downgrade protection levels include:
- New information indicating that the situation is less hazardous than was originally thought
- Change in site conditions that decreases the hazard
- Change in work task that will reduce contact with hazardous materials

The National Fire Protection Association (NFPA) has developed standards for chemical-protective suits. The standards cover certification, documentation requirements, design and performance requirements, and test methods. NFPA 1991 applies to vapor-protective suits used for chemical protection in the hot zone. NFPA 1992 applies to liquid-splash B protective suits used in the hot zone. NFPA 1994 applies to protective equipment designed for use at incidents involving the release of chemical or biological agents. These standards assist responders in understanding and selecting protective clothing.

Because NFPA 1994 sets performance requirements for protective clothing used at chemical and biological terrorism incidents, it is discussed in depth. This standard defines three classes of PPE ensembles based on the perceived threat at the emergency scene. All NFPA 1994 ensembles are designed for a single exposure (use).

CLASS 1 ENSEMBLES

Class 1 ensembles offer the highest level of protection. They consist of a vapor-tight, fully encapsulated suit and SCBA. They are intended for the worst circumstances, where the

substance involved creates an immediate threat, is unidentified, and is of unknown concentration. These situations would occur in an ongoing release with likely gas or vapor exposure where the responder is close to the point of the release and most victims in the area appear to be unconscious or dead from exposure. Stay times in the hazard zone are likely to be short and limited to the breathing air available from the SCBA.

CLASS 2 ENSEMBLES

Class 2 ensembles offer an intermediate level of protection. Class 2 ensembles are intended for circumstances where the agent or threat may be identified, when the actual release has subsided, or in an area where live victims may be rescued. Conditions of exposure include possible contact with residual vapor or gas and highly contaminated surfaces at the emergency scene. Most victims in the response area are alive and show signs of movement but are nonambulatory. For Class 2 ensembles, breathing air from the SCBA may still limit wearing time. However, Class 2 ensembles may also be configured with powered air-purifying respirators that provide longer work time.

CLASS 3 ENSEMBLES

Class 3 ensembles offer the lowest level of protection. Class 3 ensembles are intended for use long after the release has occurred, at relatively great distances from the point of release, or in the peripheral zone of the release scene for such functions as decontamination, patient care, crowd control, perimeter control, traffic control, and cleanup. Class 3 ensembles should only be used when there is very little potential for vapor or gas exposure, when exposure to liquids is expected to be incidental through contact with contaminated surfaces, or when dealing with patients or self-evacuating victims. Class 3 ensembles must cover the wearer and preferably the wearer's respirator, as well, to limit the potential for contamination. Because these ensembles are intended for longer wearing periods, the use of air-purifying respirators with these suits is likely.

FIREFIGHTER TURNOUT GEAR

In 1999 SBCCOM, with the assistance of Montgomery County (Maryland) Fire and Rescue Service, tested firefighter's protective clothing (bunker or turnout gear) for resistance to chemical agents inside a hot zone (Fig. 12-19). The following are the general guidelines for use of turnout gear at the scene of a chemical agent release.
- "Standard turnout gear with SCBA provides a first responder with sufficient protection from a nerve agent vapor hazards inside interior or downwind areas of the hot zone to allow 30 minutes' rescue time for known live victims."
- "Self-taped turnout gear with SCBA provides sufficient protection in an unknown nerve agent environment for a 3-minute reconnaissance to search for living victims (or 2-minute reconnaissance if mustard agent (HD) is suspected)."

What do these tests mean to firefighters first on scene of a chemical agent release? First, it should provide these firefighters with an added level of security when responding, whether the chemical agent comes from the primary incident or a secondary

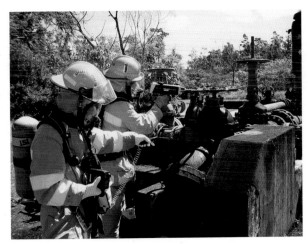

Fig. 12-19
Responders using firefighters' protective equipment.

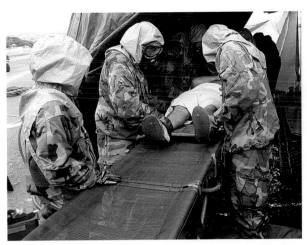

Fig. 12-20
Military responders using MOPP 4.

device. Second, it will allow incident commanders to begin rescue operations if the need is seen. Before these firefighters enter a hot zone, appropriate decontamination must be established. As always, the incident commander must do a solid risk-benefit analysis before sending firefighters in this situation into the hot zone.

Another factor that can improve protection to these first responders is the use of chemical-resistant suits under the turnout and the use of chemical-resistant tape around the boots and gloves. The tests also showed that brand-new turnout offers less protection than gear that has been used because the soot and carbon that builds up in the fabric acts as an adsorbent for chemical vapors. Finally, the use of positive-pressure ventilation inside a structure can provide first responders with a higher level of protection. More information on these studies is available on the SBCCOM website at www.ecbc.army.mil/hld/cwirp/cwirp_final_incident_command_download.htm.

MISSION-ORIENTED PROTECTIVE POSTURE

Mission-oriented protective posture (MOPP) equipment is the standard military chemical protective equipment for battlefield use (Fig. 12-20). It is worn in several configurations depending on the perceived level of threat from chemical or biological agents.
- MOPP 0: All protective equipment is carried with the individual responder.
- MOPP 1: Chemical overgarment is worn, and overboots, mask with hood, and gloves are carried, when an attack is possible.
- MOPP 2: Chemical overgarment and overboots are worn, and mask with hood and gloves are carried, when an attack is probable.
- MOPP 3: Chemical overgarment, overboots, and mask with hood are worn, and gloves are carried, when chemical or biological agents, or both, are present at a negligible risk level.

- MOPP 4: All protective equipment is worn. This provides the highest degree of protection when agents are present but the risk is undetermined.

The MOPP protective overgarments include the Saratoga suit or the joint services lightweight integrated suit technology (JSLIST) suit.

The Saratoga suit is a reusable two-piece suit made of a cotton rip-stop outer layer and a filter layer that consists of carbon spheres that adsorb the chemical agents before they can reach the inner layer of the suit. In noncontaminated environments, the suit can be laundered four times during its service life. Protective capabilities extend to 30 days, with active protection of 24 hours during that period. The suit should be discarded within 24 hours of exposure to chemicals. The Saratoga suit protects against chemical agent vapors, aerosols, and droplets and all known biological agents.

The JSLIST overgarment has raglan sleeves for more maneuverability and an integrated chemical hood that replaces the butyl rubber hood used with the Saratoga system. It is lighter than the older systems and reduces heat stress. The JSLIST suit can be laundered up to six times. It provides protection for 45 days.

In the past these suits were available only to military units. Now civilian response agencies can also take advantage of this type of garment. Protective undergarments and overgarments by Lanx Fabric Systems (Richmond, Va) are made from the same technology. They are made of polymerically encapsulated activated carbon material. They can be laundered up to 10 times. When stored in airtight containers they have a shelf life of 12 years.

CHEMICAL-PROTECTIVE CLOTHING

Unlike the military or Lanx suits that use carbon to adsorb chemical vapors, classic chemical-protective clothing relies on a chemical-resistant fabric. Selecting the correct fabric is just as important as selecting the correct level of protection. CPC materials are those that by their physical and chemical makeup

Protective Clothing Resistance

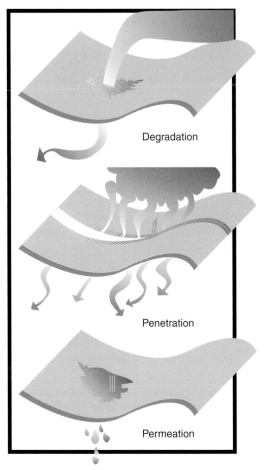

Degradation

Penetration

Permeation

Fig. 12-21
Degradation, penetration, and permeation.

are able to resist the physical and chemical hazards inherent in various hazardous substances. These products have excellent to fair resistance to selected chemicals. No material has total resistance to all chemical exposures. Very often, chemical resistance is extremely limited.

CHEMICAL RESISTANCE

Chemical resistance is the ability of a material to physically resist degradation, permeation, and penetration by a contaminant (Fig. 12-21). *Degradation* is the loss in physical properties caused by an exposure to a chemical. Damage to the material may be so slight that it may not be visible to the naked eye. *Permeation*, or diffusion, is the process by which a chemical moves through a material on a molecular level. Permeation typically is measured by the time it takes to pass from the outer side of a material (once exposed) to the inside. This is referred to as *permeation time*. *Permeation rate* is the speed at which the chemical passes through. *Penetration* is the flow of a substance or material through openings such as zippers, seams, stitches, holes, or tears in the garment.

The degree of resistance is measured by testing a particular material or substance against a specific product or chemical. To assist users of specialized protective clothing, manufacturers of materials submit their product or fabric sample to a research laboratory or agency for testing. Chemical resistance is represented by charts or tables distributed by manufacturers of protective clothing or their testing agencies. They typically show their resistance or relative effectiveness against specific classes of chemicals.

Many hazardous chemicals are mixtures for which specific data are not available for selecting chemical-resistant fabrics. Because of a lack of testing, only limited permeation data for multicomponent liquids are currently available. Mixtures of chemicals can be significantly more aggressive toward CPC materials than can any single component alone. Even small amounts of a rapidly permeating chemical can provide a pathway that accelerates the permeation of other chemicals. NIOSH is developing methods for evaluating CPC materials against mixtures of chemicals and unknowns in the field. For emergency response operations, select CPC that offers the widest range of protection against the chemicals expected at the incident. Vendors are now producing CPC material composed of two or three different materials laminated together. These multilaminate fabrics provide the best features of each material.

EMS responders should not expect any one protective fabric or gloves to provide protection against all chemicals. A selection of fabrics should be stocked and compatibility with the chemical checked before use.

HEAT-TRANSFER CHARACTERISTICS

The heat-transfer characteristics of CPC can be an important selection factor. Because most CPC is virtually impermeable to moisture, evaporative cooling is limited. The *clo value* (thermal insulation value) of CPC is a scientific measure of the capacity of CPC to dissipate heat through means other than evaporation. The larger the clo value, the greater the insulating properties of the garment and, consequently, the lower the heat transfer. A clo value of 1 is equal to the heat loss capacity of a normal business suit. Given other equivalent protective properties, protective clothing with the lowest clo value should be selected in hot environments or for high work rates. Unfortunately, clo values currently are available for only a few CPC ensembles.

Responders using Level A or Level B PPE must be monitored for the effects of heat stress and fatigue. EMS responders should anticipate that heat-stress injuries will occur. Procedures to limit heat stress should be in place. These procedures include monitoring for heat stress, using ice vests, taking frequent breaks, and taking frequent oral hydration to replace lost body fluids.

OTHER FACTORS

In addition to chemical resistance and heat transfer, several other factors must be considered during clothing selection. These factors affect not only chemical resistance but also the responder's ability to perform the required task. Included among these factors are:
- Durability
- Flexibility
- Temperature effects

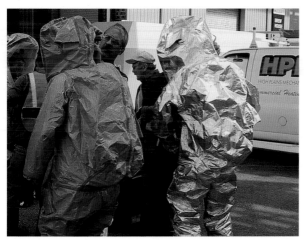

Fig. 12-22
Responder in Level A gear *(left)* and responder in Level A gear with flash suit *(right).*

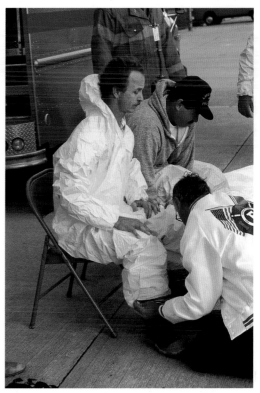

Fig. 12-23
Responders should assist in donning chemical-protective equipment to decrease the possibility of suit damage.

- Ease of decontamination
- Compatibility with other equipment
- Duration of use

Fire, explosion, heat, and nonparticulate radiation are considered special conditions that require special protective equipment. Aluminized flash suits are available for many brands of chemical-protective clothing (Fig. 12-22). These garments offer limited protection against flash fires but do not offer the protection necessary for wear in proximity to high temperatures or for firefighting operations. Additional fire protection may be obtained with the use of coveralls, gloves, and hoods made from a fire-resistant fabric such as Nomex or PBI.

DONNING AND DOFFING PERSONAL PROTECTIVE EQUIPMENT

A routine for donning PPE should be established and practiced periodically. Assistance should be provided for donning and doffing because these operations are difficult to perform alone, and solo efforts may increase the possibility of suit damage (Fig. 12-23).

Once the equipment has been donned, its fit should be evaluated. If the clothing is too small, it will restrict movement, thereby increasing the likelihood of tearing the suit material and accelerating responder fatigue and heat stress. If the clothing is too large, the possibility of snagging the material is increased, and the dexterity and coordination of the responder may be compromised.

If responders have problems with the PPE while wearing it, they should immediately exit the hot zone and report any perceived problems or difficulties. Problems include but are not limited to:
- Visible damage to the suit
- Degradation of the suit
- Respirator malfunction

- Perception of odors
- Skin irritation
- Physical discomfort
- Interference with vision or communication
- Restriction of movement
- Personal responses such as rapid pulse, nausea, and dizziness

Exact procedures for removing fully encapsulating suit and SCBA ensembles must be established and followed to prevent contaminants from migrating from the hot zone and transferring to the wearer and other responders. Doffing procedures should be performed only after decontamination. They require a suitably attired assistant. Throughout the procedures, the responder should only touch the inside suit surfaces and the assistant should only touch the outside surfaces.

Chemicals that have begun to permeate clothing during use might not be removed during decontamination and could continue to diffuse through the fabric toward the inside surface. This presents a hazard of direct skin contact to the next person who uses the clothing. Where such potential hazards could develop, clothing should be checked inside and out for discoloration or other evidence of contamination. This is especially important for multiuse, fully encapsulating suits, which are generally subject to reuse because of their cost. Level A suits must be pressure-tested annually and before each reuse.

CLOTHING REUSE

At present, little documentation exists about clothing reuse. Reuse decisions must consider both permeation rates and toxicity of the contaminants. In fact, unless extreme care is taken to ensure that clothing is properly decontaminated and that the decontamination does not degrade the material, it is not advisable to reuse CPC that has been contaminated with toxic chemicals. This is the major reason limited-use protective clothing is becoming popular. The lower cost of limited-use garments makes disposal after each incident a viable alternative. All equipment, such as SCBA, that will be reused must be carefully decontaminated.

CLOTHING MAINTENANCE

CPC should be inspected when it is received from the factory, periodically while in storage, and before and after each use. Level A suits should be pressure-tested on the same schedule (Fig. 12-24). Detailed inspection procedures are usually available from the manufacturer.

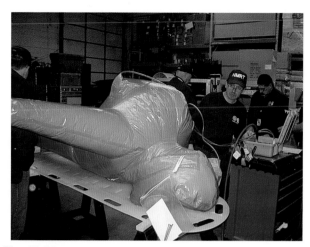

Fig. 12-24
Responders conducting Level A suit pressure-test.

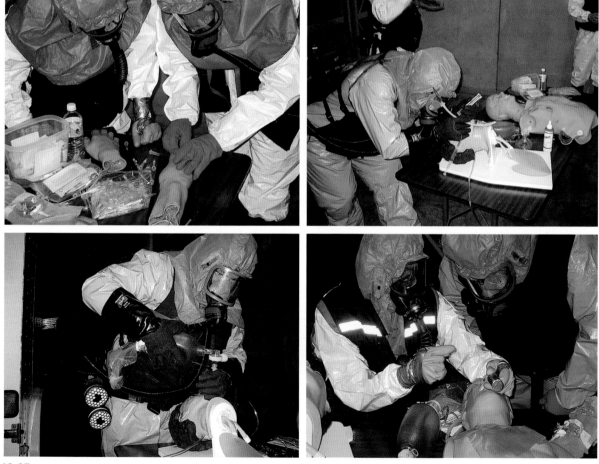

Fig. 12-25
Medical responders with the Central National Medical Response Team practice medical treatment skills while wearing protective equipment.

Suggested Protective Equipment Ensembles — Box 12-3

Chemical Agents

Hot zone
Minimum of firefighter's structural protective equipment or chemical-resistant suit and SCBA (Level B) for immediate rescue and reconnaissance activities

Level A protective equipment and SCBA for direct-contact chemical control or extended work in the hot zone

Warm zone
Minimum of PAPR/APR or SCBA and chemical-resistant suit (Level C or B) for decontamination and patient-care activities

Cold zone
Work uniform (Level D) with quick access to respiratory protection in case of wind shift or secondary device

Biological Agents

Hot and warm zones
Standard body substance isolation equipment (gloves, face shield, gloves, suit and N95 mask)

Upgrade to P100 (HEPA) for contagious agents such as smallpox, pneumonic plague, viral hemorrhagic fevers

Cold zone
Work uniform (Level D) with quick access to respiratory protection in case of wind shift or secondary device

Radiological Agents (Alpha and Beta Contamination)

Hot and warm zones
Minimum of APR/PAPR or SCBA and protective suit

Cold zone
Work uniform (Level D) with quick access to respiratory protection in case of wind shift or secondary device

---

The technical depth of maintenance procedures varies. Manufacturers frequently restrict the sale of certain PPE parts to individuals or groups who are specially trained, equipped, and authorized by the manufacturer to purchase them. Procedures should be adopted to ensure that the appropriate level of maintenance is performed only by personnel who have this specialized training and equipment.

Clothing and respirators must be stored properly to prevent damage or malfunction resulting from exposure to dust, moisture, sunlight, damaging chemicals, extreme temperatures, and impact. Many equipment failures can be directly attributed to improper storage. Different types and materials of clothing and gloves should be stored separately to prevent issuing the wrong type or material by mistake. Protective clothing should be stored according to manufacturers' recommendations.

Detailed records should be maintained for each item of PPE and clothing. This is especially true of reusable items. Records should contain the item's purchase date, inspection records, decontamination information, and the chemicals the item has been exposed to.

CHAPTER SUMMARY

Medical responders must be trained to wear protective equipment, and it is essential that they be able to provide necessary patient treatment while wearing the equipment. This will take initial training and frequent practice (Fig. 12-25).

Selection of PPE is a complex task and should be performed by personnel with training and experience. If the chemical has been identified, the following items should be considered:

- State of matter (solid, liquid, vapor) of the chemical
- Chemical and physical properties of the chemical
- Level of protection required (vapor or splash protection)
- Type of fabric that will provide the longest breakthrough time
- Type of activities to be performed
- Potential for heat stress

If the chemicals have not been identified, the task of proper equipment selection is much more difficult. Additional indicators that should be assessed include:

- Visible IDLH indicators (e.g., visible vapors, smoke, or particles; incapacitated victims or animals; dead vegetation)
- Positive readings on direct-reading instruments
- Indicators of gases or highly toxic substances (e.g., placards, labels, specific containers, signs)
- Poorly ventilated or enclosed areas

Under all conditions, equipment is selected by evaluating the performance characteristics of the equipment against the requirements and limitations of the scene- and task-specific conditions (Box 12-3).

It is unlikely that most EMS responders will ever need to wear Level A PPE. Firefighters or hazardous materials response team members are usually the only responders who enter the contaminated area and rescue patients from this area. Patient-care activities are limited by the Level A suit. In rare cases, EMS responders may be called on to perform triage in the contaminated area. Patients who are trapped may need care during extrication. EMS responders should have an understanding of PPE. At locations where EMS activities may be needed in the hot zone, training with Level A suits should be conducted. EMS responders should be able to use Level B or C PPE to carry out patient care during decontamination. Under no circumstances should responders wear any PPE without proper training, practice, and fit-testing as necessary.

REFERENCES

1. Fairfax RE: *Respiratory protection requirements for hospital staff decontaminating chemically contaminated patients*, September 5, 2002, http://www.osha.gov/pls/oshaweb/owadisp.show_document?p_table=INTERPRETATIONS&p_id=24516, retrieved November 8, 2004.

2. Fairfax RE: *Training and PPE requirements for hospital staff that decontaminate victims/patients*, December 2, 2002, http://www.osha.gov/pls/oshaweb/owadisp.show_document?p_table=INTERPRETATIONS&p_id=24523, retrieved November 8, 2004.

BIBLIOGRAPHY

Agency for Toxic Substances and Disease Registry: *Managing hazardous materials incidents, emergency medical services: a planning guide for the management of contaminated patients,* Atlanta, 2001, U.S. Department of Health and Human Services.

Andrews LP, editor: *Emergency responder training manual for the hazardous materials technician,* New York, 1992, Van Nostrand Reinhold.

Bronstein AC, Currance PL: Module 4: emergency medical operations. In Ayers S, Christopher J, editors: *Medical response to chemical emergencies,* Washington, DC, 1994, Chemical Manufacturers Association.

Currance PL: *Hazmat for EMS,* St Louis, 1995, Mosby (videotape and guidebook).

Department of Transportation: *2000 North American emergency response guidebook,* Washington, DC, 2000, U.S. Department of Transportation.

Hawley C: *Hazardous materials incidents,* Albany, NY, 2002, Delmar.

Laughlin J, Trebisacci D, editors: *Hazardous materials response handbook,* ed 2, Quincy, Mass, 2002, National Fire Protection Association.

National Fire Protection Association: *NFPA 471, Recommended practice for responding to hazardous materials incidents,* Quincy, Mass, 2002, National Fire Protection Association.

National Fire Protection Association: *NFPA 1991, Vapor-protective suits for hazardous materials emergencies,* Quincy, Mass, 2000, National Fire Protection Association.

National Fire Protection Association: *NFPA 1992, Liquid splash protective suits for hazardous materials emergencies,* Quincy, Mass, 2000, National Fire Protection Association.

National Fire Protection Association: *NFPA 1994, Protective ensembles for chemical/biological terrorism incidents,* Quincy, Mass, 2001, National Fire Protection Association.

Noll GG, Hildebrand MS, Yvorra JG: *Hazardous materials: managing the incident,* ed 2, Stillwater, Okla, 1995, Fire Protection Publications.

Occupational Safety and Health Administration: *29 CFR 1910.120, hazardous waste operations and emergency response, final rule, March 6, 1989,* Washington, DC, 1989, U.S. Government Printing Office.

Schultz M, Cisek, J, Wabeke R: Simulated exposure of hospital personnel to solvent vapors and respirable dust during decontamination of chemically exposed patients, *Ann Emerg Med* 26:324-329, 1995.

Soldier Biological and Chemical Command: *Guidelines for incident commanders: final report: FFPE use in chemical agent vapor,* Washington, DC, 1999, U.S. Army, http://www.mipt.org/pdf/ffpe_scba.pdf, retrieved October 4, 2004.

Strong CB, Irvin TR: *Emergency response and hazardous chemical management: principles and practices,* Delray Beach, Fla, 1996, St Lucie Press.

United States Fire Administration: *Guidelines for public sector hazardous materials training,* Emmitsburg, Md, 1998, Federal Emergency Management Administration.

Decontamination Procedures

Phil Currance

CHAPTER OBJECTIVES

At the conclusion of this chapter the student will be able to:

- Identify the need for and the contents of a decontamination plan.
- Discuss how the decontamination area is established.
- Explain in detail how patient decontamination is carried out.
- Identify chemicals that present a major risk of secondary contamination.
- Describe the differences between ambulatory and nonambulatory patient decontamination procedures.
- Explain how patient decontamination procedures need to be modified in cases of contamination involving radiation or water- or air-reactive materials.
- Describe decontamination procedures for responder protective equipment and clothing.
- Describe how the dry decontamination process is carried out.
- Identify the need for and describe the process of equipment decontamination.
- Identify procedures to determine the effectiveness of decontamination procedures.

CASE STUDY

A small group of terrorists wearing protective equipment and using backpack-mounted pesticide sprayers ran into a crowd at a downtown street fair. Many fairgoers were sprayed with the unknown chemical. Some people were shot by the terrorists when they tried to intervene. Three of the terrorists were also shot by law enforcement officers responding to the scene. There are numerous ambulatory and nonambulatory patients. Using personal protective equipment (PPE), the fire department and hazardous materials (HAZMAT) team have started rescue and decontamination activities. A postdecontamination triage area has been established, and ambulances are ready to transport victims to appropriate medical facilities.

Which should come first, patient decontamination or primary assessment and management of airway, breathing, and circulation (ABC)?

How much patient decontamination is necessary at the scene? How much is necessary at the hospital?

What kind of decontamination procedures will the fire and HAZMAT responders need?

Will the ambulances have to be decontaminated after they are used for transport?

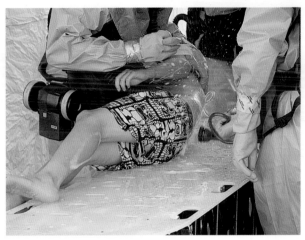

Fig. 13-1
Responders conducting patient decontamination during an exercise.

have a thorough understanding of how contamination occurs. The decontamination plan should identify procedures for avoiding contact with suspected agents. If patients, responders, or equipment become contaminated, the plan should detail the contamination control and decontamination processes.

Contamination occurs when responders, victims, or equipment come into contact with chemical, biological, or radiological agents. Direct contact with a chemical leaking from a container is an obvious way to become contaminated. However, indirect contact can be much more subtle. People may become contaminated in a number of ways, including:

• Contacting vapors, gases, mists, or particulates in the air
• Being splashed by liquid materials
• Walking through puddles or on contaminated soil
• Using contaminated instruments or equipment
• Contacting contaminated PPE
• Treating contaminated patients

SITE SELECTION AND PREPARATION

Decontamination operations should be established before allowing entrance into the contaminated area (hot zone) for any reason, including rescue. As victims or personnel exit the hot zone, they must be decontaminated. Contaminated equipment also must be decontaminated as it leaves the hot zone. A contamination reduction corridor, in which decontamination procedures are carried out, should be established in the warm zone. The decontamination corridor should contain separate areas to decontaminate patients, responders, and heavy equipment as necessary.

LOCATION

Selection of a decontamination site should be based on availability, water supply, ability to contain runoff, and the

Decontamination is the process of removing, or rendering harmless, contaminants that have accumulated on personnel, patients, and equipment (Fig. 13-1). Indications are to limit tissue damage and absorption, to prevent systemic poisoning, to confine contamination to a specified area, and to prevent secondary contamination of EMS and hospital personnel.

Decontamination is critical to the health and safety of responders at WMD incidents and should be a priority. Every agency that responds to these emergencies should have a well-developed decontamination plan. Contacts should be made with other agencies to ensure that each agency's decontamination plan will fit with those of other agencies when they work together at an incident or at a hospital facility. The plan should guide all decontamination activities during the emergency.

CONTAMINATION

The best way to ensure that things are decontaminated is to not let them be contaminated in the first place. Responders must proximity of drains, sewers, streams, and ponds. The site should be upwind and uphill from the incident. The site must be a safe distance from the incident but close enough to allow easy access from the hot zone and limit the spread of contaminants. If the decontamination site must be placed a long distance from the actual work area, transportation will be needed to move personnel and victims. Matters will be complicated if weather or other conditions mandate an off-site decontamination location.

Shelters such as schools, firehouses, garages, indoor car washes, and swimming pools may be used after initial rinse at the scene for thorough decontamination. A problem associated with indoor facility use is containment of the runoff. If contaminated runoff cannot be contained, local authorities and water treatment plants must be contacted. Remember that transport personnel, vehicles, and the facility used will be contaminated.

HOSPITAL DECONTAMINATION

Hospital decontamination can be conducted outside the emergency department (ED) by using portable equipment (Fig. 13-2). Some hospitals are constructing outside decontamination systems (Fig. 13-3). An alternative to outside decontamination is a specially designed room with a separate entrance, contained drains, and separate ventilation system. Many hospitals are building special decontamination rooms. Contingency planning should be in place to handle more patients than the indoor facility can manage.

PATIENT DECONTAMINATION

Emergency medical services (EMS) responders should be concerned with patient decontamination. If patients are transported before being adequately decontaminated, there is a risk of secondary contamination of EMS and hospital personnel,

ambulances, and the receiving emergency department. EMS responders also must know the proper way to decontaminate PPE, equipment, vehicles, and themselves.

Decontamination should be carried out in the warm zone, before transport, with simultaneous patient care provided by qualified, trained, and protected responders (Fig. 13-4). Emergency medical decontamination usually is considered a primary decontamination procedure to stop the chemical action on the patient and allow for safe patient care and transport. In other words, the purpose of field decontamination is to get the patient as clean as reasonably possible, depending on scene conditions and patient presentation. If time, patient presentation, and scene conditions permit, a secondary detailed decontamination can be carried out. This secondary process,

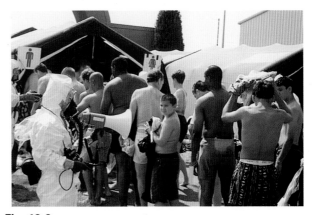

Fig. 13-2
Patients lining up outside the hospital for ambulatory decontamination.

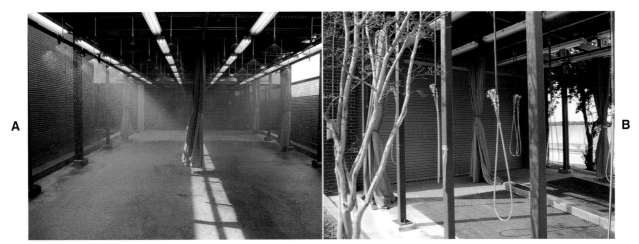

Fig. 13-3
Example of a hospital fixed outside decontamination system. This system is found at the Noble Training Center in Anniston, Alabama. **A,** Ambulatory patients. **B,** The setup for nonambulatory patients.

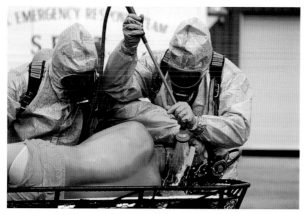

Fig. 13-4
Responders carrying out patient decontamination.

depending on scene conditions and number of patients, may be performed at a prepared and properly equipped hospital emergency department. Hospitals are poor choices for the primary decontamination process. The chemical will continue to affect the patient during transport, and vehicles and personnel may be contaminated.

In inclement weather, a decontamination shelter will be a major asset. Other shelters, such as local facilities, may be used for detailed decontamination after an initial rinse at the scene.

MASS CASUALTY DECONTAMINATION

Mass casualty decontamination procedures are the major bottleneck in WMD response. Prehospital decontamination of contaminated patients should be carried out to limit tissue damage and absorption and prevent systemic poisoning. Contamination must be confined in a specified area to prevent secondary contamination of EMS and hospital personnel. A major consideration in determining the need for decontamination is the risk of secondary contamination of responders, equipment, and hospital staff. Entire systems can be put out of operation by secondary contamination.

Above all, decontamination should be considered an essential part of patient management. If the patient was injured by the affects of the chemical, he or she will not respond to treatment until the exposure is terminated. The patient decontamination procedure should be a planned and practiced event so that it does not take undue time and trouble to implement.

PATIENT DECONTAMINATION PROCESS

FACTORS IN DECONTAMINATION

The process of patient decontamination starts with identifying the product, life threat, route of exposure, and need for decontamination. If the exposure is from an unknown material, a worst-case scenario should be considered. The decision to carry out decontamination procedures on injured patients is not always easy. Whether first to provide patient management or decontamination has always been controversial. Treating the patient before decontamination places EMS personnel at risk. On the other hand, delaying primary attention to ABC concerns for complete decontamination can severely compromise the patient. Having trained, protected responders manage essential treatment at the same time as decontamination solves most of this problem.

Other factors can be used to assist in making patient decontamination decisions. If known, the nature, state of matter, potential toxicity, and concentration of the chemical should be assessed. Liquids, mists, and solids tend to have a longer duration of action because patient exposure is continual. Once the patient is removed from a gas or vapor exposure, the exposure usually stops. In some cases, gases or vapors may be trapped in clothing or turn into solution on moist areas of the patient's skin, necessitating decontamination. Extremely concentrated or high-toxicity agents mandate a higher degree of decontamination.

The route of exposure also must be assessed. Products that attack the body only through inhalation present a minimal risk of further exposure once patients are removed from the area. The duration and extent of exposure also are important considerations. Patients exposed in a peripheral area for a very short time will need minimal, if any, decontamination.

SECONDARY CONTAMINATION

Gases, such as simple asphyxiants and carbon monoxide (CO), are examples of agents with a low risk of secondary contamination. Some gas exposures may react with skin moisture and create acidic or alkaline conditions (e.g., chlorine, anhydrous ammonia). These exposures may need to be decontaminated for the proper care of the patient. Inhalation-only exposure to volatile liquids or vapors requires minimal decontamination. However, responders must be aware of any concurrent liquid or solid exposure.

Examples of agents with a high risk of secondary contamination include corrosive products, nerve agents, blister agents, asbestos, any highly toxic products, high-viscosity liquids, oily or adherent products, dusts, and powders. Patients contaminated with a product that carries a high risk of secondary contamination should always undergo decontamination before transport.

In reality, the decision to decontaminate is not easily made. Consider that several million chemicals are listed in the Chemical Abstracts Service (CAS) index, and we have given suggestions for only a handful. In cases of large exposure, if there is a continuing effect or an exposure to an unknown product, decontamination is indicated. Toxicity is not the only concern. Flammable products may cause fire hazards, and patients exposed to these products should be decontaminated. If any visible product or odor remains on the patient, decontaminate. In all cases, when in doubt, decontaminate!

TYPES OF DECONTAMINATION

Decontamination in mass casualty situations is usually broken down into two major parts, emergency decontamination and technical decontamination.

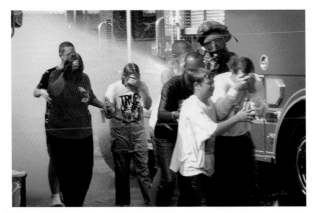

Fig. 13-5
Simple drench drill emergency decontamination system.

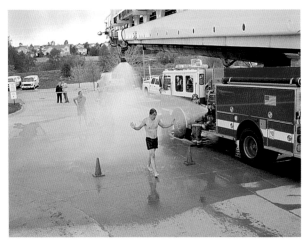

Fig. 13-6
Overhead drench drill emergency decontamination system.

EMERGENCY DECONTAMINATION

Emergency decontamination, or what some agencies call the drench drill, is designed to provide immediate decontamination of large numbers of patients. This procedure uses fire department apparatus or hoses to decontaminate extremely large numbers of patients in a very short time. The major focus of an emergency decontamination system is speed. The idea is to remove the agent from the patient as rapidly as possible. This reduces or stops the agent's action on the victims.

Procedure. The decontamination area should be in a visible location to attract patients. In one common system, two fire engines are parked side by side approximately 15 to 20 feet apart (Fig. 13-5). This establishes a corridor for ambulatory patients to walk through. Fog nozzles are placed on the discharge gates on the sides of the engines facing each other. A 30% fog setting on the nozzles usually provides an adequate pattern. Patients then walk through the corridor. You may want to consider using a third engine to pump water and shut down the motors on the two decontamination engines to reduce patient exposure to diesel exhaust. Another way to establish the drench drill is to use an elevated stream (ladder, squirt, tower), providing an overhead shower (Fig. 13-6). Numerous units can be used to provide multiple overhead sprays.

If time allows, a more private emergency decontamination system can be established with similar techniques. The two fire engines are parked side by side approximately 20 feet apart as in the first system. Ground ladders are placed on top, spanning the distance between the two engines. Hose lines (1½ or 1¾ inch) are placed on top of the ladders, with fog nozzles pointing down to form overhead showers. Tarps are then draped over the ladders to provide privacy. Tarps can also be used to establish different corridors for sex segregation in the showers. A third engine can be used to pump into the two primary decontamination engines to reduce patient exposure to diesel exhaust. Although this type of emergency decontamination system provides a bit more privacy, it does take longer to establish. Responders may want to establish a simpler system with the first arriving engines and have later-arriving units set up the more private system.

For chemical contamination, patients should strip off clothing before they enter the water spray. This will remove the contaminants before they are driven to the skin by the water flow. If the situation involves radiation or biological contamination, patients should be sprayed with water before removing clothing. This will reduce the chance of the contamination's becoming airborne as patients remove their clothing.

Patients are triaged for decontamination priority and moved into the emergency decontamination system. They should remove their clothes and isolate them in plastic bags. They then move through the water rinse and redress or cover up on the other side. If conditions permit, patients should be monitored with detection equipment for decontamination efficacy before they redress.

Problems. Although this procedure does move a lot of people through the decontamination process, some concerns must be addressed. With all of these systems, privacy and weather concerns present problems. Also, the drench drill might not totally decontaminate the patients. Cold water is used, so hypothermia is a concern even in temperate weather. If clothes are left on during the drench drill, chemical contamination could be driven to the skin; patients should disrobe before going through the decontamination process. This presents a problem due to lack of privacy and the patient's unwillingness to disrobe. Adding to this concern is the probable presence of media at the incident site.

This procedure is not effective with nonambulatory patients. Because they must be carried through the water spray, only the front of the patient is cleaned, and patient care during the process is next to impossible.

Another problem is that the system may move too many patients through. Because of the psychological effect of the incident there may be far more patients with no contamination than there are contaminated patients. So many patients may go through the drench drill that responders on the clean side will be overwhelmed. If this includes a large number of patients who didn't really need decontamination, we may be causing more problems due to hypothermia. An emergency decontamination system must take this into consideration and have towels, blankets, suits or gowns for redressing, and transportation to move the patients to a holding area.

TECHNICAL PATIENT DECONTAMINATION SYSTEMS

Because of the concerns associated with emergency decontamination systems, many teams are using decontamination trailers or special tents and patient roller systems or carts to establish a technical patient decontamination system. In a technical patient decontamination system, the decontamination process is more detailed. Decontamination solutions and scrubbing can also be added to the process.

Many mass casualty decontamination systems are commercially available. Some teams have made mass-casualty shower units from free-standing shelters or tarps, PVC pipes, and shower nozzles (Fig. 13-7). There are many portable commercial units on the market. Some of the Metropolitan Medical Response Systems (MMRSs) and other special operation teams such as the National Medical Response Teams (NMRTs) are equipped with portable commercial systems (Fig. 13-9).

Some MMRSs and fire departments use decontamination trailers. Trailers usually are self-contained and quick to get into operation. They have water and air heaters, decontamination solution injection into the water spray, and a runoff holding tank. Newer units are usually set up so that ambulatory decontamination takes place inside the trailers with gender segregation; nonambulatory decontamination is carried out on roller systems outside the trailer under awnings (Fig. 13-8).

Although decontamination trailers provide good mass decontamination that is quick to set up and offers protection from weather, there are some tradeoffs. If the trailer is not pre-positioned, it may be difficult to get it to the venue when everybody else is trying to escape. Also trailers do not provide the flexibility that some portable units do.

Decontamination lines for both ambulatory and nonambulatory patients should be established. A triage point is established in front of the decontamination system to establish decontamination priority. Patients needing immediate treatment or those with heavy contamination are decontaminated first. A treatment area may also be established to provide essential care (airway, ventilation, hemorrhage control, administration of antidotes by self-injectors) while patients are waiting to enter the decontamination system.

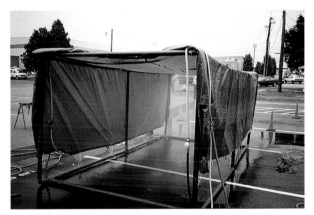

Fig. 13-7
Free-standing mass casualty decontamination system made from PVC pipe and tarp.

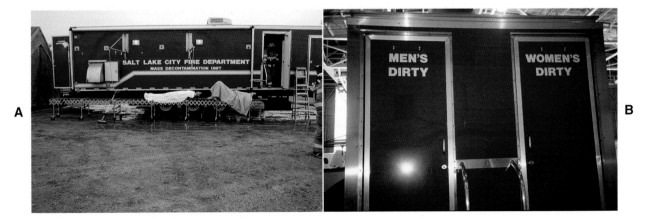

Fig. 13-8
A, Decontamination trailer with nonambulatory decontamination. **B,** Decontamination trailer with ambulatory decontamination.

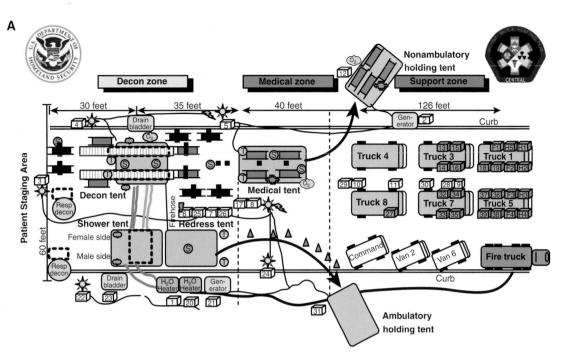

Fig. 13-9
A, Standard decontamination setup footprint of the Central U.S. NMRT-WMD mass casualty decontamination system.
B, All ambulatory decontamination setup footprint of the Central U.S. NMRT-WMD mass casualty decontamination system.

Setup No.1–Standard

NMRT-Central
National Medical Response Team
Weapons of Mass Destruction

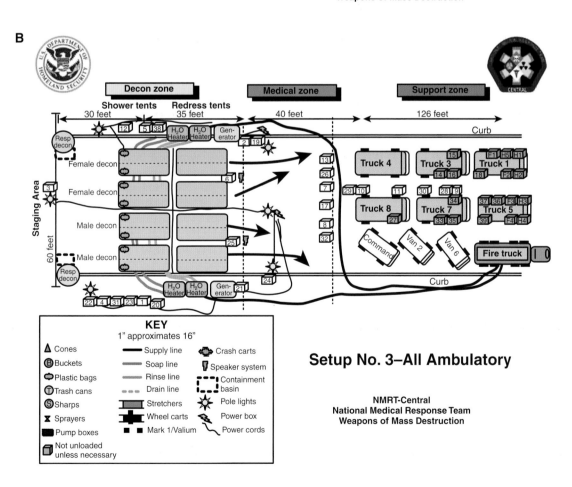

Setup No. 3–All Ambulatory

NMRT-Central
National Medical Response Team
Weapons of Mass Destruction

DECONTAMINATION PROCEDURES FOR AMBULATORY PATIENTS

This discussion focuses on mass casualty decontamination, but the same procedures apply to single-patient decontamination procedures. The ambulatory side of the system requires minimal responder support. Ambulatory patient decontamination procedures start with the patients exiting the contaminated area. Ambulatory patients should be directed to enter the decontamination area (Fig. 13-10).

The ambulatory system should provide gender segregation. Small children should be allowed to accompany either parent. Children should walk if they are able. If the parent is carrying the child, neither one will receive adequate decontamination.

Patients should quickly undress (for radiological or biological contamination, patients should be rinsed before they remove their clothing, if possible) and isolate their clothes and personal possessions in plastic bags marked to identify the patient. Many teams use triage tags with tear-off labels for this purpose. All personal possessions should be removed. If the patient must wear glasses, the glasses should be decontaminated during the process. Contact lenses should be removed after the patient has decontaminated his or her hands. The lenses should be isolated for disposal.

Patients should then move through a minimum two-stage decontamination process. The first stage should consist of a decontamination solution spray followed by the second stage water rinse. Water heater–decontamination solution mixer units are available to supply heated (90° F to 95° F [32° C to 35° C]) decontamination solution and rinse water through fixed shower nozzles to improve decontamination efficiency and reduce the effects of hypothermia (Fig. 13-11). Avoid use of hot water, which may increase absorption. Use low water pressure and a gentle spray to avoid aggravating any soft-tissue injuries. Special attention should be paid to areas of gross contamination, injured areas, hair, and opposing body surfaces such as the underarms

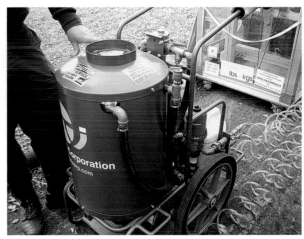

Fig. 13-11
Warm water heater and decontamination solution injector.

and groin. Soft brushes and sponges may be used. Be careful not to abrade the skin, and use extra caution over bruised or broken skin areas. Damaged skin areas can enhance the dermal absorption of toxic products. Large boards with instructions or speaker systems with recorded messages can be used to instruct patients on decontamination procedures as they progress through the system.

Patients should be checked for residual contamination using monitoring equipment, and then they should move into dressing areas (one for each gender) and redress in disposable clothing. As much privacy as possible should be maintained during the decontamination process. Responders assisting in this process should be trained to use PPE and should wear appropriate respiratory protection and protective clothing. After decontamination and redressing, all patients should be checked by medical personnel and treated, transported, or transferred to another area as necessary.

DECONTAMINATION PROCEDURES FOR NONAMBULATORY PATIENTS

For the nonambulatory patient, responders must carry out decontamination after the patient is removed from the contaminated area. Responders providing initial care or carrying out decontamination operations should wear appropriate PPE.

The nonambulatory patient should be placed on a backboard or stretcher, then on something to elevate the patient to a convenient position. Plastic sawhorses, stretcher stands, chairs, or wood blocks can be used. Patient decontamination will be much easier if the nonambulatory patient is elevated to the decontamination personnel's waist height. Some teams use patient roller systems or stretcher carts to more effectively move patients through the decontamination process (Fig. 13-12). The patient's clothing, jewelry, and shoes should be quickly removed and isolated for further decontamination or disposal. Plastic bags marked to identify the patient should be used.

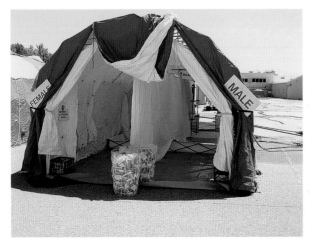

Fig. 13-10
Ambulatory decontamination tent.

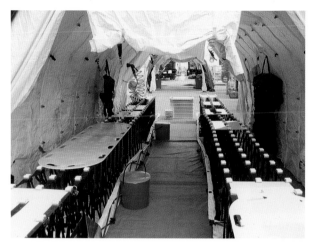

Fig. 13-12
Nonambulatory decontamination rollers.

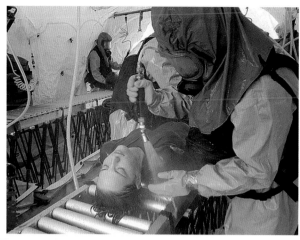

Fig. 13-13
Responders using hand decontamination spray during an exercise.

To reduce the likelihood of a chemical reaction with water, visible solid or particulate contaminants should be brushed off as completely as possible before rinsing. Visible liquid contaminants also should be blotted from the body, using absorbent material, before rinsing. Because skin damage increases the chemical absorption rate, use care not to damage the protective dermal barrier.

The patient is then flushed with a decontamination solution or water. As in the ambulatory system, combination water heater and decontamination solution mixers can be used to supply heated solution and rinse water (90° F to 95° F [32° C to 35° C]) to spray nozzles. Low water pressure and gentle spray nozzles on hose lines should be used to control the spray and prevent aggravating any soft-tissue injuries. Handheld shower massage sprayers work very well (Fig. 13-13).

Try to avoid overspraying and splashing. Patients are sprayed with decontamination solution and washed with sponges or soft brushes. Be careful not to abrade the skin, and use extra caution over bruised or broken skin areas. If the sprayer system cannot mix decontamination solution in the spray, small squeeze or spray bottles work very well. Special attention should be paid to hair, nail beds, and skin folds.

The decontamination procedure should be carried out in a systematic fashion. To protect the airway, the head and face should be decontaminated first. Brush or blot visible contaminants away from the eyes, mouth, and nose, then wash in the same manner. If conditions permit, the patient's airway should be isolated and protected with an oxygen mask or a bag-valve-mask with chemical cartridge. If eye irrigation is necessary, use gentle running water from the nose to the lateral face. If possible, contact lenses should be removed.

Areas of skin damage or gross contamination should be decontaminated next. Use care not to allow contamination into areas of tissue damage. Lightly covering damaged tissues after decontamination with a plastic cover or wrap will help prevent recontamination.

The rest of the patient's body, including the back, then can be decontaminated. When the patient is rolled on his or her side to clean the back, you should also decontaminate the board or stretcher the patient is lying on. Trained and properly protected medical personnel should provide essential medical care during the decontamination process. The process is then repeated with a warm water rinse. Finally, patients are checked for contamination using monitoring equipment. Adequate blankets should be available to reduce the effects of hypothermia. Patients are then triaged for treatment or transport.

Some WMD decontamination teams use video cameras to photograph both ambulatory and nonambulatory patients' faces as they leave the decontamination area. The videotape is then given to local or federal law enforcement agencies to document the identity of the patients who were decontaminated.

PATIENT DECONTAMINATION SOLUTIONS

There has been much discussion about the type of solution that should be used for patient decontamination. Many people believe that water is the best decontamination solution. Water removes the agent by mechanical action. If the patient has been contaminated with agents mixed in organic substances, water might not be adequate. A mild soap used with the water will help improve the results by ionic degradation of the chemical.

Many different types of soap are available. Some agencies use liquid hand dishwashing soaps. Many teams are switching to baby shampoo as the solution of choice. It helps remove the agent and will not burn the patient's eyes when dispersed out of a sprayer system.

For years, the military has been using a dilute bleach solution for decontamination. Standard household bleach is 5% calcium hypochlorite or sodium hypochlorite. The 5% solution is used on equipment, and a 0.5% solution (1 part bleach diluted in 10 parts water) on skin. Although the bleach solution works to deactivate many chemical and biological agents, it does have its limitations. Even the 0.5% solution can cause skin and eye irritation. Care should be taken to avoid getting the solution in the patient's eyes or open wounds. Also, a study conducted by the army[1] found that the use of the hypochlorite solution, at all concentrations, resulted in increased tissue damage.

A great deal of research is being carried out on patient decontamination procedures and solutions. Other solids, soaps, solvents, foams, and UV light are showing promise. While decontamination efficiency can be increased with the proper use of solutions, patient decontamination should never be delayed to obtain or mix the solutions. Water can be used for the initial decontamination and solutions used when they are available.

RUNOFF CONTAINMENT

As in standard decontamination operations, runoff should be collected, if possible. If the incident does not involve mass casualties, the runoff from the decontamination process (ambulatory or nonambulatory) should be contained. Children's wading pools, commercially manufactured units or tables, draft tanks, or makeshift plastic-and-frame units may be useful for containing runoff. The contaminated runoff can be pumped from the pools into barrels or containment basins. Some teams successfully pump the runoff into waterbed mattresses. Hand pumps, sump pumps, or boat bilge pumps can be used.

In all situations, patient decontamination should not be delayed to allow for runoff containment. If no containment pools or tanks are immediately available, try to channel the runoff to a containment area.

With mass casualties, runoff containment may not be feasible because of the large volume of water that must be used. The EPA says that during a true mass casualty incident, runoff is of secondary concern; the primary concern is decontaminating the victims (Fig. 13-14). This policy can be found on the EPA website at http://yosemite.epa.gov/oswer/ceppoweb.nsf/vwResourcesByFilename/onepage.pdf/$File/onepage.pdf. The EPA will not pursue hazardous waste violations against first responders who are not able to contain runoff during mass casualty decontamination operations. Remember to contact local authorities and water treatment plants if the runoff cannot be contained.

SPECIAL DECONTAMINATION SITUATIONS

BIOLOGICAL AGENTS

In cases of covert biological agent release, decontamination is usually not needed. During the incubation phase the patient has probably removed clothing and decontaminated numerous times with home showers. In case of an overt release (agent is visible; agent has been detected by monitoring equipment) involving a small number of patients, decontamination can usually be accomplished by having the patients remove and isolate their clothing and wash areas of the skin that were exposed with soap and water. They should take a full body shower as soon

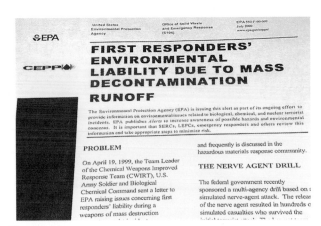

Fig. 13-14
EPA mass casualty decontamination letter.

as possible. In cases of a large number of patients in an overt release or dissemination by an explosive device, standard mass casualty decontamination procedures should be followed.

REACTIVE CHEMICALS

Patient decontamination procedures may need to be modified in cases of water-reactive or air-reactive products that are embedded in the skin. If water-reactive products (e.g., lithium, magnesium, potassium) are embedded in the skin, no water should be applied to that area. The embedded products should be covered with a light oil (mineral or cooking oil) until the pieces can be surgically removed. If the products are not embedded, gently brush away the contaminant as much as possible, then flush with copious amounts of water to rapidly remove any residual product and follow standard patient decontamination procedures.

Phosphorus is air reactive. It spontaneously ignites when in contact with air. If phosphorus particles are embedded in the skin, continuous water irrigation, water immersion, or sterile, water-soaked dressings should be applied until the embedded pieces can be surgically removed. Do not use oil for phosphorus exposure because it may promote dermal absorption.

RADIOACTIVE SUBSTANCES

Transportation incidents where radioactive materials are the only significant hazard can present a special decontamination concern. Packages for large-quantity or high-level radioactive shipments are designed to withstand accident conditions and therefore are unlikely to release their contents when involved in an accident. Small-quantity radioactive shipments, such as a medical imaging isotope, are much more likely to be involved in a radiation release.

Life-threatening conditions are unlikely from the radioactive material released in these situations. The trauma that the patient sustained is a much greater risk. Prolonged field decontamination of patients with life-threatening injuries may delay needed trauma care. In addition, alpha and beta particles may be difficult to remove from the skin. Effective, complete decontamination may require radiological monitoring equipment that may not be available in the field. Most important, improper decontamination methods may facilitate absorption (internalization) by transferring contamination to areas of tissue damage or by converting contaminants to a form that could be more readily absorbed through the skin.

Decontamination procedures should be modified for a small number of victims of transportation accidents in which releases of small quantities of radioactive materials are the only significant hazard. When removed from the area of contamination, patients with only electromagnetic radiation (gamma) exposure will require no further decontamination. The clothing, jewelry, and shoes of patients with particle (alpha and beta) or liquid exposure should be removed quickly and isolated. The patient should then be packaged using reverse isolation procedures such as specially designed patient transportation bags, plastic, or blankets. This will help prevent the spread of contamination during transport. EMS personnel should ensure adequate ambulance ventilation by using both intake and exhaust fans of proper size.

PPE, such as air-purifying respirators (APRs) and outer protective garments, should be used if they are available and EMS personnel have received adequate training. Transportation should be to a receiving hospital that is capable of decontaminating a patient exposed to radioactive products. This should be established in preplanning.

Notify the hospital emergency department that a potentially contaminated patient is en route and provide all available information concerning the identity and nature of the contaminant. This allows the facility to prepare the radiation decontamination area. Preparation might include covering the floor with butcher paper or plastic, allowing for easier cleanup. Infrequently used equipment within the area can be covered or removed as needed. This also allows time to gather special equipment such as radiation survey meters and to call for specialty consultations. Complete decontamination of the patient should be carried out at the emergency department, guided by radiological monitoring devices and under the direction of a physician or health physicist.

During decontamination, extreme care should be exercised to keep contaminants away from areas of tissue damage and body cavity openings. Assistance and advice on patient decontamination and management concerns may be obtained 24 hours a day from the Oak Ridge Radiation Emergency Assistance Center and Training Site by calling 615-576-3131 or 615-481-1000 and asking for the REAC/TS team.

Standard field and emergency department decontamination guidelines should be followed in cases involving a dirty bomb, improvised nuclear device detonation, nuclear device detonation with fallout, or transportation incidents involving a large-quantity shipment in which the container has been breached; in a large release at a fixed facility; or if other chemical contaminants besides radioactive materials are suspected. In cases involving mass casualties, many victims will self-rescue and present themselves to the nearest hospital facility. These patients

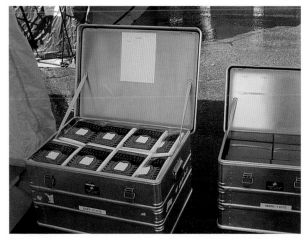

Fig. 13-15
Personal decontamination kit with paper poncho, foot covers, and bags for isolating contaminated clothing.

in addition to the transported contaminated patients can quickly overwhelm the EMS and hospital systems. In these cases patient decontamination should take place prior to transport to the hospital.

DECONTAMINATION IN COLD WEATHER

Severe weather poses several problems during patient decontamination. If cold water must be used in these circumstances, hypothermia will be a major concern. Many technical patient decontamination systems include water heaters to heat the decontamination water. Air heaters are also available to heat the decontamination structures. Some teams use a dry decontamination process for these situations.

Many references state that a majority of the contamination (80% to 90%) can be removed with the clothing, especially in cold weather climates where people wear multiple clothing layers. This may be true in some cases, but there is no guarantee. Certain agents may have passed through the clothing and contaminated the skin.

Many manufacturers are marketing kits that contain a large paper poncho, shoes, and plastic bags to place contaminated clothing in (Fig. 13-15). The idea is to have patients place the poncho over their heads and then remove their clothing under the poncho. In some situations this may be adequate. If there is any doubt, the patient should undergo a conventional decontamination. The kits can also be incorporated into the standard decontamination systems. Many teams use these in all weather conditions to allow privacy as patients undress while they are waiting to enter the decontamination system.

An absorptive solid such as flour or dirt can be used to absorb the agent on the patient's skin. This may not provide complete decontamination but will get the process started (Fig. 13-16). Setting up the decontamination system in an indoor location such as a parking structure, gymnasium, or locker room

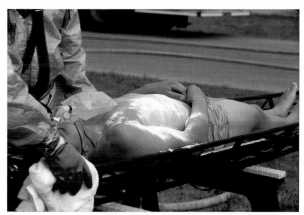

Fig. 13-16
Dry decontamination technique using an absorbent powder.

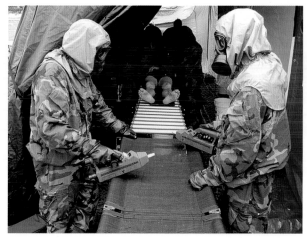

Fig. 13-17
Responders waiting to check a nonambulatory patient for residual contamination.

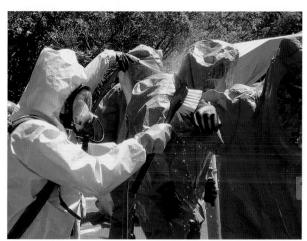

Fig. 13-18
Responder decontamination.

may be useful. The entrance into a building can be used to begin decontamination by opening a fire control sprinkler and having patients move through the sprinkler into the building.

SBCCOM conducted tests on the efficiency of swimming pools for ambulatory patient decontamination. An Olympic-sized swimming pool can be used to decontaminate hundreds of thousands of ambulatory patients by having them walk through the shallow end of the pool. The research can be found at the SBCCOM website at www.ecbc.army.mil/hld/cwirp/cwirp_cold _weather_mass_decon_download.htm.

If patients are going to be moved to an indoor decontamination location, mass transportation must be available. Most large cities already have memoranda of understanding with the local mass transit systems to move patients from standard mass casualty situations. These should be extended to include chemical incidents. Buses that are used to move patients to off-site locations will be contaminated and will need to be isolated and decontaminated as necessary. School buses should be avoided due to the public relations aspect of using those buses to later transport children.

POSTDECONTAMINATION PROCEDURES

After decontamination, nonambulatory patients should be checked for residual contamination. Clean patients should be transferred on a clean backboard (plastic backboards should be used whenever possible) or stretcher to triage or a non-contaminated transport team in the cold zone (Fig. 13-17). Ambulatory patients should be checked for residual contamination and moved to a holding area and triaged to identify any delayed onset of symptoms.

All articles that might be contaminated must be isolated for further decontamination, testing, or proper disposal according to federal, state, and local regulations. These items may include patient clothes or personal possessions, any contaminated patient-care equipment, and the responders' contaminated uniforms or PPE. Disposal of hazardous waste is strictly regulated. Contact the local or state health department for assistance. Any equipment

that was used on the patient before decontamination must be considered contaminated and left in the warm zone until it can be decontaminated or disposed of properly.

RESPONDER DECONTAMINATION

All responders who were contaminated at the scene must also be decontaminated (Fig. 13-18). The best protection for responders is to avoid contact with the agent and with anything that has been in contact with the agent because then responder decontamination is unnecessary. In addition, standard operating procedures should be established that maximize worker protection. For example, following proper procedures for donning and doffing PPE will minimize the potential for contaminants to bypass the protective clothing and escape decontamination. In general, all fasteners should be used (i.e., zippers fully closed, all buttons fastened, all snaps closed).

Inner and outer gloves should be used. Disposable boot covers will help protect reusable boots. If responders are contaminated, they should follow a procedure that will ensure proper decontamination.

DECONTAMINATION PLAN

The original decontamination plan must be adapted to specific conditions found at each incident. The plan should be revised whenever the type of PPE or scene conditions change or whenever the hazards are reassessed based on new information. Depending on numerous factors, these conditions may require more or less personnel decontamination than planned.

DETERMINING THE EXTENT OF RESPONDER DECONTAMINATION

CONTAMINANT PROPERTIES

First, the extent of personnel decontamination will depend on the hazards associated with the agent and its physical and chemical properties. If the agent is suspected to be highly toxic or destructive to skin, full decontamination procedures for personnel who were contaminated should be followed. If permeable garments, such as firefighter gear, are contaminated, detailed decontamination or disposal is essential. Solids and liquids will require more detailed decontamination than gas or vapor exposure. The substance's vapor pressure will significantly affect the extent of decontamination needed. If equipment is contaminated with a high-vapor-pressure liquid, then the majority of the product will evaporate, reducing the need for detailed decontamination.

LOCATION

The location of the contamination is an important factor in determining the extent of decontamination. If contamination is isolated to gloves and boot covers, gross decontamination can be accomplished by removing the contaminated items. If the entire suit is contaminated, more in-depth decontamination is called for.

PERSONAL PROTECTIVE EQUIPMENT

The level of protection and type of protective clothing worn also are factors to be considered. Each level of protection incorporates different problems in decontamination and doffing of the equipment. For example, decontamination of the harness straps and backpack assembly of a SCBA is difficult. Encapsulated Level B or Level A suits will protect the SCBA from contamination. However, these suits will require almost complete decontamination when changing air tanks. If nonencapsulated Level B clothing is worn, a change of air tanks can be accomplished after the back and SCBA connections have been decontaminated.

The type of protective clothing (limited use or multiuse) also will be a factor. For limited-use garments the decontamination must be adequate to remove the responder safely from the garment. The garment is then isolated and disposed of as hazardous waste. If multiuse garments are used, delayed permeation is a factor. Because these garments will be used again, decontamination must be complete.

DEGREE OF EXPOSURE

The task that each responder performs determines the potential for contact with the agent. If tasks do not bring the responder into contact with the agent, minimal, if any, decontamination is appropriate. Anybody with the potential for direct contact with the agent will require a more thorough decontamination.

The quantity of contaminants on equipment and protective clothing also will determine the extent of decontamination needed. If there is visible contamination or obvious discoloration or degradation of PPE, then decontamination is needed. The problem is that many contaminants are invisible to the eye. Therefore, the responder's work function and the type of release that has occurred must be assessed, and if it is possible that either responders or equipment may have had contact with the agent, then thorough decontamination is required.

REASON FOR LEAVING THE HOT ZONE

The reason for leaving the hot or warm zone also determines the need for and extent of decontamination. A responder going to the edge of the contaminated area to pick up or drop off patients, tools, or instruments in a designated area and immediately returning to work may not require decontamination. A worker leaving to get a new SCBA cylinder will require some degree of decontamination. Personnel departing the hot or warm zone at the end of the response must be thoroughly decontaminated to prevent migration of the agent.

RESPONDER DECONTAMINATION PROCEDURES

All personnel, clothing, and equipment leaving the hot or warm zone must be decontaminated to remove any harmful chemicals or infectious organisms that may have adhered to them. Decontamination methods result in:
- Physical removal of contaminants
- Inactivation of contaminants by chemical detoxification or by disinfection or sterilization
- Removal of contaminants by a combination of both physical and chemical means

REMOVAL METHODS

Dilution involves rinsing off the contaminant with water. Dilution often is used because water is readily available. However, this method has many disadvantages. Dilution does not change the hazards associated with the substance, but it does increase the volume of the substance. Containing the contaminated runoff also is a problem. This runoff is hazardous waste and must be disposed of properly. Also, many substances may not be readily removed by dilution.

Absorption is a process that usually is used for equipment, tools, and flat surfaces. In cases of gross contamination of protective clothing or equipment, absorbent pads or sheets may be used to physically remove as much contaminant as possible before another method is used. The disadvantages of absorption are that the absorbent must be picked up and the absorption process does not change the hazards of the chemical.

Hazardous contaminants sometimes can be removed by brushing or wiping away the substance. This is called *physical removal*. Special vacuums also may be used. The vacuums must have special high-efficiency filters on the exhaust. Physical removal may cause solid contaminants to become airborne as dusts and pose further threats of contamination and respiratory exposure.

Solidification is a process of turning a liquid into a solid. Solidifying liquid or gel contaminants can enhance their physical removal. Mechanisms of solidification include moisture removal through the use of adsorbents, chemical reactions via catalysts or chemical reagents, and freezing by using ice water or dry ice. Because of the associated hazards, these methods are restricted to tools and equipment. Technical assistance will be needed to determine the proper solidifying agent. The resulting product also must be considered hazardous waste and must be disposed of properly.

Chemical disinfectants are a practical means of inactivating infectious agents on tools and equipment. Unfortunately, standard sterilization techniques generally are impractical for large equipment and for PPE.

Chemical *neutralization* or *degradation* may be used in the decontamination process. Chemical methods of decontamination require that the contaminant be identified. A decontamination chemical then is needed that will change the contaminant into a less harmful substance. Especially troublesome are unknown substances or mixtures from known or unknown substances. Because of the potential hazards, using chemicals for decontamination should be done only by experienced personnel and only if recommended by an experienced chemist, industrial hygienist, or other qualified health professional.

Chemical removal of surface contaminants sometimes can be accomplished by dissolving them in a solvent. The solvent must be chemically compatible with the equipment being cleaned. In addition, care must be taken in selecting, using, and disposing of any organic solvents that may be flammable or potentially toxic. Surfactants can be used to reduce adhesion forces between contaminants and the surface being cleaned. Household detergents are among the most common surfactants. Neutralization may be used to reduce the hazard potential of specific hazardous substances (acids and alkalis). This process may reduce the chemical hazard but may cause an exothermic reaction, toxic gas production, and suit degradation.

Chemical decontamination will require the use of decontamination solutions. The solutions are usually composed of water and chemical compounds that are designed to react with specific contaminants. Standard solutions are used for decontaminating PPE and equipment (Box 13-1).

EQUIPMENT DECONTAMINATION SOLUTIONS

Decontamination solutions should be used for equipment only. Only in extremely rare circumstances (e.g., very dilute solution B [0.5%] for nerve agent or biological agent exposure,

---

Equipment Decontamination Solutions   Box 13-1

Solution A: 5% Sodium Carbonate and 5% Trisodium Phosphate

Useful for: Inorganic acids, metal-processing wastes, heavy metals, solvents, polychlorinated biphenyls
To prepare: Add 4 pounds of sodium carbonate (soda lime) and 4 pounds of trisodium phosphate (TSP) to 10 gallons of water. Stir until evenly mixed.

Solution B: 10% Calcium Hypochlorite

Useful for: Pesticides (especially organophosphates), fungicides, chlorinated phenols, phencyclidine (PCP), cyanides, ammonia
To prepare: Add 8 pounds of calcium hypochlorite to 10 gallons of water. Stir with plastic or wooden stirrer until evenly mixed.

Solution C: 5% Trisodium Phosphate

Useful for: Solvents, other lipid-soluble organic compounds
To prepare: Add 4 pounds of trisodium phosphate to 10 gallons of water. Stir until evenly mixed.

Solution D: Diluted Hydrochloric Acid

Useful for: Oily, greasy, unspecified substances; alkali and caustic substances
To prepare: Add 1 pint of concentrated hydrochloric acid to 10 gallons of water. Stir with a plastic or wooden stirrer until evenly mixed.

Solution E: A Concentrated Solution of Laundry Detergent and Water

Useful for: Radioactive substances and adhesive chemicals
To prepare: Mix into a paste and scrub with a brush. Rinse with water.

---

and solution D for last-resort radionuclide contamination) should they ever be applied to skin surfaces. Using chemical decontamination on skin may cause skin damage, thermal burns from the exothermic neutralization reaction, or increased absorption from the solvent. Unless otherwise specifically advised by a knowledgeable physician, the only thing that should be used for skin decontamination is mild soap and copious amounts of water. The chemical manufacturer or the Agency for Toxic Substances and Disease Registry (ATSDR) or CHEMTREC (Chemical Transportation Emergency Center) may be consulted for specific recommendations on equipment decontamination.

At times, equipment might not be able to be safely and completely decontaminated. Instead of trying to decontaminate these items, it may be better to isolate and dispose of them as hazardous waste. Porous items, such as fire hoses, ropes, and canvas stretchers, are extremely difficult to decontaminate. In some cases limited-use protective clothing may be carefully

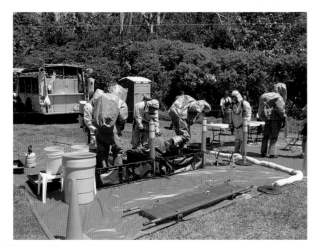

Fig. 13-19
Responder decontamination line.

stripped away, avoiding skin contact. Articles should be isolated and treated as hazardous waste.

The appropriate procedure will depend on the contaminant and its physical properties. Thorough research of the chemical involved, its properties, and expert consultation are necessary to make appropriate decontamination decisions. Many factors, such as cost, availability, and ease of implementation, influence the selection of a decontamination method. Care must be taken to ensure that decontamination methods do not introduce new hazards into the situation. Additionally, the residues of the decontamination process must be treated as hazardous wastes. From a health and safety standpoint, two key questions must be addressed:

- Is the decontamination method effective for the specific substances present?
- Does the method itself pose any health or safety hazards?

DECONTAMINATION LINE

Decontamination procedures must provide an organized process by which levels of contamination are reduced (Fig. 13-19). The decontamination process should consist of a series of procedures performed in a specific sequence (Box 13-2). For example, outer, more heavily contaminated items (e.g., outer boots and gloves) should be decontaminated and removed first, followed by decontamination and removal of inner, less-contaminated items (e.g., jackets and pants). Each procedure should be performed at a separate station to prevent cross-contamination. The sequence of stations is called the *decontamination line.*

The responder decontamination line usually is set up in the same general area but separately from the patient decontamination area. Stations in the decontamination line should be separated physically to prevent cross-contamination and should be arranged in order of decreasing contamination, preferably in a straight line. Entry and exit points should be well marked.

The EPA has established suggested decontamination setups. They range from a maximum layout of 19 stations to a minimum layout of 7 stations. The number of stations will

---

Sample Decontamination Setup Box 13-2

A typical emergency response decontamination setup for responders in Level B protection might include:

1. *Equipment drop:* A tarp or plastic sheet should be placed just inside the hot zone at the exit point to the warm zone. Equipment that will be needed again should be left at the equipment drop.
2. *Primary decontamination:* This step may actually entail many intermediate steps. Personnel should undergo water rinsing and soap or solution washes as necessary to remove as much contaminant as possible.
3. *Secondary decontamination:* The number of washes will depend on the nature of the contaminant. If the worker will be returning to the hot zone and needs only an air bottle change, this can be done after primary decontamination.
4. *Removal and isolation of chemical-protective clothing:* Outer protective clothing, including outer gloves and overboots, is removed at this station.
5. *Removal and isolation of respiratory-protective equipment:* The SCBA harness should be removed, but the mask should remain connected and in place on the worker's face. The protective clothing then can be removed, using special care to reduce the risk of contaminating the worker. Once the outer clothing is removed, the SCBA mask can be removed. Inner gloves are the last piece of PPE to be removed. (See Fig. 13-21.)
6. *Removal of personal clothing:* With extremely hazardous substances, removal and isolation of the responder's personal clothing may be necessary. All clothing should be isolated for later cleaning or disposal.
7. *Field wash or personnel shower:* Personnel should wash their face and hands. To ensure complete decontamination, all personnel should shower as soon as possible. In cases of PPE failure or exposure without PPE, this shower should be conducted in the field.
8. *Drying off and redressing:* Disposable towels should be used for drying. Clean clothes then can be donned. Many teams use disposable coveralls or hospital scrubs.
9. *Medical evaluation:* All personnel involved in mitigation activities must undergo a medical evaluation. Entry personnel should have received a pre-entry baseline examination. Vital signs, indications of exposure, and signs of heat stress all should be evaluated.
10. *Rehabilitation:* A clean area in the cold zone should be established as a rehabilitation area. Food and liquid supplements should be provided in this area. The welfare of response personnel is a vital step and should not be overlooked.

---

depend on the extent of decontamination required (Figs. 13-20 and 13-21). Personnel will work their way through the decontamination corridor, becoming cleaner as they progress. The object is to be absolutely clean by the time they leave the contamination reduction corridor.

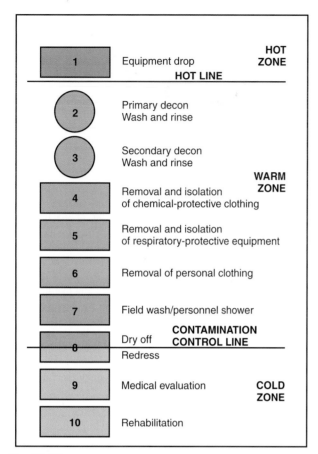

Fig. 13-20
Individual stations in a responder decontamination line.

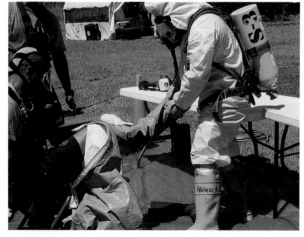

Fig. 13-21
Responder is assisted in personal protective equipment (PPE) removal by a decontamination worker wearing PPE.

Responder Dry Decontamination Procedure   **Box 13-3**

1. Remove the tape securing the gloves to the suit.
2. Remove the outer gloves, turning them inside-out as they are removed.
3. Remove the suit, turning it inside-out. Avoid shaking it.
4. Remove the plastic shoe cover from one foot, and step over the "clean line." Remove the other shoe cover, and put that foot over the line.
5. Remove the mask. The last staff member to doff protective gear may want to wash all masks with soapy water before removing his or her suit and gloves. Place the masks in a plastic bag, and hand the bag over the clean line and into a second bag held by another staff member. Send the masks for further decontamination and proper inspection or disposal.
6. Remove the inner gloves and discard them in a drum or bag inside the dirty area.
7. Close off the dirty area until the level of contamination is established and the area is properly cleaned.
8. Move to the shower area, remove the uniform, and place it in a plastic bag.
9. Shower and dress in clean attire.

DRY DECONTAMINATION

The trend is toward dry decontamination in cases where the contamination is minimal. Dry decontamination involves using disposable clothing and systematically removing these garments in a manner that prevents contact with the contaminant (Box 13-3). Dry decontamination will probably be the method of choice for EMS personnel who transported patients to the hospital.

EQUIPMENT DECONTAMINATION

In selecting equipment, consider whether the equipment itself can be decontaminated for reuse or can be disposed of easily. For example, canvas stretchers are extremely difficult to decontaminate. There are specially designed decontamination stretchers, such as the Raven stretcher, designed for this purpose. Wooden handles cannot be decontaminated. Plastic-handled tools are a better choice, but some substances may degrade or decompose the plastic. Painted and bare metal surfaces usually can be decontaminated by solutions or steam cleaning.

Firefighters structural firefighting protective clothing (turnout) must be carefully decontaminated. Never use an oxidizer solution such as calcium hypochlorite. Oxidizers will severely reduce the strength and fire resistance of the fabric. Use only soap and water, or contact the clothing manufacturer for specific recommendations.

Leather is extremely difficult to decontaminate, and therefore leather items, including turnout gear with leather trim, gloves, boots, belts, watchbands, and wallets must be disposed of properly. SCBA straps and harnesses may be difficult to decontaminate. Refer to the manufacturer for specific advice.

Heavy equipment and vehicles (ambulances) used at the scene may come into contact with the agent. If so, the equipment must be decontaminated before it is removed from the scene. Accessible areas on the equipment can be washed with water and decontamination solutions. All runoff must be contained as hazardous waste. Pay close attention to tires, wheel wells, and exposed surfaces. In extreme cases, steam cleaning or sand blasting may be needed.

The ambulance used for transport may have a contaminated patient compartment. Returning the unit to service prematurely will prolong the exposure of EMS personnel and create a hazard for other patients. The unit should be isolated until it can be decontaminated. This includes a thorough decontamination of the patient compartment as well as mechanical and exterior decontamination as necessary. Tests should be carried out to verify proper decontamination. In most cases soap and water are adequate for vehicle decontamination. CHEMTREC, ATSDR, and the local health department can assist with decision making.

This is another reason to ensure adequate decontamination occurs before transport. If the patient is clean, then the ambulance and everything that the patient touches also will be clean. If the substance was released as an airborne contaminant, then air filters and vehicle interiors may need to be decontaminated.

EQUIPMENT USED FOR DECONTAMINATION

All equipment used for decontamination also must be decontaminated or disposed of properly. Buckets, brushes, clothing, tools, and other contaminated equipment should be collected, placed in containers, and labeled. Clothing that is not completely decontaminated should be placed in plastic bags, pending further decontamination or proper disposal.

All spent solutions and wash water should be collected and disposed of properly. The local health and environmental regulatory agencies should be contacted for advice. In some cases decontamination water may be disposed of by discharging it into a sanitary sewer. Approval from the local regulatory agencies and wastewater treatment facility is mandatory. In other cases the water must be placed in containers and disposed of as hazardous waste.

DECONTAMINATION PERSONNEL

Decontamination workers who come in contact with personnel, victims, and equipment leaving the hot zone will require protection from contaminants. Generally, decontamination personnel may be sufficiently protected by wearing protective clothing that is one level lower than that of responders in the hot zone (e.g., decontamination personnel wear Level B protective clothing when responders in the hot zone are wearing Level A protective clothing) (Fig. 13-22). Supplied-air respirators (air lines) can increase the efficiency of the decontamination team by allowing them an extended time in protective equipment. Air-purifying respirators (APRs) may be used if all requirements for the use of such equipment are met. Even decontamination

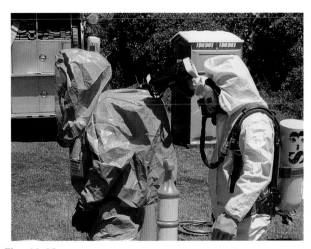

Fig. 13-22
Responder decontamination personnel wearing appropriate personal protective equipment.

workers assisting in removing protective clothing that has been decontaminated should take precautions by using, at a minimum, chemical-protective gloves and protective eyewear.

All decontamination workers are in a contaminated area and must be decontaminated before entering the cold zone. The extent of their decontamination should be determined by the type of contaminants they may have contacted and the type of work they performed. Generally, the decontamination worker closest to the hot zone should progress through the other stations, following the station that they were staffing, to be decontaminated. They are followed by the next closest person and so on down the decontamination line. The last person (closest to the cold zone) decontaminates himself or herself at the last station.

TESTING THE EFFECTIVENESS OF DECONTAMINATION PROCEDURES

Decontamination methods vary in their effectiveness for removing different substances. The effectiveness of any decontamination method should be assessed throughout the response. If contamination is not being removed or if it is penetrating protective clothing, the decontamination plan must be revised.

The problem is that no reliable test exists to determine immediately how effective decontamination is. In some cases, effectiveness can be estimated by visual observation. Discolorations, stains, corrosive effects, visible products, or alterations in the fabric of protective clothing may indicate that contaminants have not been removed. However, not all contaminants leave visible traces. Certain contaminants fluoresce and can be detected visually when exposed to ultraviolet light. Exposure to ultraviolet light might be harmful, and appropriate safety precautions must be followed. If an air-monitoring device is available that will detect the presence of the contaminant, it may be useful to determine if gross contamination still is present.

Wipe testing provides after-the-fact information on the effectiveness of decontamination. In this procedure, a dry or wet cloth, glass fiber filter paper, or swab is wiped over the surface of the potentially contaminated object and then analyzed in a laboratory. Both the inner and outer surfaces of protective clothing should be tested. Skin also may be tested, using wipe samples.

Another way to test the effectiveness of decontamination procedures is to analyze for contaminants left in the cleaning solutions. Elevated levels of contaminants in the final rinse solution may suggest that additional cleaning and rinsing are needed.

Reusable PPE also may be tested for permeation. Testing for the presence of permeated chemical contaminants requires that pieces of the protective garments be sent to a laboratory for analysis.

CHAPTER SUMMARY

Decontamination procedures will help protect responders from agents that may contaminate individuals, PPE, tools, vehicles, and other equipment used at the scene. Because decontamination stops the chemical's action on the victim, it also is a valuable part of patient treatment. Decontamination protects personnel by minimizing the transfer of harmful materials into clean areas. Decontamination also will help protect the community by preventing uncontrolled migration of contamination away from the scene.

REFERENCE

1. Gold MB et al: Hypochlorite solution as a decontaminant in sulfur mustard contaminated skin defects in the euthymic hairless guinea pig, *Drug Chem Toxicol* 17:499-527, 1994.

BIBLIOGRAPHY

Agency for Toxic Substances and Disease Registry: *Managing hazardous materials incidents, emergency medical services: a planning guide for the management of contaminated patients,* Atlanta, 2001, U.S. Department of Health and Human Services.

Andrews LP, editor: *Emergency responder training manual for the hazardous materials technician,* New York, 1992, Van Nostrand Reinhold.

Bowen JE: *Emergency management of hazardous materials incidents,* Quincy, Mass, 1995, National Fire Protection Association.

Bronstein AC, Currance PL: Module 4: emergency medical operations. In Ayers S, Christopher J, editors: *Medical response to chemical emergencies,* Washington, DC, 1994, Chemical Manufacturers Association.

Buck G: *Preparing for biological terrorism,* Albany, NY, 2002, Delmar.

Carroll TR: *Contamination and decontamination of turnout clothing,* Emmitsburg, Md, 1993, Federal Emergency Management Agency, U.S. Fire Administration.

Currance PL: *Hazmat for EMS,* St Louis, 1995, Mosby (videotape and guidebook).

Goldfrank LR et al, editors: *Goldfrank's toxicological emergencies,* ed 6, Norwalk, Conn, 1998, Appleton & Lange.

Gosselin RE, Smith RP, Hodge HC: *Clinical toxicology of commercial products,* ed 5, Baltimore, 1994, Williams & Wilkins.

Hawley C: *Hazardous materials incidents,* Albany, NY, 2002, Delmar.

National Fire Protection Association: *NFPA 471, Recommended practice for responding to hazardous materials incidents,* Quincy, Mass, 2002, National Fire Protection Association.

Noll GG, Hildebrand MS, Yvorra JG: *Hazardous materials: managing the incident,* ed 2, Stillwater, Okla, 1995, Fire Protection Publications.

Olson KR, editor: *Poisoning and drug overdose,* ed 3, East Norwalk, Conn, 1998, Appleton & Lange.

Ricks RC, Leonard RB: *Hospital emergency department of radiation accidents,* Washington, DC, 1984, Emergency Management Institute, National Emergency Training Center.

Strong CB, Irvin TR: *Emergency response and hazardous chemical management: principles and practices,* Delray Beach, Fla, 1996, St Lucie Press.

United States Fire Administration: *Guidelines for public sector hazardous materials training,* Emmitsburg, Md, 1998, Federal Emergency Management Administration.

Chapter **14**

Psychological Preparedness and Response

PATRICK F. DEMARCO

CHAPTER OBJECTIVES

At the conclusion of this chapter the student will be able to:

- Discuss the basic psychological issues that a medical team is likely to face when responding to a weapons of mass destruction (WMD) incident.
- Identify the psychological difficulties presented in a disaster caused by a WMD agent.
- Recognize the psychological issues that extend beyond a medical team to their families and significant others before, during, and after a deployment to a WMD incident.
- Identify the need for ongoing training and preparation as an aid to coping with the psychological issues of a WMD incident.

CASE STUDY

The Oklahoma City bombing was a major catastrophe. While the nation was stunned by the enormity of the attack, medical and psychological responders were quickly deployed to provide help to the victims and the responders. This was the largest response to date. Responders as well as victims were able to get help quickly. The psychological fallout of that disaster with people across the country was significant but not to the level it could have reached if the training and preparations that had been ongoing were not in place. Critical incident stress management and debriefings became standard and accepted as a significant part of deployment for medical teams and other responders.

The issue of preparedness for a WMD attack now pushes those psychological boundaries further. Trained teams of responders specific to those types of weapons are now imperative. Psychological preparation becomes a necessity for this type of deployment.

What types of emotional stress can be expected in the general population?

What types of emotional stress can be expected in the responders?

What kind of debriefing will be necessary?

How will the presence of weapons of mass destruction at a disaster change the stress factors?

This chapter focuses on the psychological issues facing the disaster team and particularly a disaster team that responds to nuclear, biological, and chemical weapons of mass destruction (WMD-NBC). Responders need to learn how to handle WMD attacks as well as how to resume a level of normalcy following a deployment to such an attack.

Weapons of mass destruction present a unique and difficult challenge because WMD have been used only a few times in the United States, so there have been very few situations in which to evaluate disaster teams and their psychological needs based on actual experiences.

HISTORY

The use of biological weapons is not new. Following the French and Indian War, Native Americans who had fought on the side of the British and colonists tried to collect the payment they were promised for providing their assistance. The repre-

sentative of the colonists, while promising he would pay them, gave them blankets he knew had been used by smallpox victims. Using smallpox as a biological agent, he destroyed the Native Americans, with the result that he did not have to pay them.

In World War I, mustard gas was used in trench warfare; in World War II, atomic bombs were dropped on Hiroshima and Nagasaki. In March 1995, terrorists attacked a Tokyo train using sarin, killing 12 people and affecting approximately 5000 people (many of whose injuries were psychological). The government of Iraq has used chemical weapons and possibly biological weapons against the Kurds in Northern Iraq.

In all but one of those situations, there was no trained WMD disaster response team to provide support and relief. In Tokyo, the victims of the attack were treated by first responders and at their local hospitals. A disaster response team that is oriented to responding to these types of weapons requires specific and detailed training. Responders are trained to anticipate a variety of circumstances.

PSYCHOLOGICAL RESPONSE TO DISASTERS

Psychological response to disasters has been studied for several years, but studies of psychological response to weapons of mass destruction have been limited. Most research about effects on responders has focused on natural disasters: fire, ice storms, hurricanes, earthquakes, volcanic activity, tsunamis, floods, tornadoes, lightning strikes, and mudslides. A trained disaster response team will be exposed to excessive stress over the course of a deployment. The training, preparation, and return (following a deployment) also results in significant levels of stress, depending on the particular task.

We live with stressors every day. Stress is brought on by events and actions of daily living. It is the degree of stress that can impede functioning. This chapter focuses on how to manage the stress of responding to a deployment related to the use of a WMD. We will explore how stress affects our bodies and the development of stress-related symptoms and illness. The issue of *secondary traumatic stress disorder* will be discussed and how members of a disaster response team can be affected by it.

People have dealt with danger, threat, violent death, and other stressful events for thousands of years. The uniqueness of WMD creates a new type of stress and stress response. It is therefore important to acquire a detailed understanding of the stress and stress response that a disaster response team faces as well as the many factors that will determine the team's success in dealing with the effects of a WMD attack.

PREPARATION AND TRAINING

Plans for anticipating and dealing with issues related to WMD attacks have only recently been developed. In March 2001 the Defense Threat Reduction Agency, the Federal Bureau of Investigation, and the U.S. Joint Forces Command released *Human Behavior and WMD Crisis/Risk Communication Workshop*, which asserts that the Defense Threat Reduction Agency's Advanced Systems and Concepts Office (ASCO) must look at ways to improve the ability of the Department of

Defense (DOD) to protect U.S. and allied forces from the threat of WMD. Their first steps were to develop strategies that focus directly on the preparedness mission and on the task of integrating various agencies, responders, media, and the DOD into a *consequence management team* prepared to respond to a WMD attack.

The impact of that report is that a clear plan for dealing with WMD was just being developed in 2001. The data on preparation and expectation of how a disaster response team can best be trained is still a relatively new concept. Overall preparation and training before an attack becomes critical in developing a disaster response team for WMD (Fig. 14-1).

Why engage in ongoing training exercises? Psychologically it becomes important to develop a repertoire of coping mechanisms. As humans build on newly learned behavior and tasks, they increase their level of confidence and competence. As a disaster response team trains for WMD attacks, new skills and awareness are developed that improve the efficiency of and confidence of individual responders. With the increase in confidence comes a reduction of stress-related illnesses. Stressful events often include adverse psychobiological responses. A disaster response team for WMD attacks needs to develop a strong sense of survival, stress management techniques, and postevent habituation or sensitization.

The training of a WMD disaster response team must focus on the management of fear. The goal of a terrorist is to cause fear, or more specifically to create fear through the threat of the use of WMD. To many, the idea of being exposed to an invisible agent is more frightening than the prospect of physical injury or death by conventional weapons (Fig. 14-2).

PSYCHOLOGICAL EFFECTS

Responders are likely to be exposed to seemingly overwhelming physical events as well as the psychological impact that these events have on others. The responder may at times feel linked

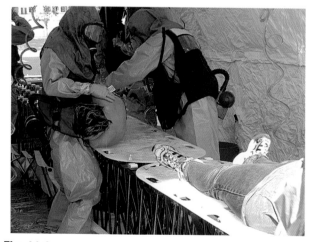

Fig. 14-1
The Central NMRT-WMD personnel participating in a training exercise.

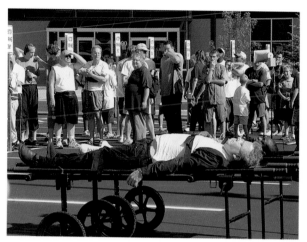

Fig. 14-2
Mass casualty incidents (here a training drill) result in a high degree of responder stress.

with those who have been exposed to a WMD attack or some aspect of the situation and develop feelings of discomfort.

STRESS-RELATED PROBLEMS IN DISASTER RESPONSE

Stress has a potential pathogenic effect; posttraumatic stress disorder (PTSD) and secondary traumatic stress disorder (STSD) are the particularly grave outcomes. Stress-related ailments are the concern not only of the responders but also of those they have come to assist. Stress-related illness hampers the overall mission of a deployment.

Stress-related problems affect the performance of a responder. Personal stress issues must be resolved as best they can before the responder is deployed. Responders with high levels of personal stress are the most likely to be affected by the deployment. A responder with high levels of personal stress is likely to experience symptoms of fatigue, headache, anger and frustration, and sleep problems. These symptoms, when combined with the stress of a deployment, increase the susceptibility to PTSD.

PERSONAL SITUATION STRESSORS

Personal situations can cause stress that may interfere with deployment. Some of these situations are difficulty with a spouse or significant other, children with behavior problems or special needs, family members in crisis, work-related problems, financial problems, and personal health problems. Psychiatric problems can impede performance during a deployment, for example, depression or anxiety. Fear of WMD attacks can also create a high stress level. Some responders find it personally stressful to leave their families and loved ones to deploy into a situation that is likely to be hazardous.

Responders can deal with these personal stressors before deployment with training and preparation that increases the responder's confidence level so that fear of deploying in a response to a WMD attack is substantially reduced. Another helpful way is through counseling (individual, couples, family, and groups).

Once deployed, a responder faces four major stress reactions: emotional, cognitive, psychosocial, and biological.

Emotional Stress. Responders face emotional stress upon a deployment. The first part of this stress is realizing the magnitude of the disaster and the limitations that are imposed on responders by the circumstances. The desire to help is tempered by the need to provide safe limits of response, which is a challenge. This stress becomes further complicated when the responder realizes that the situation may call for pulling back into a safer arena of engagement.

Emotional stress is also exacerbated by the need to maintain a professional demeanor in the face of a troubling situation. A normal response to a disaster is to behave erratically and to over-react. The responder cannot behave in such a way. Essentially, a responder must behave in this situation in a way that is not normal. Having to maintain that level of professional detachment is emotionally difficult. Remaining empathetic to the situation and treating the victims instead of responding sympathetically can put an emotional strain on a responder's resolve.

The responder will be exposed to overwhelming events as well as the psychological impact of these events on others. It is a natural desire to identify with the victims and be emotionally moved by their circumstance. A responder to a WMD attack has to keep those emotions in check.

The responder cannot react to personal levels of anger, frustration, disgust, depression, fear, and the general sense of being overwhelmed. Not responding to normal human emotions becomes emotionally stressful. During a deployment, a responder may feel anxiety, guilt, grief, denial, panic, fear, irritability, loss of control, sense of failure, blame of others, and depression. Although the responder is aware of these emotions, during a deployment to a WMD attack, the responder cannot engage those emotions. This prompts the need for debriefing following a deployment.

Cognitive Stress. Cognitive stress reactions are those of confusion, nightmares, disorientation, heightened or lowered alertness, poor concentration, memory problems, poor problem solving, and difficulty identifying with familiar objects or people.

Psychosocial Stress. Psychosocial and behavioral stress reactions include intense anger, withdrawal, emotional out-bursts, temporary loss of or increase in appetite, inability to rest, pacing, change in sexual functioning, and increased use of alcohol, tobacco, or drugs.

Biological Stress. Biological stress reactions include chest pain, difficulty breathing, shock symptoms, fatigue, nausea and vomiting, dizziness, profuse sweating, rapid heart rate, thirst, headaches, visual difficulties, jaw clenching, and nonspecific aches and pains.

Occupational Hazards. Occupational hazards add to the stress reaction that responders experience. Teams specifically trained for WMD attacks have the added stress of the nature of the disaster. The fear of exposure to these weapons and the potential for true risk creates an atmosphere of tension and stress that cannot be ignored. The magnitude of the deployment places a heavy burden on those responsible for responding to such a situation.

The work culture of responders has an impact on how stress is perceived and responded to. Responders who come from a medical background are more likely to handle the initial impact of victims who are physically affected by the WMD attack. They are likely to find the emotional impact of the disaster difficult to accept. A responder from a behavioral health background will likely experience the stress in the opposite way. Further stress is likely for responders because of their need to rescue and maintain life and to have to address the overwhelming situation of a WMD attack. Responders may view such an attack as a personal affront. This adds to the overall stress response.

CONTRIBUTING PSYCHOLOGICAL ISSUES

Three areas of stress can complicate and in some instances impede performance for a responder to a WMD attack: work and employment, family responsibilities, and financial obligations.

WORK AND EMPLOYMENT

Some employers are understanding and reasonable about the responder's deployment. They will hold the person's job and position. However, despite memoranda of understanding, as well as financial assistance in some cases, that can be given to an employer, some employers are unwilling to allow for special circumstances and will demote or terminate the employee.

Some responders are self-employed. A deployment can cause a significant financial loss for some and can affect their business. In those situations where the responder is in a medical or related field and in a private practice, a deployment may adversely affect their practice.

FAMILY RESPONSIBILITIES

For some responders, being away from their family can be quite stressful. They may have family members who are ill or have needs that require special attention. Deployment may result in increased family stress. In some personal relationships the deployment can end the relationship or set off a distancing in the relationship. These types of stressors can adversely affect the performance of the responder.

FINANCIAL OBLIGATIONS

For some disaster response teams there is no financial compensation. The time away from work and home can cause significant financial pressures. Some teams do provide financial compensation, but the amount may be below the level of income responders are used to. Also, on those teams that do provide compensation, the payment for services rendered may not be immediate. These add to the overall burden and stress of a responder.

SPECIAL STRESS PROBLEMS FOR A RESPONSE TEAM

A WMD response team has unique stress-related problems that are significantly different from those of a disaster medical response team or other disaster responders. There are five areas of focus: uniqueness of circumstances; level of physical preparedness and training; education and detailed awareness of nuclear, biological, and chemical weapons; maintaining long-standing alert-response readiness; and psychosocial pressures.

UNIQUENESS OF CIRCUMSTANCES

Facing the possibility of a WMD attack is emotionally difficult because of the unknowns about the weapon. Psychological stress studies have shown that people tend to find it much easier to face the idea of a conventional weapon. The feeling is that a person might be able to protect himself or herself against conventional weapons such as bombs, missiles, and guns. With a weapon of mass destruction, however, there is neither warning of the attack nor a clear course of action to protect oneself. This creates unusual fear and apprehension.

There have not been clear guidelines for creating a sense of personal protection in the event of a WMD attack. Personal protective equipment provides a layer of protection but it cannot provide protection from the psychological assault (Fig. 14-3). The fear becomes fear of a weapon being used without personal knowledge until exposure as well as a fear of multiple attacks that overwhelm an area and reduce medical response and services to a minimum.

LEVEL OF PHYSICAL PREPAREDNESS AND TRAINING

The level of physical preparedness and training causes additional stress. A team prepared to respond to WMD attacks must be well trained. Equipment and gear must be in a peak state of readiness, and responders needs detailed training in the use of the equipment and gear. Each team member must become familiar with all positions and the way equipment is used. In the event of an attack, each member of the team has to be able to do another person's task.

In a conventional disaster response team, the detailed training for others' tasks is not as critical. A thorough understanding of others' jobs is important in a conventional disaster response team, but in a WMD response team it becomes critical and

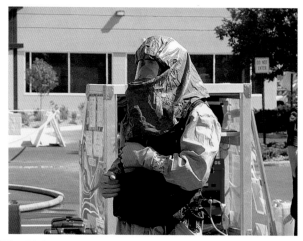

Fig. 14-3
Responder in personal protective equipment.

necessary. Frequent, thorough training is time consuming and at times feels unnecessary.

Physical training goes beyond just that of familiarity with equipment and tasks. Team members must be in good health for a deployment. A responder deploying ill or in poor health could jeopardize the entire mission. Deployment requires a fully functioning team. Each person is part of the gestalt.

EDUCATION AND DETAILED AWARENESS OF NUCLEAR, BIOLOGICAL, AND CHEMICAL WEAPONS

Education and detailed awareness of NBCs are critical to a successful deployment. Team members must understand how these weapons can be used as well as their effects. The training prepares the responder for deployment, but with the detailed education comes stress. Awareness for the responder and his or her family members and significant others about WMD and their effect provides a level of concern and fear that cannot be ignored. Education about how to protect oneself and others helps to reduce that concern and fear. Family members and significant others must be educated as well about what the team is doing to provide protection and support.

MAINTAINING LONG-STANDING ALERT-RESPONSE READINESS

Disaster teams that respond to WMD are typically on a long-standing alert response readiness. The stress level is low except for brief periods when the alert status is increased. The significant stress in maintaining long-standing alert is the continuous maintenance of equipment and gear. Each responder has to make sure that his or her personal gear is ready for deployment, and each responder has to make sure that all of the team equipment and gear is ready for deployment. For teams that are not fully prepared and maintaining a constant state of readiness, their stress level will be significantly higher upon deployment.

PSYCHOSOCIAL PRESSURES

Psychosocial pressures add to the existing stress levels for responders. Teams are aware that in a deployment, the response is to local communities where family and friends live. Before September 11, 2001, responders training to deal with WMD attacks seemed almost frivolous to most of the local communities. This attitude created a level of uncertainty for many responders about the validity of their training. Following September 11, 2001, this attitude changed. The stress level changed from lack of certainty to that of the importance of their training and preparation and a clear sense that they must be prepared for the use of WMD.

ESPRIT DE CORPS VERSUS ELITE SEGREGATION

As with any team endeavor, building a sense of esprit de corps is important. It provides a sense of cohesiveness and identity. These characteristics become important for establishing a feeling of confidence and readiness. Each team of responders must have this sense of closeness and readiness. But between teams and within teams the sense of esprit de corps can develop into elitism.

Elitism comes about when one group (whether as a team or a part of a team) believes itself to be superior to others. During training and deployment, elitism leads to dissent and contentious behavior that can negatively affect the functioning of the team or of individual responders. As with training and preparation, anything that can interfere with overall performance of the team must be resolved. Elitism has to be replaced with a solid group unity and identity that do not isolate the team or impede its efforts.

MANAGING STRESS ON DEPLOYMENT

A disaster of the magnitude caused by WMD and the close working proximity and living situation during a deployment are stressful. The American Academy of Experts in Traumatic Stress has produced the manual *Acute Traumatic Stress Management*. This manual is valuable for a disaster team that responds to WMD attacks.

MANAGEMENT OF ACUTE TRAUMATIC STRESS

In the field, response to stress is critical to success. Response to a WMD incident will be an overwhelming situation both during the deployment and afterwards. The responder must *acknowledge* that the experience is difficult. This cannot be overemphasized. By acknowledging before deployment that the situation will be difficult, during the course of the deployment the acknowledgement that it is difficult can reduce the impact of the situation.

Responders have to be *aware* of their emotional, cognitive, behavioral, and physiological reactions. If necessary, engage in some physical exercise to dissipate the stress energy. Discuss the experience with a friend or the team psychologist. Sharing the experience will help the responder to assimilate what has occurred and to gain a sense of closure. The responder who is having *sleep* problems because of continual thoughts (ruminative stress) must recognize that this is normal in a deployment. Do not fight to sleep—the difficulty will usually pass in a few days. Try to write, listen to music, or read. Often this helps. During down time, the responder should engage in nonthreatening activities (Fig. 14-4).

Try to unwind from the action. Play often becomes a good outlet for built-up tension and stress. The responder must have the strength to let go. It requires courage to face the emotions within.

HEALTH ISSUES

Health issues in the field are vital to ongoing care of victims during a deployment. This is not only the victim's health but also the responder's health. Part of stress management is managing personal health. A responder hass to take the time to eat as well as possible and drink plenty of fluids to remain hydrated. Sleep can be a difficult problem with long hours of work and long hours of down time.

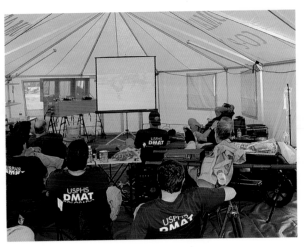

Fig. 14-4
Responders relaxing during downtime.

Down time is that period of time in which there is no direct responder activity for treating victims. This becomes crucial time for responders to rest, relax, and take care of personal needs. Down time is an excellent opportunity to begin to manage the stress of a deployment. One effective technique is to make a list of the emotions that are being experienced without trying to qualify them. Write about such feelings as anger, rage, anxiety, fear, guilt, humiliation, frustration, panic, agitation, withdrawal, insecurity, hopelessness, helplessness, or worry. Consider physical symptoms such as excessive humor, silence, shortness of breath, nausea, vomiting, sweating, chills, dry mouth, diarrhea, or increased urination, all of which can be signs of stress reaction.

Down time is also an excellent opportunity to write about different situations and describe what was learned, what action was taken, what personal insight was achieved, and the negative and positive issues in the situation. Writing these types of things down provides an outlet for stress reactions. Reducing stress reactions can improve performance and functional behavior.

Becoming comfortable with uncertainty is also a method for managing stress during a deployment. This reduces performance anxiety and increases confidence. Uncertainty can be managed by imagining the worst outcome and then imagining a scenario that allows for a positive resolution. Visualizing this helps to decrease the associated anxiety of the situation.

Responders can consult with their teammates and leaders about the stress they are experiencing and how they feel it is affecting their performance. The goal is to develop coping strategies that are effective for the deployment situation. This will vary from disaster site to disaster site. It is important to provide opportunities for emotional disclosure and cognitive reframing. This will help to mitigate long-term stress reactions, which can include posttraumatic stress disorder. Sharing feelings and other stress issues during a deployment not only helps to reduce the internalized stress reactions but also helps to improve readiness for another field deployment.

The level of stress that must be managed is directly affected by the level of intensity in the disaster situation. A WMD attack will probably create a high level of intensity. Managing stress becomes more complex because of the difference in responding to the disaster. A disaster that is not a WMD attack allows responders to work in shifts and rotate out. Once a team is deployed to a WMD incident, all personnel may be needed to handle the incoming victims. Shifts could become long and uncomfortable. Therefore, down time becomes critical and brief breaks to rest become crucial to maintaining focus in the field of response.

SUPPORT AND COUNSELING

Debriefing in the field of response and during down time becomes a significant tool for managing stress during a deployment. These debriefings are meant to be brief and timely, allowing for as much personal time as needed. Each disaster team that is deployed to a WMD attack should have at least one mental health worker to provide this type of support. This will help in reducing compassion fatigue, which is common with responders. Compassion fatigue can lead to secondary traumatic stress disorder (STSD), which is similar to posttraumatic stress disorder (PTSD). The primary difference is that PTSD affects the victims of a disaster and STSD affects the responders.

Another area that helps to decrease personal stress is providing the responder's families with support and counseling during a deployment. The family members and significant others are also affected by the deployment, and their unresolved stress issues and lack of stress management can be visited upon the responder and increase the stress load in the field. Effective stress management in the field requires management of stress at home. This can be achieved with counseling, information regarding the deployment, and communication between the responders and their families as often as practical.

DEBRIEFINGS

Debriefing refers to a defusing process that is intended to facilitate opportunities for responders and their families and significant others to express their thoughts and feelings about the deployment situation without feeling obligated to do so. Debriefing gives the responders and their families and significant others the opportunity to better understand their own reactions and to assess indications of being at risk for long-term stress reactions.

Who attends a debriefing is important. Attendance is nearly always voluntary. It is not unusual for some people to continue talking with each other about the incident for months following a deployment. In most cases this is therapeutic and helps to decrease the internalized stress reactions. However, there are those who struggle with the events and have significant difficulty coping with the deployment. In those circumstances additional professional support is likely to be beneficial.

The process of debriefing usually takes about 4 hours. The process of stress management during a deployment takes about 10 to 30 minutes.

TYPES OF DEBRIEFING AND STRESS MANAGEMENT

Four types of debriefing are the focus of this section. These are team critical incident stress management, family critical incident stress management, team critical incident stress debriefing, and family critical incident stress debriefing.

Team Critical Incident Stress Management. Debriefing in the field is important for reducing stress and keeping performance at a high level. Debriefing in the field is called team critical incident stress management. In a WMD incident, the scenario may change and change quickly due to the type of weapon used and whether or not multiple weapons were used. The debriefing process in the field will allow responders an immediate outlet for coping with the situation and circumstances. This type of debriefing can be provided on a regular basis and shaped to meet the needs of the team and individual responders. The debriefing during a deployment is an ongoing process that is not rigid or forced. Time is provided to the team and individual responders to meet their emotional needs.

Family Critical Incident Stress Management. The second type of debriefing occurs while a team is in the field. This debriefing is for the families and significant others of the responders. The family's debriefing may not occur as frequently as the team's, but it is vital that family critical incident stress management be conducted as often as practical. This debriefing should be provided by an experienced mental health professional who has a disaster-response background. This debriefing will provide assurances and support for the emotional strain that the families and significant others are experiencing.

Team Critical Incident Stress Debriefing. Team critical incident stress debriefing is a formal process that occurs after a deployment. Debriefing is a structured process that helps responders understand and manage intense emotions, further understand effective coping strategies, and receive the support of peers (Box 14-1). *Defusing* refers to a process intended to facilitate opportunities for responders and their families and significant others to express their thoughts and feelings about the deployment (Boxes 14-2 and 14-3).

Family Critical Incident Stress Debriefing. Family critical incident stress debriefing follows the same guidelines as the team critical incident stress debriefing, except that the families and significant others are already in the community and workplace. However, they should be allowed to discuss their view of the community and workplace and to explore what type of support they received and where they perceived support lacking.

RESTORATION OF NORMAL ACTIVITIES

Following a deployment, it is necessary to focus on restoring normal daily routines and moving beyond the psychological problems. A disaster does not leave just a trail of property destruction in its wake; it also damages people.

The victims of a disaster, especially one involving a WMD attack, are not the only ones affected by this destruction. The destruction of human life is always difficult, but mass destruction of life becomes overwhelming. Responders are not immune to

Debriefing Protocol   Box 14-1

The protocol for debriefing consists of eight steps:
1. Preparation: Make the necessary arrangements with the incident commander or team commander and obtain information about the conditions of the deployment and if there are particular concerns about the responders.
2. Introduction: Debriefers begin with self-introductions, a including brief description of their disaster mental health experience and the purpose of debriefing. They explain that debriefing is an opportunity to talk about personal impressions of the recent experience and to learn about stress reactions and stress management strategies, and that it is not psychotherapy. Confidentiality is discussed and group rules are explained.
3. Fact Phase: The debriefer asks the responders to describe the experience from their own perspective. They should describe what happened, where they were, what they did, and what they experienced.
4. Thought Phase: Responders describe their cognitive reaction or thoughts about their experience.
5. Reaction Phase: Responders are encouraged to discuss the emotions they experienced during the course of the deployment.
6. Symptom (Stress Reaction) Phase: Stress reactions are reviewed in the context of what responders experienced at the scene, what stress reactions have lingered, and what they are experiencing at present.
7. Teaching Phase: Definitions are given of traumatic stress, common stress reactions, factors associated with adaptation to trauma, and self-care and stress management.
8. Reentry Phase: The final phase of the debriefing is allotted to discussing unfinished issues, giving reactions to the debriefing, giving a summation of the debriefing, and describing the referral process.

Defusing Protocol   Box 14-2

There are seven key parts to defusing:
1. Assess the impact of the critical incident(s) on responders.
2. Identify immediate issues surrounding problems involving safety and security.
3. Use defusing to allow for the ventilation of thoughts, emotions, and experiences associated with the event and provide validation of possible reactions.
4. Predict events and reactions to come in the aftermath of the event.
5. Conduct a systematic review of the critical incident and its impact emotionally, cognitively, and physically on the responders. Look for maladaptive behavior or responses to the crisis or trauma.
6. Bring closure to the incident. Orient responders to community resources to initiate the rebuilding process. Help identify possible positive experiences from the deployment.
7. Debriefing assists in reentry back into the community or workplace. Debriefing can be done in large or small groups or one-to-one depending on the situation. Debriefing is not a critique but a systematic review of the events before, during, and after the crisis.

Defusing Topics   Box 14-3

Topics for defusing include:
Exposure to unpredictable physical danger
Encounter with human remains
Stress reactions of significant others
Encounter with suffering of others
Perception of the cause of the disaster
Perception of assistance offered to victims
Long hours, erratic work schedules, extreme fatigue
Cross-cultural differences between responders and community
Interagency and intraagency struggles over authority
Time pressures
Lack of adequate housing
Equipment failure and perception of control
Personal injury
Injury or death of loved ones, friends, or associates
Self-expectations
Level of personal and professional preparedness
Property loss
Preexisting stress
Encounter with mass death
Encounter with death of children
Role ambiguity
Difficult choices
Communication breakdowns
Allocation of resources
Perception by community
Weather conditions
Overidentification with victims
Human errors
Perceived mission failure
Proximity to scene of impact
Prior disaster experience
Level of social support
Previous trauma

this destruction, and secondary trauma becomes a response to this destruction.

Following a debriefing, responders have to return to their daily lives. The impact of the deployment will linger. Therefore responders and their families and significant others must develop guidelines that will assist them in achieving a semblance of normalcy that existed before the deployment (Box 14-4).

The keys to restoration are trying to find a balance in life and setting boundaries and limits. Reach out to receive support from others and in turn give back that support. Engage in relaxation exercises and in spiritual practices if these help you. Find outlets that let you express yourself in a creative manner. Allow yourself to be quiet at times and to pursue quiet activities, whether alone or with someone special.

Upon return to work, plan regular breaks, if possible. Take the time after work to travel home less frantically. Make the trip home a time to begin to unwind. Talk with others about your experiences. Recognize that your family and significant

Following a Deployment — Box 14-4

Some of the approaches that help to restore a balance to life following a deployment are:

Reach out to others.

Reconnect with family and friends.

Consider keeping a journal.

Do not make major life decision in the first few weeks.

Make as many daily decisions as possible to give yourself a sense of control.

Do things that you enjoy doing, things that refresh and recharge.

Be aware that you may feel fearful for your family. This is normal and will pass in time.

Remember that restoration takes time. Gradually work back into routines.

Appreciate a sense of humor in yourself and others. It is okay to laugh.

Remember that your family and significant others experienced the disaster too. Support each other.

Avoid overuse of alcohol or drugs.

Get plenty of rest and normal exercise. Eat well-balanced meals.

You decide when and how much you want to talk about the deployment.

Walk, eat, and talk more slowly.

Avoid the automatic "yes" answer. Say, "I'll check my schedule and get back to you." Avoid the automatic "no" answer. This comes from the fear to do anything. These indicate possible problems in your current state of mind.

Make a stress-free sanctuary in your home where you can let go and unwind.

Get a massage.

Embrace and celebrate life.

It is acceptable to sometimes do nothing.

Nurture relationships and be nurtured by relationships.

Be extra patient with yourself and others.

Don't expect things to instantly restore themselves.

---

others will need to share with you their experiences during the deployment as well as to hear how you are doing.

Acknowledge to yourself and your teammates that you did all that you could do on the deployment. Not everyone will have a significant problem with a deployment. That is also acceptable. Problems may come up that are related to the deployment, but not always. In other words, it's all right not to have problems. If problems do develop, do not hesitate to seek out professional help.

CHAPTER SUMMARY

A WMD incident has a tremendous psychological impact on the medical response team. Each person responds to this stress in individual ways. Recognizing symptoms of this psychological stress in others, acknowledging signs of stress in oneself, and taking steps to cope with stress reactions are vital to recovery after responding to a WMD incident.

A disaster response team must develop strong survival instincts, stress and fear management techniques, and postevent coping mechanisms. This psychological preparedness and training is a critical part of any WMD training program.

BIBLIOGRAPHY

American Psychiatric Association: *Coping with a national tragedy,* Washington, DC, 2001, American Psychiatric Press.

American Psychiatric Association: *Executive summary: chemical and biological terrorism: research and development to improve civilian medical response,* Washington, DC, 1999, American Psychiatric Press.

American Psychiatric Association: *Managing the stress of those who must recover the bodies,* Washington, DC, 2001, American Psychiatric Press.

American Psychiatric Association: *Nuclear/biological/chemical (NBC) accidents and terrorism,* http://www.psych.org/disaster/dpc_nbc.cfm?pf=y, retrieved October 7, 2004.

American Psychiatric Association: *Posttraumatic stress disorder,* http://www.psych.org/public_info/ptsd.cfm, retrieved October 7, 2004.

American Psychiatric Association: *Stress management for health care providers,* http://www.psych.org/public_info/stressmgmt_health91801.cfm, retrieved October 7, 2004.

American Psychiatric Association: *When disaster strikes...,* http://www.psych.org/public_info/disaster.cfm, retrieved October 7, 2004.

Ben-David A, Lavee Y: Families in the sealed room: interaction patterns of Israeli families during SCUD missile attacks, *Fam Process* 31:35-44, 1992.

Bleich A et al: Israeli psychological casualties of the Persian Gulf War: characteristrics, therapy, and selected issues, *Isr J Med Sci* 27:673-676, 1991.

Bleich A et al: Post-traumatic stress disorder in Israel during the Gulf War, *Isr J Psychiatry Relat Sci* 29:14-21, 1992.

Carmeli A, Liberman N, Mevorach L: Anxiety-related somatic reactions during missile attacks, *Isr J Med Sci* 27:677-680, 1991.

Davis JA: *Providing critical incident stress debriefing (CISD) to individuals and communities in situational crisis,* Commack, NY, 1998, American Academy of Experts in Trauma Stress, http://www.aaets.org/arts/art54.htm, retrieved October 7, 2004.

Defense Threat Reduction Agency, Federal Bureau of Investigation, U.S. Joint Forces Command: *Human behavior and WMD crisis/risk communication workshop,* www.au.af.mil/au/awc/awcgate/dtra/human-behavior-wmd.pdf, retrieved October 7, 2004.

Department of Justice: *OVC handbook for coping after terrorism: a guide to healing and recovery,* http://www.ojp.usdoj.gov/ovc/publications/infores/cat_hndbk/welcome.html, retrieved October 7, 2004.

Figley CR: *Compassion fatigue: coping with secondary traumatic stress disorder in those who treat the traumatized,* New York, 1995, Brunner/Mazel.

Fullerton CS et al: Debriefing following trauma, *Psychiatr Q* 71:259-276, 2000.

Lerner MD, Shelton, RD: *Acute traumatic stress management (ATSM),* Commack, NY, 2001, American Academy of Experts in Trauma Stress.

National Institute for Occupational Safety and Health: *Traumatic incident stress: information for emergency response workers,* Atlanta, 1996, Centers for Disease Control and Prevention.

Neudeck-Dicken M: *Cumulative stress management for search and rescue: a workbook for all emergency personnel,* Palmer Lake, Colo, 1997, Filter Press.

Potter D: *Debriefing the trauma team: taking care of your own,* American Academy of Experts in Trauma Stress, http://www.aaets. org/arts/art89.htm, retrieved October 7, 2004.

Shalev AY: Biological responses to disasters, *Psychiatr Q* 71:277-288, 2000.

Solomon Z et al: In the shadow of the Gulf War: psychological distress, social support and coping among Israeli soldiers in a high risk area, *Isr J Med Sci* 27:687-695, 1991.

Stern M: *Thoughts of a therapist on the Gulf War,* Tel Aviv University, Sackler Faculty of Medicine, Department of Psychotherapy, Ramat, Tel Aviv, Israel. (Free)

Virginia Cooperative Extension: *Dealing with stress after a disaster,* http://www.cdc.gov/nasd/docs/d001201-d001300/d001280/ d001280.html, retrieved October 7, 2004.

Young BH et al: *Disaster mental health services: a guidebook for clinicians and administrators,* National Center for Post Traumatic Stress Disorder, http://www.ncptsd.org//publications/disaster/, retrieved October 7, 2004.

APPENDIX A

Summary of Chemical Agents

Agent Name	Volatility Persistence	LD_{50} mg on skin	LCt_{50} mg/min/m³ (ppm)	ICt_{50} mg/min/m³ (ppm)	IDLH ppm	Hazard	Symptoms	Physical Characteristics
Tabun (GA)	Volatile, nonpersistent	1000	400 (60)	300 (45)	0.08	Respiratory, skin, eyes	Pinpoint pupils, blurred vision, running nose, salivation, chest tightness, difficulty breathing, vomiting, tachycardia, muscle twitching, paralysis, loss of consciousness, seizures	Colorless to light colored liquid at normal temperatures; slightly less volatile than water
Sarin (GB)	Volatile, nonpersistent	1700	100 (12)	75 (8)	0.03	Respiratory, skin, eyes		
Soman (GD)	Volatile, nonpersistent	50	70 (90)	50 (8)	0.08	Respiratory, skin, eyes		
VX	Nonvolatile, persistent	10	30 (3)	24 (3)	0.0018	Respiratory, skin, eyes		Consistency of motor oil
Mustard (H, HD)	Volatile, persistent	100 mg/kg	1500 (231)	150 (23)	0.003	Respiratory, skin, eyes	Erythema, blisters, eye pain, airway irration and damage	Oily, light yellow to brown, strong odor of garlic or mustard
Nitrogen mustard (HN)	Volatile, persistent	unk	1500 (231)	200 (23)	0.003	Respiratory, skin, eyes		
Phosgene oxime (CX)	Nonvolatile, persistent	unk	3200 (687)	3 (0.6)	unk	Respiratory, skin, eyes	Immediate burning, skin lesions, eye and airway irritation and damage	Solid below 95° F (35° C), but vapor can result
Lewisite (L)	Nonvolatile, persistent	40 mg/kg	1200 (165)	<300 (unk)	0.0004	Respiratory, skin, eyes	Immediate pain or irritation of skin	Oily, colorless liquid with odor of geraniums
Hydrogen cyanide (AC)	Volatile, nonpersistent	unk	2000 (3600)	Varies (unk)	45	Respiratory	Cherry red skin and lips, rapid breathing, nausea, dizziness, headache, seizures, death	Rapidly evaporating liquid
Cyanogen chloride (CK)	Volatile, nonpersistent	unk	11,000 (4375)	7000 (2784)	unk	Respiratory		
Phosgene (CG)	Volatile, nonpersistent	unk	3200 (791)	1600 (395)	2	Respiratory	Coughing, choking	Odor of newly mown hay

LD_{50}, Lethal dose, 50th percentile; *LCt_{50}*, lethal concentration per unit time, 50th percentile; *ppm*, parts per million; *ICt_{50}*, incapacitating concentration per unit time, 50th percentile; *IDLH*, immediately dangerous to life or health; *unk*, unknown.

APPENDIX B

Internet Resources

Resources on the World Wide Web on Bioterrorism and Disaster Preparedness*

Many of the following links come from The AMA Disaster Preparedness and Medical Response website (http://www.ama-assn.org/go/DisasterPreparedness).

DISASTER PLANNING RESOURCES

AHA Chemical and Bioterrorism Preparedness Checklist http://www.aha.org/Emergency/Content/MaAtChecklistB1003.doc
AHA Hospital Preparedness for Mass Casualties http://www.ahapolicyforum.org/policyresources/Modisaster.asp
APIC Mass Casualty Disaster Plan Checklist: A Template for Healthcare Facilities http://www.apic.org/bioterror/checklist.doc
JCAHO Hazard Vulnerability Analysis Tool http://128.11.25.81/ahj/hazardvulnerabilityanalysis.doc
State of Wisconsin Preparedness Plan http://www.dhfs.state.wi.us/rl_dsl/hospital/hospitaldisastrplng.htm

PHYSICIAN RESOURCES

AAFP Biochemical Terrorism Defense: The Role of the Family Physician http://www.aafp.org/hssa/biochem
AAFP Bioterrorism Online Lecture Series http://www.aafp.org/assembly/2001/lectures
ACP-ASIM Bioterrorism Resources http://www.acponline.org/bioterro/index.html
ACS—Unconventional Civilian Disasters: What the Surgeon Should Know http://www.facs.org/civiliandisasters/intro.html
Center for the Study of Bioterrorism and Emerging Infections Clinical Slide Sets: Anthrax http://bioterrorism.slu.edu/quick/pps/anthrax.pps
Center for the Study of Bioterrorism and Emerging Infections Clinical Slide Sets: General Bioterrorism http://bioterrorism.slu.edu/quick/pps/BT_general.pps
Center for the Study of Bioterrorism and Emerging Infections Clinical Slide Sets: Smallpox http://bioterrorism.slu.edu/quick/pps/Smallpox.pps
City and County Public Health Telephone Numbers http://www.naccho.org/general8.cfm
Medical Management of Biological Casualties Handbook http://www.usamriid.army.mil/education/bluebook.html

*From Colorado BNICE Training Center.

Medical Management of Chemical Casualties Handbook http://ccc.apgea.army.mil/reference_materials/handbooks/RedHandbook/001TitlePage.htm
State Public Health Contact Telephone Numbers http://www.statepublichealth.org/directory.php
The Textbook of Military Medicine—Medical aspects of chemical and biological warfare http://ccc.apgea.army.mil/reference_materials/textbook/HTML_Restricted/index.htm http://chemdef.apgea.army.mil/textbook/contents.asp (for downloading PDF files of each chapter)
UCLA Center for Public Health and Disasters—Bioterrorism: Are You Prepared? A slide presentation for primary care physicians http://www.ph.ucla.edu/cphdr/bioterrorism/slidepresentation.html
Virtual Naval Hospital—Biological, Chemical and Nuclear Warfare and Radiation Safety http://www.vnh.org/Providers.html#NBC
World Health Organization Slide Set on the Diagnosis of Smallpox http://www.who.int/emc/diseases/smallpox/Smallpox-English.ppt

DISEASE-SPECIFIC RESOURCES

National Library of Medicine

MEDLINEplus Health Topic on Anthrax http://www.nlm.nih.gov/medlineplus/anthrax.html
MEDLINEplus Health Topic on Biological and Chemical Weapons http://www.nlm.nih.gov/medlineplus/biologicalandchemicalweapons.html
MEDLINEplus Health Topic on Smallpox http://www.nlm.nih.gov/medlineplus/smallpox.html

Journal of the American Medical Association Consensus Statements

Anthrax as a Biological Weapon May 12, 1999 http://jama.ama-assn.org/issues/v281n18/ffull/jst80027.html
Botulinum Toxin as a Biological Weapon February 28, 2001 http://jama.ama-assn.org/issues/v285n8/ffull/jst00017.html
Plague as a Biological Weapon May 3, 2000 http://jama.ama-assn.org/issues/v283n17/ffull/jst90013.html
Smallpox as a Biological Weapon June 9, 1999 http://jama.ama-assn.org/issues/v281n22/ffull/jst90000.html
Tularemia as a Biological Weapon June 6, 2001 http://jama.ama-assn.org/issues/v285n21/ffull/jst10001.html

PATIENT RESOURCES

Advice for communicating with children about disasters from the AAP http://www.aap.org/advocacy/releases/disastercomm.htm
APA—Coping with Disaster (pdf file) http://www.psych.org/disaster/bioterrorism102201.pdf
Facts about Anthrax, Botulism, Pneumonic Plague, Smallpox (Centers for Disease Control and Prevention) http://www.bt.cdc.gov/DocumentsApp/FactsAbout/FactsAbout.asp
FAQs from Johns Hopkins http://www.hopkins-biodefense.org/faq.html

Helping Children Cope after a Terrorist Attack (AMA) http://www.ama-assn.org/ama/pub/category/6174.html
Helping Children Cope with War and Terrorism (AMA) http://www.ama-assn.org/ama/upload/mm/415/helpingchildren.doc
The Patient Education Institute—Anthrax and Bioterrorism http://www.patient-education.com/anthrax

NATIONAL RESOURCES

Federal

Association of State and Territorial Health Officials (ASTHO) http://www.astho.org/phiip/responds.html
Centers for Disease Control and Prevention (CDC) http://www.bt.cdc.gov/
National Association of County and City Health Officials (NACCHO) http://www.naccho.org/files/documents/explanatory.html
U.S. Army Medical Research Institute of Chemical Defense (USAMRICD) http://chemdef.apgea.army.mil/
U.S. Army Medical Research Institute of Infectious Diseases http://www.usamriid.army.mil/education/index.html
USAMRICD Chemical Casualty Care Division http://ccc.apgea.army.mil/

National Organizations

American Academy of Family Physicians (AAFP) http://www.aafp.org/btresponse/index.xml
American Academy of Pediatrics (AAP) http://www.aap.org/advocacy/releases/cad.htm
American College of Physicians-American Society of Internal Medicine (ACP-ASIM) http://www.acponline.org/bioterro/index.html
American Hospital Association (AHA) http://www.aha.org/Emergency/EmIndex.asp
Association for Professionals in Infection Control and Epidemiology (APIC) http://www.apic.org/bioterror
Center for Nonproliferation Studies—Monterey Institute of International Studies http://cns.miis.edu/index.htm
Center for the Study of Bioterrorism and Emerging Infections, St. Louis University School of Public Health (CSBEI) http://www.bioterrorism.slu.edu/
Infectious Diseases Society of North America (IDSA) http://www.idsociety.org/PA/PS&P/BT_Preparedness_10-2-01.htm
Johns Hopkins Center for Civilian Biodefense http://www.hopkins-biodefense.org/
National Medical Association (NMA) http://www.nmanet.org/nonflash.htm

Rapid Response Information System http://www.rris.fema.gov/
University of Alabama Center for Bioterrorism http://www.bioterrorism.uab.edu/
University of South Florida Center for Biological Defense http://www.bt.usf.edu
World Health Organization-Communicable Disease Surveillance and Response (WHO-CSR) http://www.who.int/emc/deliberate_epi.html

Peer-Reviewed Literature

Biological and Chemical Terrorism Defense: A View From the "Front Lines" of Public Health (Adobe pdf format) *American Journal of Public Health* Vol. 91 No. 5 May 2001
Bioterrorism articles from the Journal of the American Medical Association (free of charge) *Journal of the American Medical Association*
Bioterrorism articles from the New England Journal of Medicine (free of charge) *New England Journal of Medicine*
Bioterrorism updates from the Morbidity and Mortality Weekly Report *Morbidity and Mortality Weekly Report*
Bioterrorism-Related Inhalational Anthrax: The First 10 Cases Reported in the United States *Emerging Infectious Diseases*—November/December 2001
Developing New Smallpox Vaccines *Emerging Infectious Diseases*—November/December 2001
Good Intentions and the Road to Bioterrorism Preparedness (Adobe pdf format) *American Journal of Public Health* Vol. 91 No. 5 May 2001
Hospital Preparedness for Victims of Chemical or Biological Terrorism (Adobe pdf format) *American Journal of Public Health* Vol. 91 No. 5 May 2001
Medical Progress: Anthrax *New England Journal of Medicine* 1999; 341:815-826, September 9, 1999
Preemptive Biopreparedness: Can We Learn Anything From History? (Adobe pdf format) *American Journal of Public Health* Vol. 91 No. 5 May 2001
Recognition and Management of Anthrax—An Update *New England Journal of Medicine*—Published online on November 6, 2001
Terrorism, Biological Weapons, and Bonanzas: Assessing the Real Threat to Public Health (Adobe pdf format) *American Journal of Public Health* Vol. 91 No. 5 May 2001

APPENDIX C

Assessment of Risk and Vulnerability

Developing an emergency management plan starts with knowing what risks you must plan for first, remembering that the assessment can change from month to month and year to year. The assessment is a continual process that must be reviewed and revised as necessary. Use all local resources to identify risks that might not be obvious to the civilian eye. The following are points to consider and questions to ask as you begin the assessment when planning for a response to weapons of mass destruction. This is not an all-inclusive list.

If your community has any of the following, the threat risk increases:

- Political gatherings or protests
- Visits from national or international dignitaries
- Activists
- National sporting events, festivals, concerts, or religious activities
- Special events involving celebrities or national or international political figures

Here are some risk and vulnerability planning questions. Other general emergency planning questions for any disaster can also apply. For example, are there seasonal challenges that may apply to your facility? Points to consider in your plan:

- What is the location of your health care facility in regard to local hazards or high-profile buildings such as public safety facilities, schools, religious institutions, or computer centers?
- Could the utilities (water, sewer, telephone, power stations) in your area be identified as targets?
- Are there fuel refineries or chemical plants in the area?
- Is there a state capitol, or are there other political buildings such as federal mints or national monuments in your community? What is their proximity to your facility?
- What highways or major airports are located near your facility or in your community?
- Are there research facilities that might house investigational medications or chemicals?
- What happens if your facility is disabled in the disaster or your facility becomes contaminated?
- Do you have sufficient backup power and lighting to handle a mass casualty incident?
- Do you have local agreements with other facilities or clinics during a mass casualty incident?
- Do you have appropriate downtime procedures?
- Can you evacuate your facility in a disaster?
- Do you have agreements with local government agencies for disasters?
- Are there any military, nuclear, or chemical sites that your facility may serve?

APPENDIX D

Essentials of Facility Emergency Management Plan

Suggested sections of the Emergency Managment Plan:
Assessment of mitigation, vulnerability, and risk
Incident Command System
HEICS organizational positions
- Use of designated checklists
Activation and deactivation procedures
Communication procedures during a mass casualty incident
- Internal and external communication systems
- Redundancy in communication model
Coordinated patient care
- Standing orders for management and rapid discharge

Evacuation policy and procedures
- Internal and external procedures
Resource management for the mass casualty incident
- Immediate and progressive needs (over 72 hours)
- People management
  - Personnel
  - Family and friends
  - Media
  - Volunteers
Data management for the mass casualty incident
- Victim and patient tracking
- Personnel tracking (current and oncoming)
- Sharing of data between staging areas
  - Computerized versus hand-collected data
Security measures for the mass casualty incident
- Internal and external security measures
Facility property management
- Internal and external management
Identification of local, state, and federal resources
- Accessing available resources
Critical incident stress management plan
Extensive educational planning
Evaluation of the plan annually or as needed
Committee and procedure for annual evaluation

APPENDIX E

Education Training Plan—Suggested Topics (not all inclusive)

I. Overview of the Emergency Management Plan (EMP)
  A. Start education in orientation (immediate needs)
    1. Introduction of the EMP
      a. Activation and deactivation of plan
      b. Training expectations of staff
      c. Staff call down list, reporting duties, and holding area
    2. Introduction of the Incident Command System (ICS)
    3. Introduction to roles and responsibilities
II. Operations Level of OSHA training
  A. For staff members involved in decontamination processes and planning
  B. Regulations

III. Communication
  A. Entire communication model
    1. Backup communication systems
  B. Call signs or codes, if used (keep simple)
  C. Practice with all available tools
  D. Radio communication
IV. Personal protective equipment
  A. Classroom and hands-on training
  B. Fit testing and physical exam requirements
V. Incident Command System
  A. Process
  B. Roles
VI. Decontamination process
  A. Ambulatory and nonambulatory victim decontamination
  B. Hands-on training with decontamination unit
VII. Drills and table-top exercises
VIII. Special situations related to weapons of mass destruction
  A. Nuclear, biological, and chemical (NBC) agent information
  B. Treatment and diagnosis of NBC
  C. Evidence collection and preservation
IX. Data Management tools and processes
X. Security measures during a mass casualty incident (MCI)
XI. Triage in an MCI
XII. Critical incident stress management

APPENDIX F

Strategic National Stockpile

The following is a brief overview of the Strategic National Stockpile (SNS) that can provide you with information that will assist in long-term planning.

A decision to deploy the stockpile is based on the best epidemiologic, laboratory, and public health information regarding the nature of the threat. The mission of the Centers for Disease Control and Prevention (CDC) Strategic National Stockpile program (SNSP) is to ensure the availability of lifesaving pharmaceuticals, antibiotics, and chemical interventions; medical, surgical and patient support supplies; and equipment for prompt delivery to the site of a disaster, including a possible biological or chemical terrorist event anywhere in the United States.

STOCKPILE CONTENTS

- Because anthrax, plague, and tularemia can be effectively treated with antibiotics that are immediately available, purchasing these products for the SNS formulary was given first priority.
- The SNS also has a cache of vaccine available to address smallpox threats.
- In addition to medications and supplies for intravenous administration, the SNS includes medical equipment that would be essential for treatment, including airway supplies, bandages and dressings, and other emergency medications. These are items that local clinicians may find in short supply in the event of a terrorism incident.

STRATEGIC NATIONAL STOCKPILE COMPONENTS

- The SNS has two basic components. The first component consists of eight 12-hour push packages for immediate response. The 12-hour push packages are fully stocked, positioned in environmentally controlled and secured warehouses, and ready for immediate deployment to reach any affected area within 12 hours of the federal decision to release the assets.
- A 12-hour push package is a preassembled set of supplies, pharmaceuticals, and medical equipment ready for quick delivery to and use in the field. Each package consists of 50 tons of material intended to address a mass casualty incident. These packages will permit emergency medical staff to treat a variety of different agents, because the actual threat may not have been identified at the time of the stockpile deployment.
- The second component is composed of vendor-managed inventory (VMI) material. If the incident requires a larger or multi-phased response, follow-on VMI packages will be shipped to arrive within 24 to 36 hours.
- The follow-on VMI packages are composed of pharmaceuticals and supplies that can be tailored to provide pharmaceuticals, supplies and/or products specific for the suspected or confirmed agent or combination of agents.

Glossary

Abscess Accumulation of purulent material in tissues or organs; usually associated with an infection.

Absorb To physically penetrate into the porous surface of another material.

Absorbed contamination A chemical, biological, or radioactive agent that has penetrated into the material; not just sitting on the surface.

AC Hydrogen cyanide.

ACADA-M22 Automatic chemical agent detection alarm.

ACGIH American Conference of Governmental and Industrial Hygienists.

Acute respiratory distress syndrome A clinical syndrome that includes pulmonary insufficiency. Formerly called *adult respiratory distress syndrome*.

Adenosine triphosphate A compound used for energy in living cells.

Adsorbents Materials that adhere liquid and vaporous hazardous materials on their surfaces.

Aerosols Solids or liquids suspended in air.

Afebrile Without a fever.

Alpha particle A positively charged particle emitted by certain radioactive materials.

Alphaviruses Group A arboviruses, which are serologically related. They are transmitted by mosquitoes.

American Conference of Governmental and Industrial Hygienists A private consortium of scientists from government, universities, and industry that has developed the threshold limit values system.

Anemia A reduction in the number of circulating erythrocytes or hemoglobin in the blood.

ANFO Ammonium nitrate and fuel (such as diesel fuel) mixed together to create an explosive.

Anthrax An acute bacterial infection caused by inhalation of, contact with, or ingestion of *Bacillus anthracis* organisms. There are three forms of anthrax disease; the form depends on the route of exposure. Inhalational anthrax disease occurs from inhaling anthrax spores. Cutaneous anthrax is the most common form and occurs following the exposure of compromised skin to anthrax spores. Gastrointestinal anthrax occurs following the ingestion of live *B. anthracis,* usually in contaminated meat.

Anticholinesterase An agent, such as an organophasphate, that blocks nerve impulses by inhibiting the enzyme cholinesterase.

Anxiety The physiological and psychological reaction to an expected danger, either real or imagined.

APD Advanced portable detector.

APR Air-purifying respirator.

ARDS Acute respiratory distress syndrome.

***Arenaviridae* (Arenaviruses)** A family of viruses including the causative agents of Lassa fever and Machupo.

Arthralgia Pain in the joints.

Asphyxiant A substance that can cause death by depriving the body of oxygen. Asphyxiants may be classified as either simple or chemical.

Asphyxiant, chemical Chemicals that have systemic actions that impair the body's ability to supply oxygen to the tissues or to prevent oxygen from being used during metabolism. Examples include cyanide and carbon monoxide.

Asphyxiant, simple Chemicals that deprive the body of oxygen by displacing oxygen in ambient air. The simple asphyxiant has no chemical action. Examples include argon, neon, and helium.

Asphyxiation Oxygen deprivation within the body. Simple asphyxiants displace oxygen, and chemical asphyxiants interfere with oxygen transportation or use inside the body.

ATP Adenosine triphosphate.

Awareness Level Responders who may be the first on the scene of a hazardous materials emergency. Awareness Level responders are trained to recognize the presence of hazardous materials, protect themselves, call for help, and secure the area.

Bacillus anthracis A gram-positive, spore-forming bacterium that causes anthrax disease in humans and animals.

Bacteremia The presence of bacteria in the blood. Fever, chills, tachycardia, and tachypnea are common manifestations of bacteremia.

BAL British anti-lewisite (dimercaprol).

Beta particle A negatively charged particle emitted by certain radioactive materials.

Biological agent A disease-causing pathogen or a toxin that can be used as a weapon to cause disease or injury to people.

Blepharospasm Spasm of the eyelids.

Blister agent A chemical used as a weapon, designed specifically to internally and externally injure the body tissue of people who are exposed to its vapors or liquid. The method of injury is to cause painful skin blisters or tissue destruction of the exposed surface area. Examples: mustard, lewisite.

Blood agent Hydrogen cyanide (AC) and cyanogen chloride (CK).

BNICE Biological, nuclear, incendiary, chemical, and explosive.

Botulism A severe neurological illness caused by a potent toxin produced by *Clostridium botulinum*. There are three forms of botulism disease: foodborne, wound, and infant (also called intestinal) botulism.

Breakthrough The point at which chemical permeation of a protective barrier is first detected.

Breakthrough time The time needed for a specific chemical to permeate a protective barrier material to a detectable concentration.

British anti-lewisite (dimercaprol) An antidote for lewisite exposure.

Brucella A family of gram-negative aerobic organisms that can infect humans including: *Brucella abortus, Brucella canis, Brucella suis*, and *Brucella melitensis*. They are commonly found in hoofed animals such as dairy cattle, sheep, and swine but can also be found in other animals.

Brucellosis A bacterial infection caused by inhalation or ingestion of one of four species of *Brucella*, a family of gram-negative aerobic organisms. Human disease is divided into three stages: acute, subacute, and chronic. The acute stage (exposure to 2 months) is characterized by a flulike illness with nonspecific symptoms. The subacute stage (2 to 12 months) manifests with similar symptoms. The chronic stage (longer than 12 months) has predominately neuropsychiatric symptoms. It is also known as undulant fever, Malta fever, and Mediterranean fever.

BSA Body surface area.

Bubonic Relating to an inflamed, enlarged lymph gland.

Buddy system Personnel organization system in which each responder is working with and observed by at least one other employee in the response group.

Bulbar palsy A neurological disease marked by progressive weakness of the muscles stimulated by cranial nerves. Clinical manifestations include dysarthria, dysphagia, facial weakness, tongue weakness, and fasciculations of the tongue and facial muscles.

Burkholderia mallei An aerobic, gram-negative, non–spore-forming bacillus that naturally occurs in horses, donkeys, and mules; causes glanders in humans.

Burkholderia pseudomallei A species of gram-negative aerobic bacteria that causes melioidosis. It has been isolated from soil and water in tropical regions.

CAM Chemical agent monitor.

Capillaroscopy Examination of capillaries for diagnostic purposes.

CBN Chemical, biological, and nuclear.

Central nervous system syndrome Ataxia, seizures, lethargy, and coma that follow an acute radiation dose of up to 2000 rads or more. These symptoms occur within minutes of an acute exposure. Neurologic syndromes indicate a dose high enough to cause permanent damage to multiple organ systems.

CG Phosgene.

CGI Combustible gas indicator.

Chill A feeling of cold with shivering and pale skin; usually a prodrome of an infection.

Chlamydia psittaci An intracellular pathogen infecting primarily birds. Human disease usually results from inhalation of dried droppings, secretions, and dust from the feathers of infected birds. Sequelae may include endocarditis, hepatitis, and neurological complications.

Choking agent An industrial chemical used as a weapon to kill people who inhale the vapors or gases. The method of injury or death is by asphyxiation from lung damage from hydrochloric acid burns. Examples: chlorine, phosgene.

Cholera A serious, acute diarrheal disease caused by *Vibrio cholerae*; usually caused by consumption of contaminated water; can lead to severe dehydration in a matter of hours unless quickly treated.

CK Cyanogen chloride.

CL Chlorine.

Clo value The insulation value of clothing. Clo for no clothing (i.e., a nude person) is 0.0; clo for a business suit is 1.0. One clo unit is the amount of clothing required to keep a resting person comfortable at normal room temperature.

Clostridium botulinum A bacterium that produces a powerful toxin that causes botulism in humans, waterfowl, and cattle.

Cold zone The safe area that is isolated from the area of contamination. This zone has safe and easy access. It contains the command post and the staging areas for personnel, vehicles, and equipment. EMS personnel are stationed in the cold zone.

Combustible liquids Liquids having a flash point above 141° F (60.5° C) and below 200° F (93° C). Examples include brake fluid, glycol ethers, and camphor oil.

Compassion fatigue Feeling the same results of trauma as the victims of trauma feel. The responder absorbs the victims' emotional response while caring for the victims. Compassion fatigue is a stress disorder.

Contamination The deposition or absorption of chemical, biological, or radiological materials onto personnel or other materials.

Coping strategies Methods of relating to stress. Coping responses are influenced by personal history.

Corrosive substance Any liquid or solid that can destroy human flesh on contact or has a severe corrosion rate on steel.

Coxiella burnetii A ubiquitous rickettsia organism found on every continent and causing a common disease in farm and domestic animals (e.g., goats, sheep, cows, dogs, cats). Infection of humans may occur through inhalation of aerosolized particles from body fluids, tissues, or excreta of infected animals, through direct contact with contaminated materials, or through drinking contaminated milk.

CPC Chemical-protective clothing.

Crimean-Congo hemorrhagic fever (CCHF) A severe hemorrhagic fever syndrome caused by viruses of the *Nairovirus* group.

Critical incident stress management A comprehensive stress-management program involving the entire organization and possibly the community during an MCI.

Cryogenics Gases that have been liquefied and that have a boiling point of less than −60° F (−51° C). Cryogenic liquids have a great expansion ratio and will vaporize rapidly when heated.

Cryptosporidiosis A mild diarrheal disease caused by *Cryptosporidium parvum*, a parasitic protozoan. Illness results from consumption of contaminated water.

Cryptosporidium parvum A species of parasitic protozoan that infects humans and domestic mammals. It is the causative agent of cryptosporidiosis, a mild diarrheal disease.

CS Chloroacetophenone (tear gas).

CX Phosgene oxime.

Cyanosis A bluish-purple discoloration of the skin and mucous membranes caused by increasing amounts of deoxygenated hemoglobin in the blood.

Cytotoxin A type of biological toxin that poisons the cells.

Debriefings A defusing process that allows responders and their significant others to express their thoughts and feelings about the deployment.

Decon Decontamination.

Decontamination The physical and chemical process of reducing and preventing the spread of contamination from persons and equipment at a hazardous materials incident. Also referred to as *contamination reduction.*

Defensive actions Actions carried out at a hazardous materials incident that do not involve direct intentional contact with the material; actions carried out from a safe distance that are focused on slowing down the progression of the incident.

Defusing A process that allows responders and their families to express their thoughts and feelings about the deployment.

Degradation The physical breakdown of chemical-resistant clothing because of use, exposure to chemicals, or improper storage conditions.

Detonate Burn faster than the speed of sound.

DIC Disseminated intravascular coagulation.

Diplopia Double vision.

Dirty bomb A conventional explosive device that disperses radiological agents.

Disseminated intravascular coagulation A complication of septic shock in which endotoxins cause systemic clotting of the blood.

DMAT Disaster Medical Assistance Team.

DMORT Disaster Mortuary Operations Team.

DNA Deoxyribonucleic acid, which makes up the genetic material found in all living cells.

Dusts Solid particles of various sizes.

Dyspnea Shortness of breath, difficulty breathing.

Eastern equine encephalitis (EEE) A form of arboviral encephalitis (primarily affecting equines) endemic to eastern North America; causative organism (eastern equine encephalitis virus) is transmitted to humans via mosquito bite; human infections may result in influenza-like illness followed by altered mentation, seizure, coma, and sometimes death.

Ebola A viral hemorrhagic fever illness caused by an Ebola virus (Filovirus family). It is seen mostly in Africa and is transmitted by person-to-person contact with body fluids of infected individuals. There is no specific treatment, and it is often fatal within several days.

ED$_{50}$ Effective dose (50th percentile). ED$_{50}$ is the dose required to produce a specified effect in 50% of the animal population.

EDS Emergency decontamination system.

EHS Extremely hazardous substances.

Elitism The belief by one group (whether as a team or a part of a team) that it is superior to others.

Emergency decontamination Process of decontaminating people exposed to and potentially contaminated with hazardous materials by rapidly removing most of the contamination in order to reduce exposure and save lives, with secondary regard for completeness of decontamination.

Emergency management plan A statement of overall policies and procedures regarding response to mass casualty incidents.

Emergency medical services (EMS) Organizations that provide emergency medical care for ill or injured persons by trained providers.

EMP Emergency management plan; electromagnetic pulse.

EMS Emergency medical services.

Encephalitis Inflammation of the brain due to infection, toxins, and other conditions.

Endocarditis Inflammatory alterations of the endocardium, characterized by the presence of vegetations on the surface of the endocardium or in the endocardium itself. Endocarditis most commonly involves a heart valve, but sometimes it affects the inner lining of the cardiac chambers or the endocardium elsewhere.

Enterotoxin A type of biological toxin that poisons the digestive system.

EPA Environmental Protection Agency.

Epidemiology The science of investigating the incidence, distribution, and control of diseases.

Epistaxis Bleeding from the nose.

Erythema Redness of the skin resulting from congestion of the capillaries.

***Eschericia coli* O157-H7** A bacterium that has been shown to cause severe food-borne disease. It is a verocytotoxin-producing serogroup belonging to the O subfamily of *E. coli* and has been linked to human disease outbreaks resulting from contamination of foods from bovine origin.

Esprit de corps A feeling of unity created by common ideals and goals in and by group of individuals.

Etiology The cause or origin of a disease or disorder.

Evaporation The process of a liquid turning into a gas.

Explosive substance Any chemical compound, mixture, or device, the primary or common purpose of which is to function by detonation or rapid combustion (i.e., with substantial instantaneous release of gas and heat). Explosives are found in liquid or solid forms and include dynamite, TNT, black powder, fireworks, and ammunition.

Extremely hazardous substances Chemicals that the Environmental Protection Agency, in the Superfund Amendment and Reauthorization Act, has determined to be extremely hazardous to a community during an emergency spill or release because of their toxicities and physical and chemical properties.

Family critical incident stress debriefing A structured therapy process that helps responders' families understand and manage intense emotions during a mass casualty incident.

Febrile Pertaining to or characterized by a fever.

Fever An abnormal elevation of body temperature (>100° F [38° C]), usually as a result of an infection.

FID Flame ionization device.

***Filoviridae* (Filoviruses)** A family of viruses that includes the causative agents of Ebola and Marburg.

Flammable The capacity of a substance to ignite.

Flammable gas Any compressed gas that meets requirements for lower flammability limit, flammability limit range, flame projection, or flame propagation as specified in CFR Title 49, Sec. 173.300(b). Examples include acetylene, butane, hydrogen, and propane.

Flammable liquid Any liquid having a flash point below 141° F (60.5° C). Examples include benzene, gasoline, and acetone.

Flammable solid A solid material other than an explosive that is liable to cause fires through friction or through retained heat from manufacturing or processing or that can be ignited readily. Examples include phosphorus, lithium, magnesium, titanium, and calcium resinate.

Fluorimeter A biological detection instrument that measures the amount of DNA in a sample.

Francisella tularensis A hardy, slow growing, highly infectious aerobic organism. Human infection may result in tularemia, also known as rabbit fever or deer fly fever.

Fulminant Sudden, intense occurrence.

G agent Nerve agent, including tabun (GA), sarin (GB), soman (GD), and GF.

GA Tabun.

Gamma radiation A type of electromagnetic radiation.

Gas chromatograph and mass spectrometer An instrument that uses a combination of laboratory analysis processes to identify and quantify the chemical contents of a sample.

Gastrointestinal syndrome Desquamation of the mucosal layer of the gastrointestinal tract that results in significant nausea, vomiting, diarrhea, and dehydration secondary to a radiation exposure.

GB Sarin.

GC Gas chromatography.

GC/MS Gas chromatograph and mass spectrometer.

GD Soman.

GF Cyclohexyl methyl phosphonofluoridate, a nerve agent.

Glanders An equine disease caused by the aerobic, gram-negative non–spore-forming bacillus *Burkholderia mallei*. Human disease has been reported in four forms: pulmonary disease, a localized form (mucous membranes), a rapidly fatal septicemic illness, or a chronic disease condition (farcy).

H Sulfur mustard.

H agent A blister agent, including sulfur mustard (H) or distilled sulfur mustard (HD).

Habituation The decrease in response to a stimulus due to repetition.

Hantavirus A virus in the Bunyaviridae family that causes a severe, rapid respiratory illness. The primary reservoir is the deer mouse.

Hantavirus pulmonary syndrome Acute respiratory illness in humans caused by one of three pathogenic Hantaviruses; it was first identified in the southwestern United States. This syndrome is characterized by rapid onset of fever, myalgias, headache, cough, and respiratory failure.

Hazardous material A substance (solid, liquid, or gas) capable of posing an unreasonable risk to health, safety, environment, or property.

HD Distilled sulfur mustard.

HEICS Hospital Emergency Incident Command System.

Hematemesis Vomiting of blood.

Hematochezia Bleeding in the gastrointestinal tract.

Hematopoietic syndrome Temporary or permanent damage to the bone marrow by radiation exposure.

Hemolytic uremic syndrome Syndrome of hemolytic anemia, thrombocytopenia, and acute renal failure leading to renal necrosis.

Hemorrhagic Related to bleeding or hemorrhage.

HEPA filter High-efficiency particulate air filter.

Hepatomegaly Enlargement of the liver.

Hepatosplenomegaly Abnormal enlargement of the liver and spleen.

High explosives Explosives whose detonation is accompanied by a pressure wave.

HN Nitrogen mustard, a family of blister agents, usually written as HN-1, HN-2, or HN-3 to denote specific chemical compounds.

Hospital Emergency Incident Command System An emergency management system that employs a logical management structure, defined responsibilities, clear reporting channels, and a common nomenclature to help unify hospitals with other emergency responders.

Hot zone The hot (exclusion) zone is the area where contamination exists. Patients are removed from this area to the warm zone for decontamination. Entrance to the hot zone requires proper personal protective equipment.

Hypotension Abnormally low blood pressure; it is seen in shock.

Hypothermia A breakdown in temperature regulation of the body. Core body temperature is below 95° F (35° C). First sign is uncontrollable shivering. Rapid rewarming of the patient is necessary.

Hypoxia Lack of an adequate amount of oxygen in inspired air; reduced oxygen concentration or tension.

IC Incident commander.

ICAM Improved chemical agent monitor.

ICt_{50} Incapacitating concentration per unit of time (50th percentile); the concentration that will predictably cause incapacitation of 50% of those exposed for a specific unit of time, usually fixed at 1 minute.

ID_{50} Incapacitating dose (50th percentile); the dose that will predictably cause incapacitation of 50% of those exposed.

IDLH Immediately dangerous to life or health. The maximum air concentration of a chemical from which one could escape within 30 minutes without symptoms of impairment and without irreversible health effects.

IED Improvised explosive device.

IMS Incident management system; ion mobility spectrometry.

Incendiary device A device that is designed to ignite a fire.

Incident Command Level Responders who will assume control of an incident scene beyond the level of the first responder operations.

Infectious substance A viable microorganism, or its toxin, that can cause human disease. Examples include anthrax, rabies, tetanus, botulism, polio, and specimens obtained from patients with acquired immunodeficiency syndrome (AIDS).

Inorganic compound Chemical compounds that do not contain carbon.

Intrinsically safe Equipment that is not capable of releasing sufficient electrical energy to cause the ignition of a flammable mixture.

IP Ionization potential.

IR Infrared spectroscopy.

Irritating material A liquid or solid substance that on contact with fire or when exposed to air gives off dangerous or intensely irritating fumes but that does not include any poisonous material.

JCAD Joint chemical agent detector.

JCAHO Joint Commission on Accreditation of Healthcare Organizations.

JSLSCAD Joint services lightweight standoff chemical agent detector.

L Lewisite.

Lassa fever A viral hemorrhagic fever illness caused by the Lassa virus (Arenavirus family).

LC$_{50}$ Lethal concentration (50th percentile); the inhaled dose of a substance that causes death in 50% of the test animal population.

LD$_{50}$ Lethal dose (50th percentile); the absorbed dose (oral or dermal) of a substance that causes death in 50% of the test animal population.

LEL Lower explosive limit.

Leukopenia Abnormal decrease in white blood cells.

Level A personal protective equipment Fully encapsulated vapor-tight suit with self-contained breathing apparatus or positive-pressure air line and chemically resistant boots and gloves. Level A provides protection against vapors and skin-toxic chemicals.

Level B personal protective equipment Chemical splash suit with self-contained breathing apparatus or positive-pressure air line and chemical-resistant boots and gloves. Level B provides protection against inadvertent chemical splash and particulates.

Level C personal protective equipment Chemical splash suit with air-purifying respirator and chemical-resistant boots and gloves. Level C rovides protection against known chemical concentrations below IDLH concentrations.

Level D personal protective equipment Work uniform; provides no protection against chemical exposure.

Limited-use garments Chemical-protective clothing that is used and then discarded as hazardous waste. Although limited-use garments can be worn several times based on use and exposure patterns, they commonly are discarded after one wearing.

Liquefied gas A gas at normal temperature and under enough pressure to force them into a liquid state.

LOC Level of concern; level of consciousness; loss of consciousness.

Low explosive An explosive that rapidly burns or deflagrates. Unless the explosion is confined, a low explosive produces no pressure wave.

Lymphocyte White blood cell responsible for much of the body's immune protection.

M256A1 detector kit Military chemical agent detector kit.

Machupo fever A viral hemorrhagic fever illness caused by Machupo virus (Arenavirus family).

Macular Related to or marked by spots.

Maculopapular A rash consisting of both spots (macules) and elevations of the skin (papules).

Malodorant A riot control agent that acts by producing an extremely offensive odor.

Marburg fever A viral hemorrhagic fever illness caused by Marburg virus (Filovirus family).

Mark 1 nerve agent antidote kit Nerve agent antidote kit consisting of self-injectors of atropine and pralidoxime chloride.

Mass casualty incident Any large number of casualties produced in a relatively short period of time that exceeds local logistical support capabilities.

Material safety data sheet A document that contains information about the specific identity of a hazardous chemical. Information includes exact name and synonyms, health effects, first aid, chemical and physical properties, and emergency telephone numbers.

MCI Mass casualty incident.

Melioidosis A disease of humans and animals caused by the aerobic, gram-negative bacillus *Burkholderia pseudomallei.* The disease may range from a dormant infection to a condition that causes multiple abscesses, pneumonia, and bacteremia.

Meningitis Inflammation of the membranes surrounding the brain and spinal cord.

Meningoencephalitis Inflammation of both the brain and meninges.

Mil-spec Military specifications.

Miosis Constricted pupils.

Mission-oriented protective posture A type of military chemical-protective equipment. MOPP levels indicate how the equipment is used.

Mist Condensation of liquid droplets on particles.

Mitigation The part of the emergency management plan that helps the facility avoid becoming a part of the disaster.

MMRS Metropolitan Medical Response System.

MOPP Mission-oriented protective posture.

MOPP 0 All protective equipment is carried with the responder.

MOPP 1 Chemical overgarment is worn, and overboots, mask with hood, and gloves are carried, when an attack is probable.

MOPP 2 Chemical overgarment and overboots are worn, and mask with hood and gloves are carried, when an attack is probable.

MOPP 3 Chemical overgarment, overboots, and mask with hood are worn, and gloves are carried, when chemical agents, biological agents, or both are present at a negligible risk level.

MOPP 4 All protective equipment is worn to provide the highest degree of protection when agents are present but the risk is undetermined.

MRI Magnetic resonance imaging.

MSDS Material safety data sheet.

Mydriasis Prolonged or excessive dilation of the pupil.

National Fire Protection Association International voluntary membership organization to promote improved fire protection and prevention and to establish safeguards against loss of life and property by fire. NFPA writes and publishes national voluntary consensus standards.

National Institute for Occupational Safety and Health The agency of the National Public Health Service that tests and certifies respirators and air sampling devices. It recommends exposure limits to OSHA for substances, investigates incidents, and researches occupational safety.

NBC Nuclear, biological, and chemical.

NDMS National Disaster Medical System.

Nephritis Inflammation of the kidney. Nephritis may be focal or diffuse proliferative or destructive process; it can involve the glomerulus, tubule, or interstitial renal tissue.

Neutropenia A decrease in the number of neutrophilic leukocytes in the blood.

NFPA National Fire Protection Association.

NIOSH National Institute for Occupational Safety and Health.

NMRT/WMD National Medical Response Team/Weapons of Mass Destruction.

Nonflammable gas Any compressed gas other than a flammable gas. Examples include ammonia, nitrogen, and carbon dioxide.

Normalcy Psychological equilibrium.

OC Oleoresin capsicum (pepper spray).

Occupational Safety and Health Administration A unit of the Department of Labor that establishes protective standards, enforces those standards, and reaches out to employers and employees through technical assistance and consultation programs.

Offensive actions Actions taken at a hazardous materials incident that involve direct, intentional contact with the hazardous material. Offensive actions are focused on mitigation of the problem.

Operations Level Training level established by OSHA 29 CFR 1910.120 for personnel who respond to a hazardous materials incident. Operations Level responders are trained to protect nearby persons, property, or the environment from the effects of the release. They respond in a defensive fashion to control the release from a safe distance and keep it from spreading.

Organic compounds Chemical compounds that contain carbon.

OSHA Occupational Safety and Health Administration.

Oxidizing substances Substances that readily yield oxygen and are thereby able to stimulate the combustion of matter. Examples include lithium peroxide and calcium chlorite.

Pancytopenia Deficiency of all three cell elements of the blood: erythrocytes, leukocytes, and platelets.

PAPR Powered air-purifying respirator.

Papular Characterized by the presence of small, circumscribed, solid elevations of the skin.

Paresthesias Abnormal sensations of the skin (e.g., cold, warmth, tingling, pressure) that are experienced without stimulation.

PEL Permissible exposure limit.

Penetration The flow of a chemical substance through openings such as zippers, seams, stitches, holes, or tears in the material of chemical-protective clothing.

Permeation The process by which a chemical moves through a chemical-resistant fabric on a molecular level; diffusion.

Permissible exposure limit Occupational exposure limits established by OSHA. These may be expressed as time-weighted average (TWA) limit, ceiling (C) limit, or short-term exposure limit (STEL). OSHA PELs are legally enforceable. These exposure limits can be different from ACGIH TLVs or NIOSH RELs.

Petechiae Purplish or brownish red discoloration, visible through the epidermis, caused by bleeding into the tissues.

PF Protection factor.

Photophobia Abnormal sensitivity or intolerance to light.

PID Photoionization device.

Plague An acute infectious disease caused by the anaerobic gram-negative bacterium *Yersinia pestis*. Plague is transmitted naturally from rodents to humans through fleabites. There are three forms of plague: bubonic (the most likely form of the disease to be seen from naturally occurring infections), pneumonic (the most likely form of the disease to result from an act of terrorism), and septicemic.

Pneumonic Related to an inflammation of the lungs.

Poisonous substances Gases, liquids, or other substances that present a danger to life or a hazard to health from exposure to a very small amount of the substance. Examples include cyanide, arsenic, phosgene, aniline, methyl bromide, insecticides, and pesticides.

Posttraumatic stress disorder An extreme, long-lasting reaction to a traumatic event. Symptoms include difficulty sleeping, irritability, poor concentration, hypervigilance, exaggerated startle response, and motor restlessness.

PPE Personal protective equipment.

ppm Parts per million.

Primary blast injury Injuries that are caused by the explosive's pressure wave.

Prodrome An early symptom of a disease.

Propellants Explosives that are designed to move an object.

psi Pounds per square inch.

Psittacosis An acute chlamydial disease caused by an intracellular pathogen, *Chlamydia psittaci,* which exists naturally in birds and is transmitted to humans by inhalation of excreta of infected birds. The illness is characterized by pneumonitis and systemic manifestations such as endocarditis, hepatitis, and neurologic complications.

PT Prothrombin time.

Ptosis Drooping of the upper eyelid.

PTT Partial thromboplastin time.

Pyrotechnics Explosives that are created to make light, sound, and smoke for fireworks displays.

Q fever An acute febrile, zoonotic disease caused by exposure to *Coxiella burnetii*. It is usually a mild, self-limiting, flulike illness.

Query fever Q fever.

rad Radiation absorbed dose.

Radiation absorbed dose The basic unit of absorbed radiation equal to the absorption of 0.01 joule per kilogram (J/kg) of absorbing material.

Radiation equivalent in man *See* Roentgen equivalent in man.

Radioactive Having the ability to emit ionizing energy.

Radioactive substance Any material (or combination of materials) that spontaneously emit ionizing radiation and have a specific activity greater than 0.002 Ci/g (curies per gram). Examples include plutonium, cobalt, uranium-235, and radioactive waste.

Rale Any noise, normal or abnormal, heard when listening to any part of the respiratory tract.

Recommended exposure limit A value developed by NIOSH to indicate the highest allowable airborne concentration of a chemical that is not expected to injure a worker. The recommended exposure limit may be expressed as a ceiling limit or as a time-weighted average (TWA), usually for 10-hour work shifts.

REL Recommended exposure limit.

rem Roentgen equivalent in man.

Respiratory distress syndrome A life-threatening syndrome of progressive pulmonary insufficiency.

Rhinorrhea Runny nose.

Ricin A highly potent cytotoxin made from castor bean–processing waste.

Ricinus communis The castor bean plant, source of the poison ricin.

Rickettsia prowazekii A rickettsial, gram-negative, small obligate intracellular coccobacillus that infects the cytoplasm of host cells, causing epidemic or louse-borne typhus.

Rickettsia typhi A rickettsial, gram-negative, small obligate intracellular coccobacillus that infects the cytoplasm of host cells, causing endemic or murine typhus.

Rickettsia tsutsugamushi A rickettsial, gram-negative, small obligate intracellular coccobacillus that infects the cytoplasm of host cells, causing scrub typhus.

Roentgen equivalent in man Measurement relative to the total effect of radioactive energy on a particular biological entity.

Salmonella A genus of gram-negative, anaerobic bacteria pathogenic for humans, causing enteric fevers, gastroenteritis, and bacteremia. Food poisoning is the most common clinical manifestation.

Salmonellosis Infections with bacteria of the genus *Salmonella*.

SAR Supplied-air respirator, also known as an air line.

SARA Superfund Amendment and Reauthorization Act.

SAW Surface acoustic wave.

SBCCOM Soldier Biological and Chemical Command.

SCBA Self-contained breathing apparatus.

Scintigraphy The injection and subsequent detection of radioactive isotopes to create images of body parts and to identify body functions and diseases.

SEB Staphylococcal enterotoxin B.

Secondary blast injury Injuries that are caused by shrapnel from the fragments of an explosive device and from things that have been attached to the explosive device.

Secondary contamination Contamination with a hazardous material acquired by contact with a contaminated victim.

Secondary device An additional explosive or other type of device that is specifically intended to harm personnel responding to the emergency.

Sensitization Exposure of a person to anxiety-provoking stimuli while relaxing. This technique allows the person to eventually confront the stress or fear without the previously associated anxiety.

Sepsis The presence of microorganisms or their toxins in tissues or in the blood. Systemic disease caused by the spread of the microorganisms or their by-products via the circulating blood is commonly called *septicemia.*

Septicemia Systemic disease associated with the presence of microorganisms or their by-products in the blood.

Septicemic Related to a systemic disease associated with the presence of microorganisms or their by-products in the blood.

Septic shock Shock due to circulatory inadequacy caused by gram-negative bacteria (bacteremia). It is less often the result of the presence of other microorganisms (fungus or virus) in the blood (fungemia or viremia, respectively).

Shigella A gram-negative flagellated bacterium of the Escherichiae group, responsible for dysentery (inflammation of the intestines) in humans. Drinking contaminated water is a common source of infection.

Shigellosis A form of bacillary dysentery (inflammation of the intestines) caused by bacteria of the genus *Shigella.*

Shock An imbalanced condition of the hemodynamic equilibrium, usually manifested by failure to oxygenate vital organs.

Short-term exposure limit A 15-minute time-weighted averate (TWA) exposure that should not be exceeded at any time during a workday, even if the 8-hour TWA is within the threshold limit value TWA (TLV-TWA). Exposures above the TLV-TWA up to the short-term exposure limit (STEL) should be for no longer than 15 minutes and should not occur more than four times a day. There should be at least 60 minutes between successive exposures in this range.

Significant other A spouse, life-partner, or close personal relation.

SLUDGE Salivation, lacrimation, urination, defecation, gastrointestinal pain, emesis.

Smallpox A disease caused by variola viruses, which are members of the orthopox virus family. It was eradicated in the 1970s; however, it still remains a threat as a bioterrorism agent.

Specialist Level Personnel who respond with and provide support to hazardous materials technicians.

Splenomegaly Enlargement of the spleen.

Staphylococcal enterotoxin B A pyrogenic toxin that is produced by *Staphylococcus aureus*. It is normally associated with foodborne illnesses that result from improper food-handling practices.

Staphylococcus aureus A bacterium found in nasal membranes, skin, hair follicles, and perineum of warm-blooded animals. It causes a wide range of infections and intoxications.

STEL Short-term exposure limit.

Stress The physical and psychological result of internal or external pressure.

Stressor Anything, internal or external, that applies psychological pressure on a person.

Superfund Amendment and Reauthorization Act An EPA regulation that reauthorized the Superfund (Comprehensive Environmental Response, Compensation and Liability Act, or CERCLA) program. It also established federal status for community right-to-know standards and emergency response to hazardous materials accidents.

Surge capacity The ability to expand care based on a sudden MCI. Surge capacity should be addressed in the emergency management plan.

Tachycardia Abnormally rapid heart rate, usually above 100 beats per minute.

Tachypnea Abnormally rapid (usually shallow) respiratory rate. Normal respiratory rate is 12 to 20 breaths per minute.

Team critical incident stress debriefing A structured therapy process that helps responders understand and manage intense emotions, further understand effective coping strategies, and receive the support of peers.

Team critical incident stress management In-the-field debriefing.

Technician Level Personnel who respond to releases of hazardous materials to control the release. They use specialized chemical-protective clothing and specialized control equipment. Technician Level responders take offensive actions.

Tertiary blast injury Injuries that are caused by the patient's being thrown like a projectile

Threshold limit value Airborne concentrations of substances to which workers may be repeatedly exposed day after day without adverse health effects. Because of wide variation in individual susceptibility, a small percentage of workers may experience ill effects at concentrations below the TLV. There are three categories of TLV: TLV-TWA, TLV-STEL, and TLV-C.

Thrombocytopenia A decrease in the number of platelets in the blood, resulting in the potential for increased bleeding.

Time-weighted average An average value of exposure over the course of a given time period.

TLV Threshold limit value.

TLV-C Threshold limit value ceiling, the airborne concentration that should not be exceeded during any part of the working exposure.

TLV-STEL Threshold limit value short-term exposure limit, the concentration to which workers can be exposed continuously for a short period without suffering irritation, chronic or irreversible tissue damage, or narcosis of sufficient degree to increase the likelihood of accidental injury, impair self-rescue, or materially reduce work efficiency, and provided that the daily TLV-TWA is not exceeded.

TLV-TWA Threshold limit value time-weighted average, the time-weighted average concentration for a normal 8-hour workday and a 40-hour workweek, to which nearly all workers may be repeatedly exposed, day after day, without adverse health effects.

TNT Trinitrotoluene.

Toxemia A generalized condition produced by toxins and other by-products of an infectious agent.

Toxicology The division of science and biology that studies poisonous substances, how to detect them, their chemistry and pharmacological actions, and antidotes and treatment methods.

Toxin A product that can cause injury to biological tissue.

Tularemia A disease resulting from infection of *Francisella tularensis*. It is normally transmitted through handling infected small mammals such as rabbits or rodents or through the bites of ticks, deer flies, or mosquitoes that have fed on infected animals. It is also known as rabbit fever or deer fly fever.

TWA Time-weighted average.

Type IV blast injuries Miscellaneous injuries that are caused by an explosive device.

Typhus A disease resulting from infection of *Rickettsia prowazekii, Rickettsia typhi,* or *Rickettsia tsutsugamushi.* It is transmitted from person to person in body lice bites, flea bites, or chigger bites. Severity of illness depends upon the type of organism and route of transmission.

Vapor pressure The ability of a material to evaporate in air. Vapor pressure is proportional to temperature. The vapor pressure increases with increasing temperature.

Variola major A member of the orthopox virus family that causes the most common form of smallpox. It is the most likely form of the organism to be used as a weapon.

Variola minor A member of the orthopox virus family that causes a less common form of smallpox with a much lower mortality than variola major.

Venezuelan equine encephalitis A form of arboviral encephalitis. Venezuelan equine encephalitis is transmitted to humans and horses via mosquito bite. Human infection may be asymptomatic or a mild flulike illness.

Vesicants Chemical weapons also known as blister agents or mustard agents; they are named due to the most obvious injury they inflict on a person. These agents burn and blister the skin or any other part of the body they contact.

Vibrio cholerae A free-living, gram-negative bacterial organism, the etiologic agent of cholera.

Viral encephalitis Inflammation of brain parenchymal tissue as a result of viral infection.

Viral hemorrhagic fevers A group of viral diseases of diverse etiology (arenaviruses, filoviruses, bunyaviruses, and flaviviruses) having many similar characteristics including increased capillary permeability, leukopenia, and thrombocytopenia, resulting in a severe multisystem syndrome.

VMAT Veterinary Medical Assistance Team.

VX Most toxic of the nerve agent class of military warfare agents.

Warm zone The area surrounding the hot zone. It functions as a safety buffer area, as a decontamination area, and as an access and egress point to and from the hot zone.

Warning property An odor, taste, or mucous membrane irritation from chemical exposure that is detectable below the PEL and persists to above the IDLH air concentration. A chemical that meets this definition is said to have adequate warning properties.

Western equine encephalitis A form of arboviral encephalitis (primarily affecting equines) endemic to western and central regions of North America. The causative organism (western equine encephalitis virus) may be transferred to humans via mosquito bite *(Culex tarsalis* and others); clinical manifestations include flulike symptoms followed by alterations in mentation, seizure, coma, and in rare cases death.

Yersinia pestis The anaerobic, gram-negative bacterium that causes plague disease in humans and rodents.

Credits

Cover photo T. Schumacher (Veterans Administration)

Chapter 1

Fig. 1-1 Phil Currance
Fig. 1-2 Phil Currance
Fig. 1-3 Phil Currance
Fig. 1-4 Phil Currance
Fig. 1-5 Phil Currance
Fig. 1-6 Phil Currance
Fig. 1-7 Phil Currance
Fig. 1-8 Phil Currance
Fig. 1-9 Phil Currance

Chapter 2

Fig. 2-1 Phil Currance
Fig. 2-2 Phil Currance
Fig. 2-3 Phil Currance
Fig. 2-5 Courtesy National Audio Visual Center
Fig. 2-7 Phil Currance
Fig. 2-10 Phil Currance

Chapter 3

Fig. 3-1 Courtesy Securesearch.inc
Fig. 3-2 Courtesy Securesearch.inc
Fig. 3-3 Courtesy Securesearch.inc
Fig. 3-4 Gary Christman
Fig. 3-5 Gary Christman
Fig. 3-6 Courtesy Securesearch.inc
Fig. 3-7 Gary Christman

Chapter 4

Fig. 4-1 Phil Currance
Fig. 4-2 Phil Currance
Fig. 4-3 Phil Currance
Fig. 4-4 Phil Currance
Fig. 4-5 Courtesy National Audio Visual Center
Fig. 4-6 Courtesy National Audio Visual Center
Fig. 4-7 David Johnsrud
Fig. 4-8 Phil Currance

Chapter 5

Fig. 5-1 Courtesy Centers for Disease Control/Public Health Image Library
Fig. 5-2 Courtesy Centers for Disease Control/Public Health Image Library
Fig. 5-3 Courtesy Centers for Disease Control/Public Health Image Library
Fig. 5-4 Courtesy Centers for Disease Control/Public Health Image Library
Fig. 5-5 James Gathany, courtesy Centers for Disease Control/Public Health Image Library
Fig. 5-6 Courtesy Centers for Disease Control/Public Health Image Library
Fig. 5-7 Courtesy Centers for Disease Control/Public Health Image Library
Fig. 5-8 Source: Morbidity and Mortality Weekly Report (© 2002 CDC)
Fig. 5-9 Courtesy Centers for Disease Control/Public Health Image Library
Fig. 5-10 C. Goldsmith, courtesy Centers for Disease Control/Public Health Image Library

Chapter 6

Fig. 6-1 Courtesy Medical Management of Chemical Casualties Version 4
Fig. 6-2 Courtesy Medical Management of Chemical Casualties Version 4
Fig. 6-3 Phil Currance
Fig. 6-4 Chris Mailliard
Fig. 6-5 Phil Currance
Fig. 6-6 Courtesy Medical Management of Chemical Casualties Version 4
Fig. 6-7 Courtesy Medical Management of Chemical Casualties Version 3
Fig. 6-9 Lana Blackwell
Fig. 6-10 Lana Blackwell

Chapter 7

Fig. 7-1 Phil Currance
Fig. 7-2 Alan Colon
Fig. 7-3 Alan Colon
Fig. 7-4 Phil Currance
Fig. 7-5 Alan Colon
Fig. 7-6 Alan Colon

Chapter 8

Fig. 8-1 David Johnsrud
Fig. 8-2 Phil Currance
Fig. 8-3 Gary Christman
Fig. 8-4 Phil Currance
Fig. 8-5 Gary Christman
Fig. 8-6 Gary Christman
Fig. 8-7 Phil Currance
Fig. 8-8 Phil Currance
Fig. 8-9 Chris Mailliard
Fig. 8-10 Phil Currance

Chapter 9

Fig. 9-1 David Johnsrud
Fig. 9-2 Phil Currance
Fig. 9-3 Phil Currance
Fig. 9-4 Phil Currance
Fig. 9-5 Phil Currance
Fig. 9-6 Phil Currance
Fig. 9-7 Phil Currance
Fig. 9-8 Phil Currance
Fig. 9-10 Phil Currance
Fig. 9-11 Phil Currance
Fig. 9-12 Phil Currance
Fig. 9-14 Phil Currance
Fig. 9-15 T. Schumacher (Veterans Administration)
Fig. 9-16 Phil Currance
Fig. 9-17 Phil Currance
Fig. 9-18 Phil Currance
Fig. 9-19 Phil Currance
Fig. 9-20 Phil Currance
Fig. 9-21 Phil Currance
Fig. 9-22 Phil Currance
Fig. 9-23 Phil Currance
Fig. 9-24 Phil Currance

Chapter 10

Fig. 10-1 Phil Currance
Fig. 10-2 Phil Currance
Fig. 10-3 T. Schumacher (Veterans Administration)
Fig. 10-4 Phil Currance
Fig. 10-5 David Johnsrud
Fig. 10-6 David Johnsrud
Fig. 10-7 Lana Blackwell
Fig. 10-8 Lana Blackwell
Fig. 10-9 Lana Blackwell
Fig. 10-10 Lana Blackwell
Fig. 10-11 Phil Currance
Fig. 10-12 Lana Blackwell
Fig. 10-13 Phil Currance
Fig. 10-14 Phil Currance
Fig. 10-15 Phil Currance
Fig. 10-16 Phil Currance
Fig. 10-17 Phil Currance

Fig. 10-18 David Johnsrud
Fig. 10-19 Phil Currance

Chapter 11

Fig. 11-1 Phil Currance
Fig. 11-2 Phil Currance
Fig. 11-3 Courtesy Medical Management of Chemical Casualties Version 3
Fig. 11-4 Phil Currance
Fig. 11-5 Phil Currance
Fig. 11-7 Courtesy Medical Management of Chemical Casualties Version 3
Fig. 11-8 Courtesy Medical Management of Chemical Casualties Version 3
Fig. 11-9 Phil Currance
Fig. 11-10 Phil Currance
Fig. 11-11 Phil Currance
Fig. 11-14 Phil Currance
Fig. 11-15 Phil Currance
Fig. 11-17 Phil Currance
Fig. 11-18 Phil Currance
Fig. 11-19 Phil Currance

Chapter 12

Fig. 12-1 Phil Currance
Fig. 12-2 Phil Currance
Fig. 12-3 Phil Currance
Fig. 12-4 T. Schumacher (Veterans Administration)
Fig. 12-5 Phil Currance
Fig. 12-6 Phil Currance
Fig. 12-7 Phil Currance
Fig. 12-8 Phil Currance
Fig. 12-9 Phil Currance
Fig. 12-10 Phil Currance
Fig. 12-11 Phil Currance
Fig. 12-12 Phil Currance
Fig. 12-13 Phil Currance
Fig. 12-14 Phil Currance
Fig. 12-15 Phil Currance
Fig. 12-16 Phil Currance
Fig. 12-17 Phil Currance
Fig. 12-18 Phil Currance
Fig. 12-19 Phil Currance
Fig. 12-20 Phil Currance
Fig. 12-22 Phil Currance
Fig. 12-23 Phil Currance

Index